GENETICS OF THE IMMUNE RESPONSE

NOBEL FOUNDATION SYMPOSIA PUBLISHED BY PLENUM

GENETICS OF THE IMMUNE RESPONSE

Edited by
Erna Möller
and
Göran Möller

Karolinska Institute
Stockholm, Sweden

PLENUM PRESS • NEW YORK AND LONDON

Library of Congress Cataloging in Publication Data

Nobel Symposium (55th: 1982: Saltsjöbaden, Sweden)
  Genetics of the immune response.

  "Proceedings of Nobel Foundation Symposium no. 55 on genetics of the immune
response, held June 15–17 1982, in Saltsjöbaden, Sweden"—Verso of t.p.
  Includes bibliographical references and index.
  1. Immunogenetics—Congresses. 2. Immune response—Congresses. I. Möller, Er-
na, 1940–   . II. Möller, Göran, 1936–   . III. Title. [DNLM: 1. Antibody forma-
tion—Congresses. 2. Immunity, Cellular—Congresses. 3. Genes, Immune Response—
Congresses. W3 N0368M 55th 1982/QW 541 N744g 1982]
QR184.N63 1982   599'.029   82-24695
ISBN-13: 978-1-4684-4471-1   e-ISBN-13: 978-1-4684-4469-8
DOI: 10.1007/978-1-4684-4469-8

Proceedings of Nobel Foundation Symposium No. 55 on
Genetics of the Immune Response, held June 15–17, 1982,
in Saltsjöbaden, Sweden

© 1983 Plenum Press, New York
Softcover reprint of the hardcover 1st edition 1983

A Division of Plenum Publishing Corporation
233 Spring Street, New York, N.Y. 10013

PREFACE

The 55th Nobel Symposium entitled "Genetics of the Immune Response" took place in Saltsjöbaden, Sweden, June 15 - 17, 1982.

The topic was selected for several reasons, such as the rapid progress in the genetic analysis of immunoglobulin and MHC genes and the elucidation of the mechanism of switch to different immunoglobulin classes and subclasses. The genetic advances formed a basis for discussions of problems relating to regulation of T cell subsets, mechanisms of activation and regulation of B cell differentiation and an analysis of the network hypothesis.

The format of the symposium was arranged so as to include two sessions in the morning and two in the afternoon. Each session was introduced by one speaker, followed by free discussion. The introductory lectures are included in the proceedings. The participants summarized their contributions to the discussion in written form.

In addition to the closed sessions, there was one open session at the Karolinska Institute with lectures by Drs. L. Hood, C. Milstein, D. Baltimore, J. Klein and B. Benacerraf, which are not included in these proceedings.

The symposium was sponsored by the Nobel Foundation and its Nobel Symposium Committee through grants from the Tercentenary Fund of the Bank of Sweden and the Knut & Alice Wallenberg Foundation. The Swedish Medical Research Council, the Swedish Cancer Society and the Swedish Ministry of Education and Cultural Affairs also made contributions.

Erna Möller
Göran Möller

CONTENTS

Session I

Antibody V Genes

Chairman: M. Weigert

THE FORMATION OF ANTIBODY VARIABLE REGION GENES

Philip Leder

Department of Genetics, Harvard Medical School

Boston, Massachusetts 02115 USA

The solution of the problem of how immunoglobulin genes produce antibody molecules is the result of extraordinary developments in the fields of immunology and molecular biology. The immunochemists, of course, discovered the interesting features of the structure of antibody molecules and proposed a variety models to account for the structural and organizational features of this remarkable class of proteins. The molecular biologists, on the other hand, set out to develop the genetic approaches that would--in the end--put these theories to the test. Six or seven years ago neither of these groups could have anticipated the spectacular success that the development of recombinant DNA technology has made possible. Many of the questions raised by immunologists are now answered in concrete terms. We know how immunoglobulin genes are encoded in germline DNA and how this structure is altered in antibody producing cells. We know that several powerful mechanisms exist to shuffle bits of DNA and RNA in somatic cells and we know how these mechanisms act to create diversity. We also suspect that we are viewing mechanisms that have significance beyond the immune system itself.

What I hope to do here is to review very briefly the state of settled knowledge regarding the formation of active variable (V) regions and--as I do this--to create a list of questions, some long recognized--others rather new, that now confront us. I suspect that some of these questions will be our major preoccupation for some years to come.

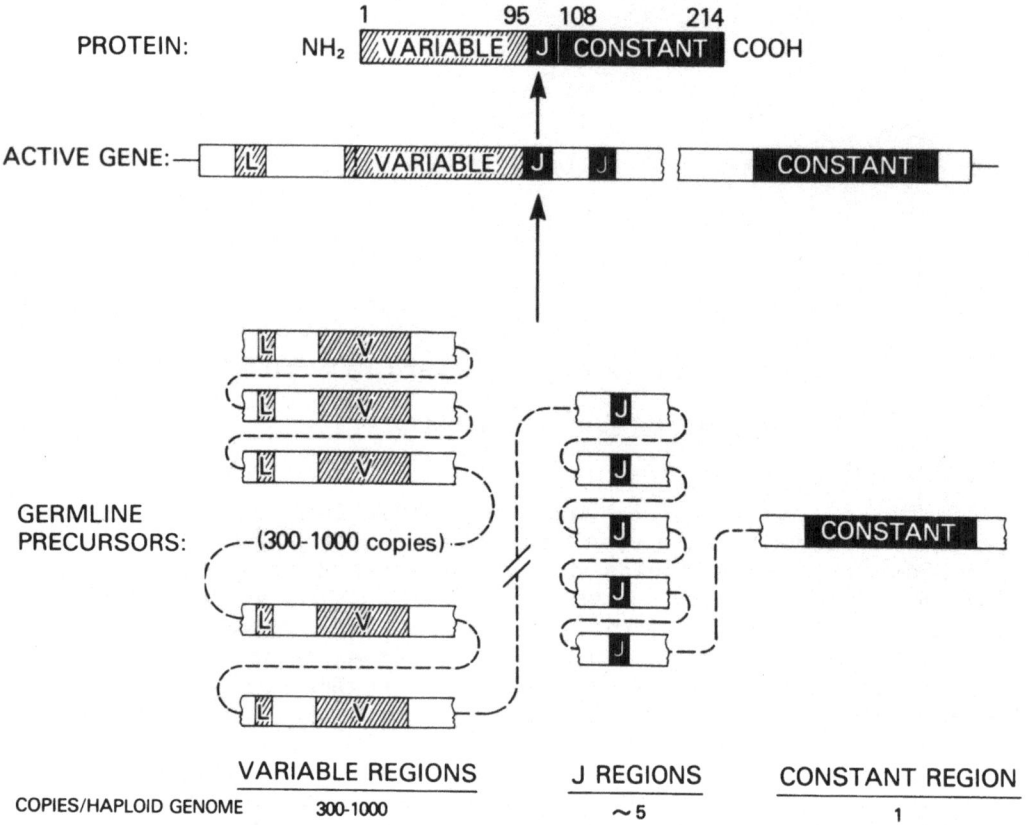

Fig. 1. Diagrammatic representation of the formation of an active
light chain gene. The flow of events occurs from bottom to
top. The bottom portion of the figure indicates diagram-
matically the germline arrangement of the immunoglobulin
light chain genes (L = leader sequence; V = variable
sequence; J = joining sequence) as described in the text
and in greater detail in Figures 2 and 3. The germline
variable regions are encoded in a tandem array at some
unknown distance (> 20,000 bp) from the J region. The J
regions are, in turn, about 2500 bp from the C_k sequence.
A somatic recombinatorial event joins one of the V's to one
of the J's to form an active gene. The gene is transcribed
in its entirety into a primary transcript (not shown); the
transcript is processed by removing its non-coding intervening sequences to a mature mRNA (not shown) and translat-
ing into the pre kappa chain form (not shown). The upper-
most diagram represents the final product, the mature kappa
light chain.

General Structure and Evolution of V Region Genes

The general scheme involved in the formation of active antibody light and heavy chain genes is by now well known (Fig. 1). There is a large number of germline V region genes (1-7) (in the case of the κ chain of the mouse, let us say about 100, though making this point immediately raises a question about their actual number). These are encoded at some unknown distance in an as yet unknown orientation with respect to the constant (C) and joining (J) region genes. The V region genes appear to be encoded in tandem arrays of related families, some of them many thousands of bases apart. Many of these genes retain significant stretches of strict homology in their coding as well as their flanking sequences. Such recurring structures and extensive homology suggest that these sequences could easily recombine with one another, that they could be amplified and or deleted by unequal mitotic crossing-over in the germline and that their sequences could be affected by powerful gene conversion mechanisms (8). Indeed, there are observations that are explicable in terms of the unequal crossing over, for example, the loss of the Vλ repertoire in the mouse or the absence of the V_{k41} subgroup in Mus phari (9). The question remains as to how these genes evolve and how they create and maintain their rich diversity in the germline.

The Detailed Structure of V Region Genes

All V region genes analyzed seem to have the same structural features regardless of whether they are components of κ, λ or heavy chains (Fig. 2). Their initial coding segment encodes a hydrophobic leader or signal peptide about 19 or 20 amino acids in length. This is separated from the main body of the V region coding sequence by a 100 or so base long intervening sequence that separates codon -4 from codon -3. The intervening sequence does not cleanly divide the two coding domains; three signal peptide amino acids occur on the main body of the V coding sequence. This variance from the Gilbert domain model (10) may be more apparent than real because the hydrophobic--and presumably functional-- portion of the V region signal sequence is entirely contained within the initial leader coding sequence.

The light chain V regions are encoded through the equivalent of κ chain codon 95 and this is, of course, very significant. Amino acid 96 forms the bottom of the antigen combining site in the crystallographic structure determined for the plasmacytoma immunologloglobulin 603 (11) and its alteration would be expected to have a very significant effect on antigen binding specificity.

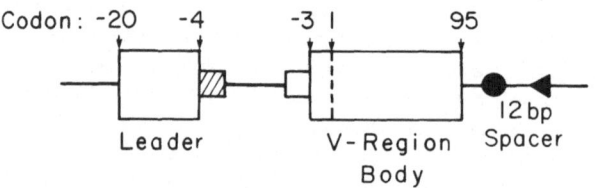

Codon: -20   -4   -3 I   95

Leader   V-Region   Spacer
                      Body

▨ = RNA Splice Donor (GT·····)

□ = RNA Splice Acceptor (·····AG)

● = A-Centered Palindrome (CACAGTG)

◀ = A-Rich Nonomer (ACATAAACC)

Fig. 2. Detailed diagrammatic representation of a germline V_k region gene. The significance of the RNA and DNA splicing signals are given in the text.

The J Segments

     The remaining portion of the V region is encoded separately and apparently at a great distance from the V region sequences (Fig. 3). These segments (called J, for joining) are also encoded redundantly. There are four active copies of J_k in the mouse (12,13) and five in man (14,15). These are encoded at rather regular intervals of about 300 bases, each about 2.5 Kb from the single constant region gene. The J genes of the κ light chains differ from one another slightly in sequence, but are of uniform length; they encode amino acids 96-108. There may be as many active J region genes encoded at the λ light chain locus, but they are encoded somewhat differently than the Jκ's. There is only one Jλ encoded adjacent to each Cλ coding region (16,17), but--in the case of man--there are five to nine (depending upon the polymorphic form) repeated copies of the J/C complex (18).

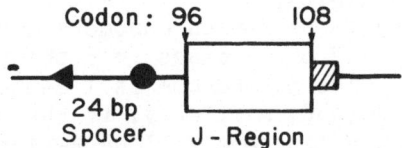

Fig. 3. Detailed diagrammatic representation of a J region gene.

This arrangement is capable of creating as much diversity as the C_k locus because it has as many or even more J regions, but it does so less economically by repeating both J and C region sequences. As we shall see below, in the case of the heavy chains of man, there are six active J genes and three pseudo-J genes (19). They differ from one another in both length and sequence. The evolutionary sources of these J regions remain entirely obscure.

The D Segments

The finding of nuleotide sequences that could not be accounted for between V and J region segments of heavy chain cDNAs led to the notion that there was yet another segment of DNA that was contributed to the H chain V region—a D (for diversity) segment (20,21).

Table 1

The "Rules" of V/J and V/D/J Recombination

Rule 1.	Complementary T- or A-centered palindromic sequences are located adjacent to segments to be joined (i.e. CACTGTG or CACAGTG).
Rule 2.	Complementary T- or A-rich nonomers are located approximately 12 or 24 bases from the palindromic sequences. If the palindrome is T centered, the nonomer will be T-rich and, similarly, if the palindrome is A centered, the palindrome will be A-rich.
Rule 3.	Recombination occurs only between segments that have dissimilar signal sequence spacing, i.e. a 12 base spaced signal joins only to a 24, and vice versa.

Moreover, it was predicted that this segment would obey certain rules (Table 1) that seemed to govern the placement of "signal" sequences thought to be important for V/J joining (see below)--namely, that these signal sequences should be separated either by a 12 basepair spacing so that they join to a segment with a 24 basepair spacing (20,21). The "rules" for V/D/J splicing are detailed above (Table 1), but sequence determinations of several gemline D segments in mouse (22) and man (23) indicate that these predictions have been fulfilled (Fig. 4).

Such sequence studies as are available in germline D segments in man and mouse indicate that they are also encoded in tandem multigene families--widely separated (by > 10 Kb) from one another in genomic DNA (22,23). Even within a family, these D genes are related--but slightly different from one another in both sequence and length. Since their sequences show segmental relationships to sequences outside their families, the question arose as to whether D's recombined with one another. There is as yet no evidence for this. These segmental homologies could be accounted for by gene conversion. The finding of a D segment just 5' to the last active J in man (23) and mouse (22) suggests that this is the relationship of the remaining D's, namely, 5' to J's. Both are presumed to be 3' to the V regions. This configuration has, however, not been established.

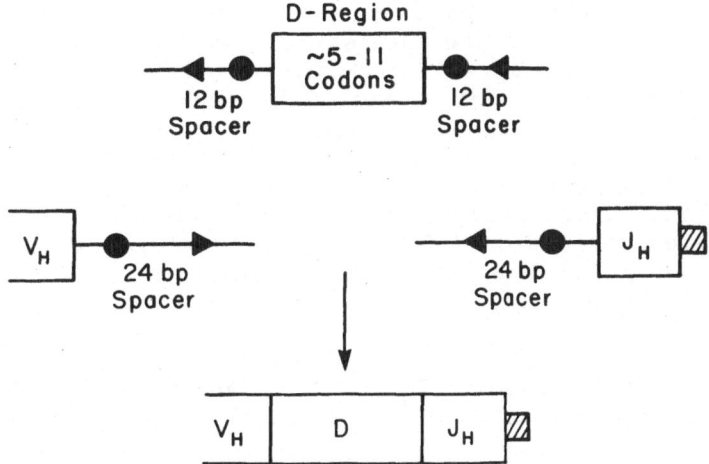

Fig. 4. Detailed diagrammatic representation of a D region gene.
The signals and spacing thought to be important for
joining of V, D and J are explained in the text.

The V/J (and V/D/J) Recombinational Event

The critical feature of V region genes is the fact that they
undergo somatic recombination—V and J (and D) regions join in
developing B cells. This means that both V and J region segments
carry two functional faces—one for DNA/DNA joining, the other for
RNA splicing.

The results of cloning and sequencing studies early identified
two small, but evidently important, structural elements encoded on
the 3' side of the V region and the 5' side of the J region
(12,13). These conserved elements are likely to be important in
the recombinatorial process and they consist of an A or T rich
nonamer separated by a short stretch of nuleotides from an A or T
centered palindrome (see Figs. 2, 3 and 4). Subsequent studies on
the heavy chain showed that the spacing between these elements was
likely to be important and resulted in the formulation of the 12/24
rule in which a set of signals with a 12 base spacing would
recombine only with a set of signals that was complementary and had
a 24 base spacing (20,21).

Early studies of V/J recombination also indicated that the segments 3' to V and 5' to J segments were deleted from myeloma cells (13). This led to the suggestion that V/J recombination could be accomplished by an intra-strand joining with deletion of the intervening DNA. Such events might have been facilitated by the formation of a weakly bonded stem-like structure that could be drawn joining V and J segments (12). Newer data that have identified back-to-back splice signals suggest a different mechanism involving reciprocal, unequal crossing-over between mitotic sister chromatids (25-29). These findings raise the issue of the precise mechanism or mechanisms of V/J and V/D/J recombination which remains one of the major questions confronting the field.

Variation in the Crossover Point of V/J and V/D/J Recombination and the Generation of Useful and Useless Diversity

The crossover point of V/J recombination appears variable, allowing diversity to accumulate at critical amino acid position 96 in the chain or its analogue in λ and heavy chains (30) (see Fig. 5). This variability together with the combinatorial power of joining one of hundreds of V regions to one of four or five J regions represents the major--but not the only--sources of variable region diversity. Such mechanisms also create nonsense recombinants and, thereby, null or aberrant genes. Such null recombinants account for some of the wastage seen among some unexpressed (allelically excluded) Ig genes and apparently represent the price to be paid for employing this powerful mechanism.

The Order of V Gene Formation

There is an order to V gene formation that was initially discerned in leukemic cells (31-34). First, the heavy chain V region is formed, then an attempt is made to form a valid κ chain gene using one or both of its alleles. If V_k/J_k recombination forms a valid gene, the cell continues its maturation as a B-cell. If this fails, rearrangement begins among the λ chain genes and continues until a valid gene is formed. Furthermore, κ genes often disappear in λ producing cells. The basis for the ordering of these events is entirely unknown, though it has been suggested that the appearance of a valid immunoglobulin on the surface of a pre-B cell may serve as a regulatory signal that brings the process of V/J recombination to an end (34). What significance (if any) of the κ gene disappearance is also entirely unknown, though its relationship to the onset of λ gene rearrangment allows us to suggest a regulatory role in this process.

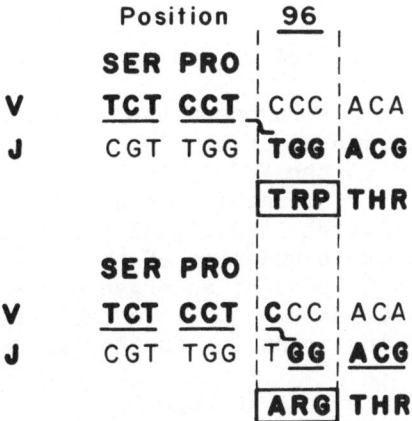

Fig. 5.   Diagrammatic representation of variation in crossover
point for V/J and V/D/J joining. V_k and J_k region
sequences are identified on their respective lines. As
shown, if joining occurs as in the upper frame, a <u>trp</u>
codon is found at amino acid position 96. If joining
occurs as in the lower frame, an <u>arg</u> codon is formed.
Such variation changes the amino acid at critical
position 96.

Somatic Point Mutations

     It is clear that certain active Ig genes are altered in a few
nucleotide positions from their germline configurations (35).
These differences occur in both their framework and hypervariable
sequences. Moreover, these alterations tend to accumulate in late
stage Ig heavy chain V regions, that is, in V regions associated
with the late-appearing IgG and IgA (36-42). The major questions

that these observations raise is what is the physiologic
significance of these somatic alterations, i.e. do they contribute
to physiologically significant diversity and, secondly, what is the
biochemical mechanism responsible for their introduction into V
region genes.

Do V/J and Switch Recombination Operate in Other Genetic Systems?

It seems reasonable to propose that a V/J-type recombination
might be used to generate diversity in some other genetic systems.
A sequence quite akin to the V/J splice signal is found close to
the site of inversion recombination seen in the flaggellar antigen
of Salmonella (43). Switch-like signal sequences are known to
occur outside the normal boundaries of the heavy chain genes (44).
While it is difficult to predict an organ system or cell type that
might possess these mechanisms, the availability of homologous Ig
probes proves a starting point for further investigation.

Epilogue

The sources of genetic diversity seen in the V regions of
antibody molecules is now understood in rough outline. Genetic
diversity arises from evolutionary processes that have generated a
large array of germline V region genes that undergo somatic
recombination with smaller arrays of J (and, in the case of heavy
chain V genes, D) region sequences to form active and diverse V
sequences. This powerful recombinational process is flexible in
that it can join these segments to different cross-over points to
create additional diversity at critical regions of the polypeptide
chain. In addition, there is a poorly understood mechanism for
introducing solitary base changes in the body of the V region gene
in the later stages of lymphocyte differentiation. All these
processes are subject to some form of regulation that ensures the
initial formation of V_H, followed by V_k, and--if V_k has not formed
a functional V sequence--V_k . The mechanisms that regulate and
catalyze these processes remain entirely unknown and constitute a
major challenge for the future.

References

1. J. Seidman, A. Leder, M.H. Edgell, F. Polsky, S.M. Tilghman, D.C. Tiemeier, and P. Leder, Multiple related mouse immuno-globulin variable region genes identified by cloning and sequence analyses. Proc. Natl. Acad. Sci. U.S.A. 75:3881 (1978).
2. J.G. Seidman and P. Leder, The arrangement and rearrangement of antibody genes. Nature 276:790 (1978).
3. G. Matthyssens, and T.H. Rabbitts, Structure and multiplicity of genes for the human immunoglobulin heavy chain variable region. Proc. Natl. Acad. Sci. U.S.A. 77:6561 (1980).
4. Bentley, D.L. and T.H. Rabbits, Human immunoglobulin variable region genes--DNA sequences of two V κ genes and a pseudogene. Nature 288:730 (1980).
5. Y. Nishioka and P. Leder, Organization and complete sequence of identical embryonic and plasmacytoma κ V-region genes. J. Biol. Chem. 255:3691 (1980).
6. D. Givol, R. Zakut, K.Effron, G. Rechavi, D. Ram, and J.B. Cohen, Diversity of germ-line immunoglobulin VH genes. Nature 292:426 (1981).
7. D.L. Bentley and T.H. Rabbitts, Human V κ immunoglobulin gene number: implications for the origin of antibody diversity. Cell 24:613 (1981).
8. J.G. Seidman, A. Leder, M. Nau, B. Norman, and P. Leder, Antibody diversity. Science 202:11 (1978).
9. P. Leder, J.G. Seidman, E.E. Max, Y. Nishioka, A. Leder, B. Norman, and M. Nau, The arrangement, rearrangement and origin of immunoglobulin genes, in "Miami Winter Symposium," Vol. 16, T.R. Russell, K. Bren, H. Faber, and J. Schalley, eds., pp. 133-145 (1979).
10. W. Gilbert, Why genes in pieces? Nature 271:501 (1978).
11. E.W. Silverton, M.A. Navia, and D.R. Davies, Three-dimensional structure of an intact human immunoglobulin. Proc. Natl. Acad. Sci. U.S.A. 74:5140 (1977).
12. E.E. Max, J.V. Maizel, Jr., and P. Leder, The nucleotide sequence of a 5.5 kilobase DNA segment containing the mouse immunoglobulin J and C region genes. J. Biol. Chem. 256:5116 (1981).
13. H. Sakano, K. Huppi, G. Heinrich, and S. Tonegawa, Sequences at the somatic recombination sites of immunoglobulin light-chain genes. Nature 280:288 (1979).
14. P.A. Hieter, J.V. Maizel, Jr., and P. Leder, Evolution of human immunoglobulin κ J region genes. J. Biol. Chem. 257:1516 (1982).

15. P.A. Hieter, E.E. Max, J.G. Seidman, J.V. Maizel, Jr., and P. Leder, Cloned human and mouse κ immunoglobulin constant and J region genes conserve homology in functional segments. Cell 22:197 (1980).

16. J. Miller, A. Bothwell, and U. Storb, Physical linkage of the constant region genes for immunoglobulins lambda I and lambda II. Proc. Natl. Acad. Sci. U.S.A. 78:3829 (1981).

17. B. Blomberg, A. Traunecker, H. Eisen, and S. Tonegawa, Organization of four mouse λ light chain immunoglobulin genes. Proc. Natl. Acad. Sci. U.S.A. 78:3765 (1981).

18. P.A. Hieter, G.F. Hollis, S.J. Korsmeyer, T.A. Waldmann, and P. Leder, Clustered arrangement of immunoglobulin λ constant regions in man. Nature 294:536 (1981).

19. J.V. Ravetch, U. Siebenlist, S. Korsmeyer, T. Waldmann, and P. Leder, Structure of the human immunoglobulin mu locus: characterization of embryonic and rearranged J and D genes. Cell 27:583 (1981).

20. P. Early, H. Huang, M. Davis, K. Calame, and L. Hood, An immunoglobulin heavy chain variable region gene is generated from three segments of DNA: VH, D and JH. Cell 19:981 (1980).

21. R. Maki, A. Traunecker, H. Sakano, W. Roeder, and S. Tonegawa, Exon shuffling generates an immunoglobulin heavy chain gene. Proc. Natl. Acad. Sci. U.S.A. 77:2138 (1980).

22. Y. Kurosawa, H. von Boehmer, W. Haas, H. Sakano, A. Trauneker, and S. Tonegawa, Identification of D segments of immunoglobulin heavy-chain genes and their rearrangement in T lymphocytes. Nature 290:565 (1981).

23. U. Siebenlist, J.V. Ravetch, S. Korsmeyer, T. Waldmann, and P. Leder, Human immunoglobulin D segments encoded in tandem multigenic families. Nature 294:631 (1981).

24. J.G. Seidman, M.M. Nau, B. Norman, S.-P.Kwan, M. Scharff, and P. Leder, Immunoglobulin V/J recombination is accompanied by deletion of joining site and variable region segments. Proc. Natl. Acad. Sci. U.S.A. 77:6022 (1980).

25. W. Altenburger, M. Steinmetz, and H.G. Zachau, Functional and non-functional joining in immunoglobulin light chain genes of a mouse myeloma. Nature 287:603 (1980).

26. M. Steinmetz, W. Altenburger, and H.G. Zachau, A rearranged DNA sequence possibly related to the translocation of immunoglobulin gene segments. Nucleic Acids Res. 8:1709 (1980).

27. A. Walfield, E. Selsing, B. Arp, and U. Storb, Misalignent of V and J gene segments resulting in a nonfunctional immunoglobulin gene. Nucleic Acids Res. 9:1101 (1981).

28. J. Hochtl, C.R. Muller, and H.G. Zachau, Recombined flanks of the variable and joining segments of immunoglobulin genes. Proc. Natl. Acad. Sci. U.S.A. 79:1383 (1982).

29. B.G., VanNess, C. Coleclough, R.P. Perry, and M. Weigert, DNA between variable and joining gene segments of immunoglobulin κ light chain is frequently retained in cells that rearrange the κ locus. Proc. Natl. Acad. Sci. U.S.A. 79:262 (1982).

30. E.E. Max, J.G. Seidman, H.I. Miller, and P. Leder, Variation in the crossover point of κ immunoglobulin gene V-J recombination: evidence from a cryptic gene. Cell 21:793 (1980).

31. P.A. Hieter, S.J. Korsmeyer, T.A. Waldmann, and P. Leder, Human immunoglobulin κ light chain genes are deleted or rearranged in λ-producing B cells. Nature 290:368 (1981).

32. S. Korsmeyer, P.A. Hieter, J.V. Ravetch, D.G. Poplack, T.A. Waldmann, and P. Leder, Developmental hierarchy of immunoglobulin gene rearrangements in human leukemic pre-B cells. Proc. Natl. Acad. Sci. U.S.A. 78:7096 (1981).

33. S.J. Korsmeyer, P.A. Hieter, J.V. Ravetch, D.G. Poplack, P. Leder, and T.A. Waldmann, Patterns of immunoglobulin gene arrangement in human lymphotic leukemias, in "Leukemia Markers", W. Knapp, ed., Academic Press, London, pp. 85-97 (1981).

34. F. Alt, N. Rosenberg, S. Lewis, E. Thomas, and D. Baltimore, Organization and reorganization of immunoglobulin genes in A-MULV-transformed cells: rearrangement of heavy but not light chain genes. Cell 27:381 (1981).

35. M. Cohn, The take home lesson, New York Academy of Sciences 190:529 (1972).

36. P. Gearhart, N.D. Johndon, R. Douglas, and L. Hood, IgG antibodies to phosphorylcholine exhibit more diversity than their IgM counterparts. Nature 291:29 (1981).

37. E. Selsing and U. Storb, Somatic mutation of immunoglobulin light-chain variable-region genes. Cell 25:47 (1981).

38. M. Pach, J. Höchtl, H. Schnell, and H.G. Zachau, Differences between germ-line and rearranged immunoglobulin V κ coding sequences suggest a localized mutation mechanism. Nature 291:668 (1981).

39. J. Sims, T.H. Rabbitts, P. Estess, C. Slaughter, P.W. Tucker, and J.D. Capra, Somatic mutation in genes for the variable portion of the immunoglobulin heavy chain. Science 216:309 (1982).

40. H.K. Gershenfeld, A. Tsukamoto, I.L. Weissman, and R. Joho, Somatic diversification is required to generate the V κ genes of MOPC 511 and MOPC 167 myeloma proteins. Proc. Natl. Acad. Sci. U.S.A. 78:7674 (1981).

41. S. Crews, J. Griffin, H. Huang, K. Calame, and L. Hood, A single VH gene segment encodes the immune response to phosphorylcholine: somatic mutation is correlated with the class of antibody. Cell 25:59 (1981).

42. A.L. Bothwell, M. Paskind, M. Reth, T. Imanishi-Kari,
     K. Rajewsky, and D. Baltimore, Heavy chain variable region
     contribution to the NPb family of antibodies: somatic mutation
     evident in a gamma 2a variable region. Cell 24:625 (1981).

43. J. Zeig, and M. Simon, Analysis of the nucleotide sequene of
     an invertible controlling element. Proc. Natl. Acad. Sci.
     U.S.A. 77:4196 (1980).

44. I.R. Kirsch, J.V. Ravetch, S.-P., Kwan, E.E. Max, R.L. Ney,
     and P. Leder, Multiple immunoglobulin switch region homologies
     outside the heavy chain constant region locus. Nature 293:585
     (1981).

DISCUSSION

Hood: In order to study the organization of V genes, we have begun to study by molecular cloning the mouse heavy chain variable region locus. There are probably at least several hundred V_H gene segments. Since the task of physically trying to link each of them to one another would be formidable, we have attempted to study the organization of a small family of closely related V_H gene segments. This set of gene segments, referred to as a T15 V_H gene family, contains four germline gene segments. All four gene segments have been previously isolated and sequenced. They differ from one another by approximately 10 per cent of their nucleotide sequences. One of these germline V_H gene sequences, the so-called T15 V_H gene segment, encodes the entire heavy chain variable region gene response to the simple hapten phosphorylcholine. One of the other V_H genes is a pseudogene, whereas the remaining two V_H genes appear to be functional V_H genes which encode other types of antibody specifities. A variety of earlier studies suggested that closely related V_H genes may be tandemly linked one to another. In order to explore this possibility we have employed our T15 cDNA probe to analyze a cosmid gene library which contains on the average 40-kilobase (kb) inserts. From the screen of the cosmid library, we isolated 16 cosmid clones which could be linked into 12 clusters or families of genes. These 12 clusters contain 21 distinct V_H genes and they encompass approximately 492 kb of DNA. The amount of DNA per V_H gene then is approximately 23 kb. This is a minimal estimate of the distance between V_H genes because in most cases the V_H genes in the clusters are not linked to their adjacent counterparts. Thus, it appears that a related family of V_H genes that can be detected by analysis with the T15 V_H gene probe are separated from one another by, on the average, more than 25 kilobases in the heavy chain chromosome. Three of these gene clusters contain the four T15 family genes mentioned above. Two of these genes were linked to one another an are separated by 16kb of DNA, whereas the remaining two genes were unlinked to any of the other genes. Preliminary analyses suggest that all four members of the T15 gene family are linked and we should be able to demonstrate this by additional chromosomal walking in the T15 gene cluster. If the T15 genes are linked, some may be 40 or even 50 kb away from adjacent V_H gene members. Thus, it appears that V_H genes even within a closely related family can be quite distantly separated one from another.

One interesting implication that arises from these calculations is that if we assume that the mouse heavy chain gene family has 250 or so V_H gene segments, each separated from one another by on an average of 25 kb of DNA, then the V_H locus encompasses some 6250 kb of DNA - a distance of enormous dimension. It will be interesting to see whether the organizational features of the T15-like genes that have been described here are typical of the many other families of V_H gene families that exist on mouse chromosome 12.

Leder: Lee (Hood), if you believe that somatic variants are selected by antigen, you could expect the variants to show a higher affinity for phosphorylcoline than the germline T15 sequences. Do they?

Hood: Unfortunately this question cannot be answered. If one measures the affinity of the variants for phosphorylcoline, as Pat Gearhart has done, some variants have higher and some lower affinities as compared with T15. However, the real question is what is the affinity for phosphorylcoline and in conjunction with its carrier determinants. This measurement cannot be made.

Mäkelä: Since the number of mutations in M167 (44) is un-expectedly large one would like to check once more that there is not a germline gene for the M167 sequence. How certain is this?

Hood: We have carried out two types of experiments to establish this point. First, we have cloned the T15 gene four times in-dependently and by sequence analysis have shown that it has in each case the T15 sequence. We never see the M167 sequence. Thus, we can conclude that the southern band representing the T15 sequence has only the T15 V_H gene. Second, the 5' flanking sequences of the M167 are very closely related to T15 (identical apart from putative somatic mutations) and quite different from the 5' sequence for the other three genes of the T15 gene family.

Cohn: Given the facts that somatic base replacements do occur in the J_{kappa} to C_{kappa} and L_{kappa} to V_{kappa} introns as well as the 5' flanking non-coding sequences, but not in C_{kappa}, provides a strong argument that a special hypermutation mechanism operates after the VJ rearrangement. However, Lee Hood's argument that this mechanism operates only after the IgM to IgG switch is weak, in fact totally unsupported on physiological grounds. The reason that you find a larger number of replacements in the IgG anti-PC than in the IgM anti-PC is due to antigenic selection not to the mutant generating mechanism. Since you are studying a germline encoded specificity, anti-PC, which is expressed antigen-independent in the B^u-class, the vast majority of B^u-cells express the unchanged germline encoded sequence. The chance of picking up a mutant in IgM hybridomas selected for their germline encoded anti-PC activity is too low given the rather cumbersome detection technique. At an incredibly high mutation rate of 10^{-1} per 1000 bp per division, more than 20 IgM hybridomas would have to be sequenced over the total 1KB stretch to detect one mutant with certainty. As the universe of non-PC antigens selects on the mutants in the $V_{kappa}V_H$ gene pair encoding anti-PC, they drive a switch to "IgG". Therefore, you cannot derive from the relative numbers of replacements per cistron in the IgM versus IgG class any conclusion concerning the stage of differentiation at which the mutational mechanism is expressed. Antigen selection is the key factor dominating your findings, which show in addition that somatic diversification is sequential and stepwise, mutation to selection to mutation to selection to etc.

Hood: Somatic variation can occur in V_H regions associated with IgM molecules. In the immune response to alpha 1-3 dextran, approximately 90% of the antibodies are of the IgM class. We have sequenced 22 of these V_H regions and found that somatic mutation can occur in IgM molecules. Indeed the two or three IgG molecules have germline sequences. Thus, we believe that somatic mutation occurs late in B cell development, and that it is not correlated directly with the class switch.

Milstein: The alternative example which suggests that the switch may not necessarily enhance somatic mutation comes from studies of the anti-oxazolone response. The anti-oxazolone response is predominantly of the IgG_1 subclass. The sequence is essentially identical.

Cohn: I would like to return to the antigenic selection pressures operating on germline v-genes. In your experiment involving the germline V-genes encoding anti-PC activity, the mutants in them were selected by environmental immunogens. No estimate of mutation rate is possible, because the number of rounds of mutation and selection to arrive at a given somatic sequence is unknown. Further, we should not forget that mutations, which create a totally new specificity and eliminate the germline encoded anti-PC activity are missed, because the hybridomas analyzed by you were screened for their anti-PC activity. However, this has revealed an important intermediate stage in somatic diversification. There exist mutants with new selectable specificities, which retain the memory of their origin in the germline, in this case anti-PC. Illustrative pathways might be

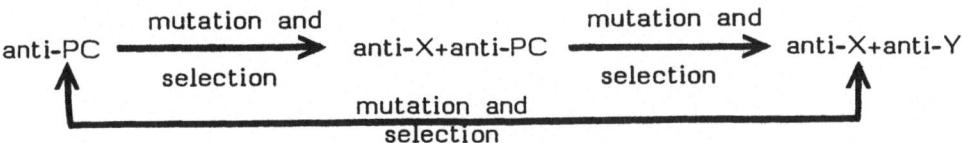

In this case we know the starting specificity, anti-PC, but not the somatically selected specificity, anti-X. When we consider the locus encoding the T cell receptor the converse will be true. The anti-X is known, but the germline encoded specificities from which it is derived are unknown, although I would argue that they are anti-allele-specific determinants on restricting elements determined by the MHC.

Sachs: I would like to ask this question to both Lee Hood and David Baltimore. You have both shown us restriction maps which distinguish the strains BALB/c and B6 for the genes you have examined. Considering the differences, is it still clear that the corresponding V genes of these strains are allelic? In this regard, have either or both of you examined recombinant inbred lines between BALB/c and B6 and, if so, do you ever see scrambling of restriction map patterns?

Hood: The T15 gene family appears to be allelic for the T15 (V1) and pseudogene (V3) in BALB/c and B10P mice, because these two genes show exactly the same linkage relationship - namely the V3 gene is 15kb 5' to the T15 gene.

Cohn: The evolution of the V-gene loci by unequal crossing over and subsequent divergence results in a rough grouping of V-genes into families, which are related by closeness of sequence. The rate of expansion and contraction of the V-gene locus must be slow compared to the rate of divergence (dispersion) of individual V-genes or else the family of V-genes would approach being identical like ribosomal genes. The degree of homology is proportional to the time of divergence. If one compares two V-genes derived from different haplotypes, but within a family they will have sequences more closely related than two V-genes in different families (by definition). However, the term "allelic", which you are using to describe this comparison has lost meaning. Maybe we should refer to them as "haplons" and use the term "haplotype exclusion".

Baltimore: You are right.

Benacerraf: Do you have an explanation for the preeminence of proline in Black and not in BALB/c mice?

Baltimore: Balb/c does not have the gene and another gene is used instead.

Session II

Antibody C Genes

Chairman: L. Hood

ORGANIZATION AND REORGANIZATION OF CONSTANT REGION GENES OF

IMMUNOGLOBULIN HEAVY CHAINS: GENETIC BASIS FOR CLASS SWITCHING

Tasuku Honjo, Norio Ishida, Tohru Kataoka,
Sumiko Nakai, Toshio Nikaido, Yasuyoshi Nishida,
Yoshihiko Noma, Masahiro Obata, Yasuhiko Sakoyama,
Akira Shimizu, Naoki Takahashi, Shunichi Takeda,
Shintaro Ueda, Yuriko Yamawaki-Kataoka & Yoshio Yaoita

Department of Genetics,
Osaka University Medical School
Osaka 530, Japan

SUMMARY

We have determined the complete organization of the mouse C_H gene family, which is comprised of the 8 C_H genes in the order $5'-J_H-6.5kb-C_\mu-4.5kb-C_\delta-55kb-C_\gamma3-34kb-C_\gamma1-21kb-C_\gamma2b-15kb-C_\gamma2a-14kb-C_\varepsilon-12kb-C_\alpha-3'$. The S regions, which contain characteristic tandemly repeated unit sequences, are located 5' to each C_H gene except for the C_δ gene. There are at least two types of repetitive sequences dispersed in this 200 kb region. No pseudogenes are present. The arrangements of the C_H genes in BALB/c and C57BL mice are similar, but the lengths of the S regions vary. The basic structures of all the C_H genes are similar in that coding sequences are interrupted at the junctions of the domains and the hinge regions. Comparison of the nucleotide sequences of the C_H genes revealed that sequence segments have been exchanged among members of the C_H gene family. Cloning and characterization of human C_γ genes, i.e. $C_\gamma1$, $C_\gamma2$, $C_\gamma3$, $C_\gamma4$ and ψC_γ, indicate that the human C_γ gene family evolved by dynamic DNA rearrangements, including gene duplication, exon duplication, and exon reassortment by unequal crossing-over. A human pseudo-epsilon gene ($C_\varepsilon3$) is a processed gene that has completely spliced out introns. The presence of movable genetic elements surrounding the $C_\varepsilon3$ gene suggests that the C_ε gene evolved by a translocation mechanism. Although S-S recombination has been shown to take place in myelomas and hybridomas secreting a large amount of immunoglobulin, analyses of the C_H gene organization in normal

spleen B cells bearing immunoglobulin on their surface suggest
that RNA splicing may be responsible for the first step in class
switching, followed by S-S recombination. The nucleotide sequences of S regions contain short common sequences, TGGG(G) and
(G)AGCT.   Comparison of nucleotide sequences surrounding recombination sites revealed common sequences TGAG and TGGG. A sister
chromatid exchange model was proposed to explain deletion of C_H
genes accompanying S-S recombination. We have found that the S
region serves as a preferred recombination site in E.coli
extracts.

I. INTRODUCTION

Church bells in western countries have a high, clear ring.
In contrast, bells in Buddhist temples in east Asia, especially
in Japan, have a low, rumbling roar.   Beautiful gardens in
European palaces are usually designed with symmetry, or at least
according to an obvious plan. In contrast, stone and sand gardens
in Zen temples look like anything you wish. They do not provide
any explanation. We love the bells and gardens in Japanese
temples because they have what we call yo-in, which may be
translated into the English words reverberation, aftertaste, or
trailing note. None of them exactly express the meaning of yo-in.
Yo-in means the state or space left unexplained or unspoken, left
for imagination. To me, yo-in is also important in science. It
is the problem full of yo-in that is really fascinating. If you
knew everything about a problem you would be bored by it.

The genetic bases of antibody diversity and class switching
have been central problems in modern immunology. These fascinating questions stimulated molecular biologists to introduce
their powerful technology, molecular genetics, into immunology.
This technology, using recombinant DNA, has been so powerful that
the outlines of the answers to the above problems have been
obtained in less than a decade. Although the organization of the
V genes is not completely known, the complete organization of the
C_λ, C_κ and C_H gene loci have been elucidated at least in the
mouse. We know that DNA rearrangements accompanied by DNA deletion play major roles in the generation of antibody diversity
as well as in class switching. The nucleotide sequences
surrounding the recombination sites have already been determined.

Rapid progress in a certain area of science often causes
people outside the area to think that everything has been solved
in that field, which would be really disappointing because of the
absence of yo-in. As was the case with many other scientific
advances, however, such achievements do not necessarily complete
the story. Instead, the introduction of new technology, in turn,
has raised more fundamental questions such as "How is the DNA

rearrangement regulated during B cell differentiation?" and "Do T cells regulate the DNA rearrangement?", thus opening a new era in contemporary immunology.

We have been working on the genetic basis of class switching. We have proposed a model in which class switching is mediated by the deletion of the intervening C_H genes between a V_H gene and the C_H gene to be expressed. We have obtained substantial evidence for this model by analysis of the germline and expressed forms of the C_H genes. In due course we have determined the complete organization of the mouse C_H genes. The complete characterization of such a complex gene family offers a unique opportunity to study evolution of a gene family in different species, thus we are currently studying the structure and organization of human C_H genes. Although S-S recombination was shown to take place in myelomas and hybridomas, analyses of the C_H gene organization in normal spleen B cells bearing immunoglobulins on their surface suggest that RNA splicing may be the first biochemical step in class switching. We have also set out to study the molecular mechanism of S-S recombination in vitro using E.coli extracts, as a step into a new era.

II. ORGANIZATION AND STRUCTURE OF THE CONSTANT REGION GENES OF THE IMMUNOGLOBULIN HEAVY CHAINS

1) Organization of Mouse C_H Genes

Hybridization kinetic analyses using cDNA have shown that specific C_H genes are deleted in mouse myelomas, depending on the C_H genes expressed (Honjo and Kataoka, 1978). The order of the C_H genes, $5'-V_H$ gene family-spacer-$C_\mu-C_\gamma3-C_\gamma1-C_\gamma2b-C_\gamma2a-C_\alpha-3'$, was consistent with the assumption that the DNA segment between a V_H and the C_H gene to be expressed is deleted, bringing these genes close to each other. Deletion of the intervening DNA segment during H chain class switch was confirmed by Southern blot hybridization analyses of myeloma DNAs in which cloned immunoglobulin genes were used (Coleclough et al., 1980 ; Cory and Adams, 1980 ; Cory et al., 1980 ; Rabbitts et al., 1980 ; Yaoita and Honjo, 1980 a,b). Such studies also support the proposed order of C_H genes.

To determine directly the order of C_H genes, we and others set out to clone mouse Ig genes using recombinant DNA technology. The strategy has been successful in isolating all the eight C_H genes of mouse and in their physical linkage (Shimizu et al., 1981, 1982a ; Takahashi et al., 1981 ; Nishida et al., 1981). As summarized in Fig. 1, we have now cloned the entire C_H region gene cluster encompassing about 200kb. Portions of the cluster were also cloned in other laboratories (Liu et al., 1980 ; Moore

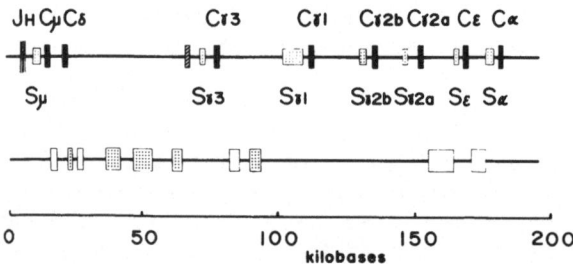

Fig. 1. Organization of the C_H gene family of BALB/c mouse.
Locations of structure genes (closed boxes) and S regions
(broken-lined boxes) are indicated on the top line. An obli-
que-lined box indicates the region which is homologous to the
$C_{\gamma 2b}$ probe. The second line indicates the location of reiterated
sequences. Taken from Shimizu et al. (1982a).

et al., 1981 ; Roeder et al., 1981). The organization of the
entire C_H gene cluster is 5'-J_H-6.5kb-C_μ-4.5kb-C_δ-55kb-$C_\gamma 3$-34kb-
$C_\gamma 1$-21kb-$C_\gamma 2b$-15kb-$C_\gamma 2a$-14kb-C_ϵ-12kb-C_α-3' in agreement with the
originally proposed order of the C_H genes (Honjo and Kataoka,
1978).

Using these isolated overlapping DNA segments, we have
characterized several stuctural features of the mouse C_H gene
loci. The results are summarized below. There are no other
J_H region segments except for those at the 5' side of the C_μ gene.
Namely, the J_H segments are shared among all the C_H genes. This
is consistent with the fact that the same V region sequence is
associated with different C region sequences in the linage of a
lymphocyte. The S region is present 5' to each C_H gene except for
the C_δ gene, and the nucleotide sequences of the S regions share
some homology as described later. There is no reasonably conserved pseudogene in the whole C_H gene cluster in contrast to the
human C_H gene family which has many pseudogenes. There are at
least two species of reiterated sequences scattered in these loci.
The distribution of such reiterated sequences in the C_H gene
family is not random, but their functional significance is not
known. Locations of reiterated sequences and S regions are schematically represented (Fig. 1).

Cloning and Southern blot hybridization analyses indicate
that the arrangements of the heavy chain gene loci of BALB/c and
C57BL/6 mice, which have many different serological markers, are
fundamentally similar but different in the length of S regions
(Fig. 2). In contrast, we found that the $C_{\gamma 2a}$ gene is duplicated
in a Japanese wild mouse Mus musculus molossinus (Shimizu et al.,

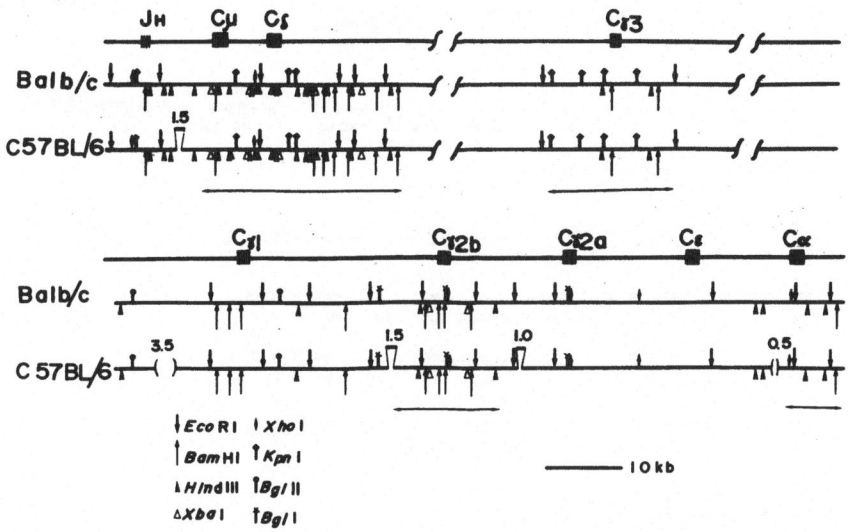

Fig. 2. Structural comparison of the C_H gene families in BALB/c and C57BL/6 mice. At the top line, structural genes are shown in closed boxes. Second and third lines show restriction maps of BALB/c and C57BL/6 mice, respectively. Only the restriction sites identified in C57BL/6 and their corresponding sites in BALB/c are shown. Numbers indicate lengths (kb) of deletions (parentheses) or insertions (bars) in C57BL/6 DNA as compaired with BALB/c DNA. Horizontal arrows below the third line indicate the regions which were cloned from C57BL/6 DNA. Taken from Shimizu et al. (1982a).

1982b). Both of these $C_{\gamma 2a}$ genes seem to be expressed because two individual mice of inbred <u>M</u>. <u>m</u>. <u>molossinus</u> have two allotypes of IgG2a (L. Herzenberg, personal communication).

2) Structure of Mouse C_H Genes

We and others have determined the complete nucleotide sequences of all the eight C_H genes of mouse. The exon-intron organization of each C_H gene is schematically shown in Fig. 3. The coding regions of these genes are split at the junctions of the domains and the hinge regions by intervening sequences (IVS). The results suggest that IVS was introduced into the C_μ gene before divergence of the H chain classes, and also support the hypothesis (Gilbert, 1978 ; Darnell, 1978) that the splicing mechanism has facilitated the evolution of eukaryotic genes by linking duplicated domains or exons of prototype peptides not directly adjacent to one another.

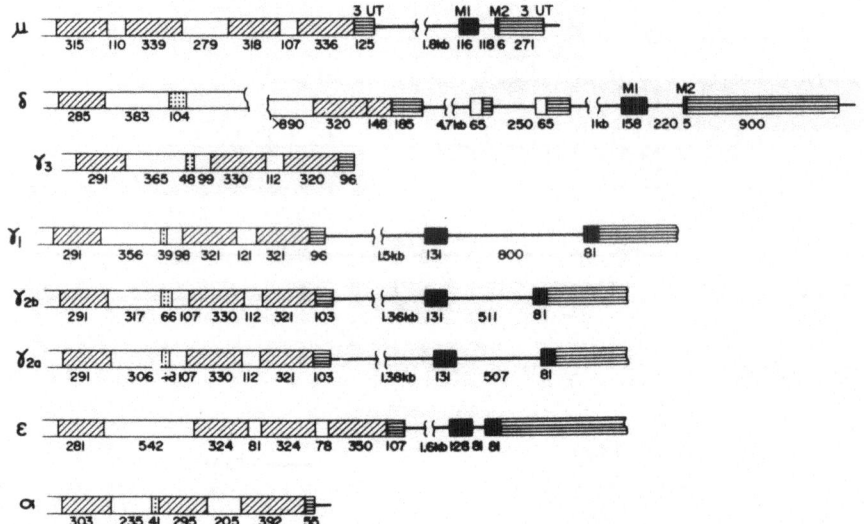

Fig. 3 Structures of mouse C_H genes. Lengths of exons, introns
and 3' untraslated sequences were determined by nucleotide
sequencing. Data are taken from various sources ; C_μ (Kawakami et
al., 1980 ; Early et al., 1980 ; Rogers et al., 1980), C_δ (Tucker
et al., 1980 ; Cheng et al., 1982), $C_{\gamma 3}$ (F. Blattner, unpublished
data), $C_{\gamma 1}$ (Honjo et al., 1979), $C_{\gamma 2b}$ (Yamawaki-Kataoka et al.,
1980), $C_{\gamma 2a}$ (Yamawaki-Kataoka et al., 1981), membrane exons of
C_γ (Yamawaki-Kataoka et al., 1982 ; Tyler et al., 1982 ; Nakai et
al., 1982 ; Roger et al., 1981) C_ε (N. Ishida and T. Honjo,
unpublished data) and C_α (Tucker et al., 1981).

Similarities in structure of C_H genes indicate that all the
C_H genes are derived from a common ancestral gene, probably a
prototype C_μ gene because some lower vertebrates can produce only
IgM.

3) IVS-mediated domain transfer

     Comparison of nucleotide sequences of C_H genes, especially
those of γ subclass genes has revealed an interesting conservation
of nucleotide sequences at limited portions of the gene (Miyata et
al., 1980 ; Yamawaki-Kataoka et al., 1981, 1982).   In order to
evaluate the divergence in the coding and non-coding segments of
the gene at the same level, the sequence divergence of the coding
region was determined by measuring two distinct types of
substitutions: one leading to the amino acid change (Ka) and the
other leading to the synonymous change (Ks). Obviously, the former
is under the influence of selective constrains at both protein and
RNA levels and the latter is under the influence of selective
constraint at the RNA level alone. The Ks values and substitution
rates at the non-coding region were used for comparison.

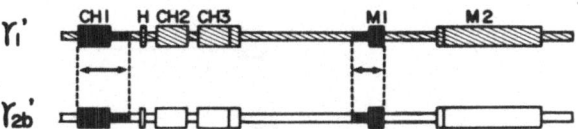

Fig. 4. Schematic representation of IVS-mediated domain exchange between ancestors of $C_\gamma 1$ and $C_\gamma 2b$ genes. Wider rectangles represent exons. Closed rectangles are homologous regions which were exchanged between the two genes. Taken from Yamawaki-Kataoka et al. (1982).

Such comparison between the γ1 and γ2b genes has shown that at least two segments, one including the CH1 domain and the 5' portion of the adjacent IVS and the other including the M1 exon and the flanking region are highly conserved as shown in Fig. 4. When the nucleotide sequences of the human γ4 and murine γ1 genes were compared, there was no particularly conserved segment in the gene. It is therefore likely that some correction mechanisms operate in the gene family. The mechanism could be either double unequal crossing-over or gene conversion (Baltimore, 1981). The exchange or transfer of genetics informations between a gene family seems to be common as growing numbers of examples were provided in immunoglobulin genes as well as in other genes (Schrier et al., 1981 ; Ollo and Rougeon, 1982 ; Slightom et al., 1980 ; Liebhaber et al., 1981 ; Lalanne et al., 1982).

4) <u>Evolution of the Human gamma Gene Family</u>

<u>Cloning and characterizaion of human γ gene clones</u> We and others have recently cloned most of the human C_H genes including C_μ, C_δ, C_γ, C_ε and C_α genes (Takahashi et al., 1980b ; Ravetch et al., 1980 ; Ellison et al., 1981 ; Ellison and Hood, 1982 ; Rabbitts et al., 1981 ; Nishida et al., 1982 ; Takahashi et al., 1982). We have isolated five human γ gene clones from phage libraries as shown in Fig. 5 (Takahashi et al., 1982). We have cloned four γ genes γ1, γ2, γ3 and γ4. The γ2 and γ4 genes were shown to be linked in this order by overlapping the flanking sequences and they are about 19kb apart. In addition, we obtained another γ gene clone called γ-11 which we think a pseudogene because of the several reasons to be discussed below. Since nucleotide sequences of human γ genes are similar to each other, we have identified these clones by determining nucleotide sequences of the hinge regions which are most divergent.

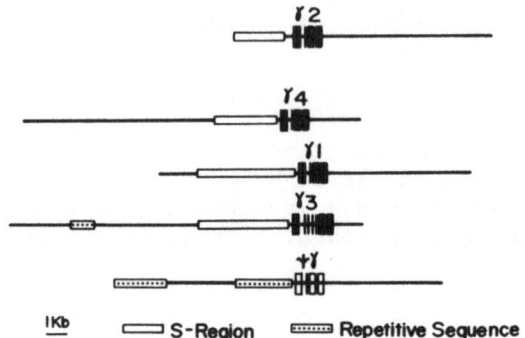

Fig. 5. Structure of human γ gene clones. Four γ genes (γ1, γ2, γ3 and γ4) and a pseudo γ gene (clone γ-11) are schematically shown. Exons are shown by closed rectangles. Taken from Takahashi et al. (1982).

As shown in Fig. 6 the amino acid sequences of the hinge regions predicted from the ńucleotide sequences of the γ1, γ2, γ3 and γ4 genes agree with the published sequences except for one residue in the γ4 gene (Edelman et al., 1969 ; Pink et al., 1970 ; Michaelsen et al., 1977 ; Wang et al., 1980). However, the amino acid sequence predicted from the nucleotide sequence of clone γ-11 does not coincide with any of the know human γ sequences.

The S regions of the μ, ε and α genes have been shown to be well conserved between human and mouse (Takahashi et al., 1980b ; Ravetch et al., 1980 ; Nishida et al., 1982). Similarly, the restriction fragments containing the 5' flanking regions of the γ1, γ2, γ3 and γ4 genes hybridized with the mouse $S_{\gamma 2b}$ probe. The γ-11 clone, however, did not have any fragment hybridizing with the mouse $S_{\gamma 2b}$ region that crosshybridized with all the S_γ regions of mouse. As the S region is essential for the class switch recombination, the γ-11 clone may not have any chance to be expressed. Furthermore, the γ-11 clone has highly repetitive sequences in the 5' flanking region where the S region is expected to be. Four gamma genes γ1, γ2, γ3 and γ4 have S region sequences at reasonable locations whereas the γ-11 clone has only repetitive sequences (Fig. 5). These observations described above, namely the absence of a known amino acid sequence, the absence of the S region and the presence of repetitive sequences, lead us to conclude tentatively that the clone γ-11 is a pseudogene.

```
γ2      GCAGAGCGCAAA------TGTTGTGTCGAG---------TGCCCACCGTGCCCAGGTAA
        GluArgLys         CysCysValGlu         CysProProCysPro

γ4      GCAGAGTCCAAA------TATGGTCCCCCA---------TGCCCATCATGCCCAGGTAA
        GluSerLys         TyrGlyProPro         CysProSerCysPro

γ1      GCAGAGCCCAAA------TCTTGTGACAAAACTCACACATGCCCACCGTGCCCAGGTAA
        GluProLys         SerCysAspLysThrHisThrCysProProCysPro

γ3H1    GCAGAGCTCAAAACCCCACTTGGTGACACAACTCACACATGCCCACGGTGCCCAGGTAA
        GluLeuLysThrProLeuGlyAspThrThrHisThrCysProArgCysPro

γ3H2    GCAGAGCCTAAA------TCTTGTGACACACCTCCCCCGTGCCCACGGTGCCCAGGTAA
        GluProLys         SerCysAspThrProProProCysProArgCysPro

γ3H3    GCAGAGCCTAAA------TCTTGTGACACACCTCCCCCGTGCCCACGGTGCCCAGGTAA
        GluProLys         SerCysAspThrProProProCysProArgCysPro

γ3H4    GCAGAGCCCAAA------TCTTGTGACACACCTCCCCCGTGCCCAAGGTGCCCAGGTAA
        GluProLys         SerCysAspThrProProProCysProArgCysPro

ψ       GCAGAGCCCAAAACCCCATGTTGTGACACAACTCACACATGCCCACCATGTGCAAGTAA
        GluProLysThrProCysCysAspThrThrHisThrCysProProCysAla
```

Fig. 6. Nucleotide sequences of the hinge regions of human γ
genes. The nucleotide sequences of the hinge regions are aligned
to maximize homology. Amino acids predicted by the nucleotide
sequences are shown below. Amino acid residue and nucleotide
sequences which are inconsistent with the published sequences are
underlined. Taken from Takahashi et al. (1982).

The γ3 gene may have been created by the exon reassortment
between the γ1 and pseudo γ genes. The structure of the γ3 gene
is interesting because there are four exons for the hinge region.
Apparently, such structure indicates that the hinge exon was
quadruplicated in the γ3 gene as proposed from the amino acid
sequence (Michaelsen et al., 1977). When we compared the
nucleotide sequences of the hinge exons of the γ3 gene with those
of the other γ genes, we realized that the fact is more
interesting than anticipated (Fig. 6). The first hinge exon (H1)
of the γ3 gene is very similar to that of the pseudogene which is
quite distinct from those of the other γ genes. However, the
other hinge exons H2, H3 and H4 of the γ3 gene are most homologous
to that of the γ1 gene. Consequently, it is most likely that the
γ3 gene was created by unequal crossing-over in the intervening
sequences (IVS) between the ancestors of the pseudo γ and γ1
genes, followed by two successive duplications of the γ1-type
hinge exon as shown in Fig. 7. Such unequal crossing-over
reassorted the exons of the ancestors of the γ1 and pseudo γ
genes, creating a new gene.

This assumption inevitably leads us to propose the order
5'-γ1-γ3-ψγ-3' in the human genome. Otherwise, the parental genes
would have been lost. The γ2 and γ4 genes are already physically

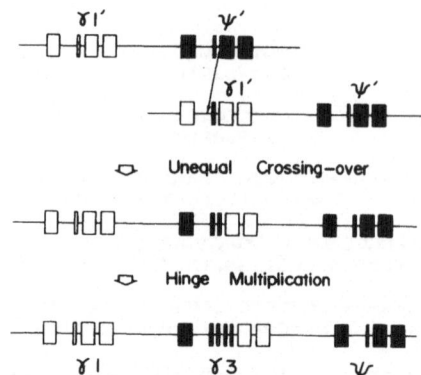

Fig. 7. An evolutionary pathway to create the γ3 gene. Open and closed rectangles indicate exons of the γ1 and pseudogene linages, respectively. Taken from Takahashi et al. (1982).

linked and their hinge region sequences are homologous to each other but different from those of the other γ genes. Two alternative γ gene orders can be proposed ; 5'-γ2-γ4-γ1-γ3-ψγ-3' and 5'-γ1-γ3-ψγ-γ2-γ4-3'. Neither of them agree with the order previously proposed on the basis of genetic studies (Natvig et al., 1967 ; Lefranc et al., 1977).

    <u>Phylogenetic trees of human gamma genes</u> From these studies we can estimate the phylogenetic tree of the human γ genes as shown in Fig. 8. There are two possibilities. In the first case (A), we assume the prototype γ gene is either γ1 or γ2 (γ4) type, both of which have deletions in the hinge exon as compared with the pseudogene. The prototype γ gene underwent duplication and segregated into the anscestors of the γ1 and γ2 genes. The γ2 gene ancestor again duplicated and evolved the γ2 and γ4 genes which are about 19kb apart. The γ1 gene anscestor also duplicated and evolved the anscestors of the γ1 and pseudo γ genes. Then, unequal crossing-over took place between these two genes and the γ3 gene anscestor was created as proposed above. In the other case (B), the prototype γ gene segregated into the ancestors of the pseudogene and all the other γ genes. Then, the γ1 gene segregated from the γ2 and γ4 gene ancestors. Like the first case, unequal crossing-over took place between the γ1 and pseudo γ genes and the γ2 and γ4 genes evolved by duplication. Had no recombination taken place among gamma genes, we could distinguish between the two models by determining whether the γ1 gene is more homologous to the pseudogene than the γ2 (or γ4) gene. Comparison of the nucleotide sequences so far determined of the pseudogene, γ2 and γ4 genes with that of the γ1 gene did not allow us to distinguish these models.

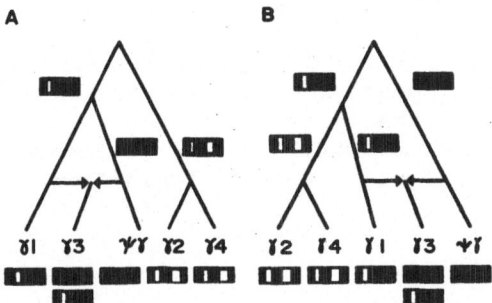

Fig. 8. Phylogenetic trees of human γ genes. The γ genes are best distinguished by the structures of the hinge exons which are schematically shown by closed boxes with deletions (see Fig. 6). Horizontal arrows indicate unequal crossing-over. Taken from Takahashi et al. (1982).

In any case, these results clearly demonstrate that human gamma genes underwent dynamic rearrangements during evolution. To create a human γ gene family there have been several types of gene rearrangement, which include at least three duplications of a complete γ gene, two duplications of the hinge exon and the exon reassortment by unequal crossing-over between two adjacent genes. Certainly many point mutations have accumulated in the γ subclass genes. Nonetheless, DNA rearrangements seem to have played a more important role for the evolution of the γ subclass genes. This might be the best example of how a gene family evolved by exon reassortments.

5) Human Pseudo Epsilon Gene Family

We have also cloned the human epsilon gene (Nishida et. al., 1982). Since the amino acid sequence homology between the human and mouse ε chains is only 43%, it is impossible to use the mouse ε gene (Nishida et al., 1981) as a probe for cloning the human ε gene. Instead, we have used the J_H probe and cloned a rearranged ε chain gene from DNA of a human ε-producing myeloma 266B1 (Nilsson, 1971).

The ε chain gene clone was identified by the complete nucleotide sequence determination. The sequence matched almost perfectly with the published amino acid sequence except for 15 residues out of 427 residues. The human ε gene has four exons, each encoding one domain just like the mouse ε gene. BamHI digestion of human DNA produced three $C_ε$ fragments of 3.0, 6.5 and

9.2kb, which were named $C_\varepsilon 1$, $C_\varepsilon 2$ and $C_\varepsilon 3$ genes, respectively (Fig. 9). We found the three C_ε gene fragments in all of the human DNA preparations from 11 individuals, excluding the possibility of polymorphysm. The C_ε gene expressed in the myeloma was identified as the $C_\varepsilon 1$ gene from the restriction map. Since the $C_\varepsilon 2$ gene is deleted from the myeloma DNA, the $C_\varepsilon 2$ is located 5' to the $C_\varepsilon 1$. The nonrearranged $C_\varepsilon 3$ gene was also cloned from the myeloma DNA.

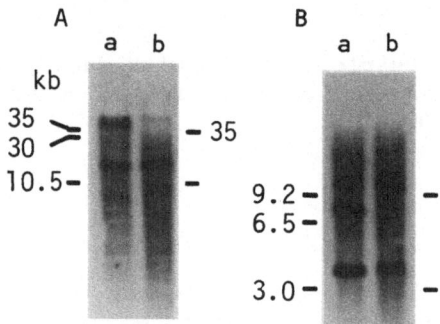

Fig. 9. Southern blot hybridization of human DNA with the C_ε probe. Human placenta and 266Bl DNAs were digested with BamHI(A) or EcoRI(B). Southern blots were hybridized with the C_ε probe. Lanes a and b contain placenta and 266Bl DNAs, respectively. Numbers indicate sizes of hybridized bands in kb. Taken from Nishida et al. (1982).

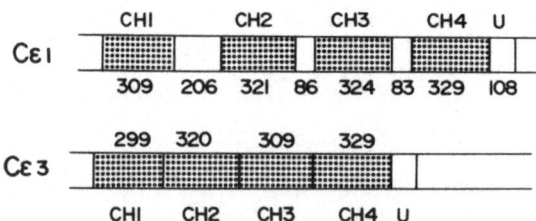

Fig. 10. Comparison of structure of the $C_\varepsilon 1$ and $C_\varepsilon 3$ genes. Dotted and open boxes indicate exons and introns, respectively. Numbers show lengths (bp) of exons and introns. U, untranslated region.

The heteroduplexes formed between the $C_{\varepsilon 1}$ and $C_{\varepsilon 3}$ genes have revealed that the $C_{\varepsilon 3}$ gene might have deleted three introns. The complete nucleotide sequence of the $C_{\varepsilon 3}$ gene was determined and compared with that of the $C_{\varepsilon 1}$ gene. Although the nucleotide sequence of the $C_{\varepsilon 3}$ gene is 83% homologous to that of the $C_{\varepsilon 1}$ gene in the exons, the introns are precisely spliced out of the $C_{\varepsilon 3}$ gene. The $C_{\varepsilon 3}$ gene does not have any J or V-like sequence at the 5' side but does have poly(A)-like sequence at the 3' side. The structures of the $C_{\varepsilon 1}$ and $C_{\varepsilon 3}$ genes are schematically shown in Fig. 10. This type of the gene was called a processed gene as previously found in the mouse α globin gene family, the human immunolobulin gene family and the human β-tubulin gene family (Nishioka et al., 1980 ; Hollis et al., 1982 ; Wilde et al., 1982).

The most exciting was the finding that movable genetic elements including LTR-like sequences flank both the 5' and 3' sides of the $C_{\varepsilon 3}$ gene as shown in Fig. 11. We can assign two sets of LTR-like sequences, both of which have an inverted repeat, a TATA box and a poly(A) signal (AATAAA). The inverted repeat of one LTR is $(T)_6-(A)_6$ and that of the other (TGAA)-(TTCA). In addition, there are short direct repeats at the 5' and 3' ends of each set. However, the 5' and 3' LTR-like sequences in each set do not constitute a direct repeat (Fig. 11A). There are multiple copies of the 3' LTR-like sequence in the human genome. The evolutional origin of the spliced gene is a fascinating question. The presence of the LTR-like structure suggests that the $C_{\varepsilon 3}$ was transcribed into RNA and that the spliced RNA might have been integrated back to the genome by way of the reverse transcription

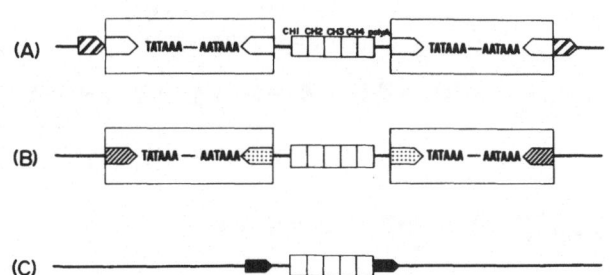

Fig. 11. The possible arrangements of movable genetic elements flanking to human immunolgobulin epsilon pseudogene $C_{\varepsilon 3}$. The sequences of direct and inverted repeats in each model are ; (A) GCT or ACC, TTTTTT or TGAA, (B) TGGCANGAG, TGGNCAAGG, (C) CCTAGAG, respectively.

as proposed previously (Hollis et al., 1982). There are several other possibilities such as the gene conversion model (Nishioka et al., 1980) and two step model (S. Ueda and T. Honjo, in preparation). Note that other types of movable genetic elements are also found in the vicinity of the $C_\varepsilon 3$ gene. We can identify two sets of large inverted repeats surrounding the $C_\varepsilon 3$ gene (Fig. 11B). It is also possible to locate the direct repeat on both sides of the $C_\varepsilon 3$ gene (Fig. 11C).

The $C_\varepsilon 2$ gene is also a pseudogene because the two exons of the C_{H1} and C_{H2} domains are deleted.

III. MOLECULAR GENETIC BASIS FOR CLASS SWITCHING

1) The S-S Recombination

During differentiation of a single B lymphocyte a given V_H region is first expressed as a μ chain, followed by the switch of the C_H region to other classes such as δ, γ, ε and α. The molecular genetic basis for this phenomenon called heavy chain class switch has been elucidated recently by cloning and characterization of immunoglobulin genes of mouse myelomas secreting various classes of immunoglobulin (Davis et al., 1980a ; Kataoka et al., 1980 ; Sakano et al., 1980). According to this model (Fig. 12) rearrangement called S-S recombination brings a

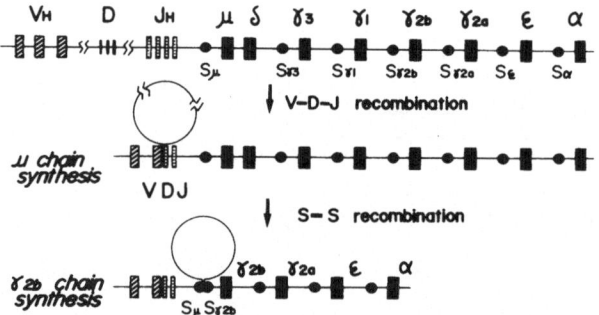

Fig. 12. Rearrangements during differentiation of B lymphocytes. Two successive recombinations V-D-J and S-S complete the expressed form of the γ2b chain gene. Both events are accompanied by deletion of intervening DNA segments which might be accomplished through looping-out or sister chromatid exchange (Obata et al., 1981). Reproduced from Honjo et al. (1981b)

completed V_H gene, which is located originally 5' to the C_μ gene, close to another C_H gene by deletion of an intervening DNA segment (Honjo and Kataoka, 1978 ; Cory et al., 1980 ; Coleclough et al., 1980 ; Rabbitts et al., 1980 ; Yaoita and Honjo, 1980). The S-S recombination takes place between S regions located in the 5' flanking region of each C_H gene. The nucleotide sequences of S regions are shown to comprise tandem repetitive sequences sharing short common sequences (Kataoka et al., 1981 ; Davis et al., 1980b ; Dunnick et al., 1980 ; Nikaido et al., 1981, 1982).

2) C_H Genes Are Not Rearranged in $\mu^+\varepsilon^+$ B Cells

It is known that resting B cells often bear two different isotypes on their surface. The most common are those bearing IgM and IgD. Some carry IgG, IgE or IgA in addition to IgM. It has been difficult to explain this type of class switching, namely from $\mu^+\delta^+$ to $\mu^+\gamma^+$ or $\mu^+\varepsilon^+$ by the S-S recombination that is accompanied by deletion of C_H genes including the C_μ gene. We have, therefore, analyzed the organization of C_H genes in sorted $\mu^+\varepsilon^+$ B-lymphocytes and found that they retain the C_μ, C_δ, C_γ and C_ε genes in the germline configulation, suggesting that the simultaneous expression of the C_μ and C_ε genes is mediated by an RNA splicing mechanism (Yaoita et al., 1982).

Borges et al (1981) found that Igh congenic strain SJA/9 (Igh^a) having SJL background cannot produce a detectable amount of IgE in the sera even after the infection of Nippostrongylus brasiliensis, which is known to stimulate polyclonal IgE production. Furthermore, Okumura and his associates (unpublished data) also found that the increase of IgE-bearing B cells after N. brasiliensis infection occurs equally in SJA/9 as well as SJL mice. Approximately 10% of the spleen cells of the N. brasiliensis-infected mice carry IgE on their surface. The advantage of SJA/9 mice is that a low IgE level in sera minimizes binding of IgE to Fc receptors of ε-negative lymphocytes, thus avoiding the contamination of ε-negative cells into sorted ε^+ B cells.

The IgE-bearing B cells were isolated from spleen cells of N. brasiliensis-infected SJA/9 mice by the fluorescence-activated cell sorter. Only brightest top 9% of the stained cells were collected. The purity of the isolated cells was examined under the fluorescent microscope, which is less sensitive and gives a lower limit value of staining. At least 86% of the sorted cells were brightly stained with anti-ε antibody. Most of the ε-bearing cells also carried the μ chain on their surface. However, they were not stained with either anti-δ, anti-γ2a or anti-γ1 antibody. The results indicate that the sorted cells are the essentially pure population of $\mu^+\varepsilon^+$ B cells.

   To confirm that IgE on the surface of $\mu^+\varepsilon^+$ B cells is endogenously synthesized, ε^+ B cells were treated with trypsin
(2.5mg/ml) for 30 min at 37°C to strip off all cell surface
immunoglobulins, then after culturing, newly synthesized immunoglobulins on the surface were reexamined by fluorescence
staining. As expected, 2hr and 5hr after the trypsin treatment,
84% and 97%, respectively, of cells were stained with anti-ε.
Furthermore, the sorted ε^+ B cells of SJA/9 were shown to secret
IgE when T cells of SJL were provided (K. Okumura, unpublished
data).

   We have extracted DNA from the sorted $\mu^+\varepsilon^+$ cells and examined
the C_H gene organization in ε-bearing cells using the Southern
blotting technique. When DNA of ε^+ B cells was digested with

Table 1 C_H Genes in $\mu^+\varepsilon^+$ B Cells

C_H genes examined	length (kb) of fragments identified*	origin of DNA	
		liver	$\mu^+\varepsilon^+$ B cell
C_μ	13 (EcoRI)	+	+
C_δ	11.5 (BamH1)	+	+
$C_{\gamma 3}$	14 (EcoRI)	+	+
	6.6 (Hind III)	+	+
$C_{\gamma 1}$	23 (Hind III)	+	+
	6.6 (EcoRI)	+	+
$C_{\gamma 2b}$	6.6 (EcoRI)	+	+
	9 (Hind III)	+	+
$C_{\gamma 2a}$	21.3 (EcoRI)	+	+
	6.2 (Hind III)	+	+
C_ε	21.3 (EcoRI)	+	+
	4.8 (Bam1)	+	+
J_H	6.4 (EcoRI)	+	− (faint)

* Restriction enzymes used are indicated in parentheses.

EcoRI, blotted and hybridized with the C_ε gene probe, it produced a 21.3 kb fragment which is identical to that produced in SJA/9 liver DNA (Table 1).   Since the EcoRI fragment (21.3kb) encompasses the whole region between the $C_{\gamma 2a}$ and C_ε genes, the above results indicate that the C_ε gene does not rearrange in the IgE-bearing lymphocytes unlike the IgE-secreting hybridoma and myeloma (Nishida et al., 1981, 1982).

EcoRI digestion of the ε^+ B cell DNA produced the germline form of the C_μ gene fragment (13 kb) as shown in Fig. 13. Inasmuch as the 13 kb C_μ fragment contains the whole S_μ region, there is no doubt about the absence of the DNA rearrangement in the S_μ region.   BamHI digestion of the ε^+ B cell and SJA/9 liver DNAs yielded the 11.5 kb fragment hybridizing with the C_μ probe. Since the 11.5 kb BamHI fragment encompasses the C_δ as well as C_μ gene, the results indicate that the C_δ gene is not rearranged in the ε^+ B cells.   Similarly, the $C_{\gamma 3}$, $C_{\gamma 1}$, $C_{\gamma 2b}$ and $C_{\gamma 2a}$ genes are not rearranged in the $\mu^+\varepsilon^+$ B cells.   In contrast, the J_H gene fragment of the IgE-bearing lymphocyte DNA drastically reduced the intensity as compared with that of SJA/9 liver DNA and appeared blurred in agreement with the interpretation that a large number of different rearrangements have generated many new EcoRI fragments of different lengths in polyclonal B cells (Nottenberg and Weisman, 1981).   From these results it is likely that the organization of the C_H gene in the IgE-bearing cells is the same with the germline gene except that the J_H is rearranged.   These data indicate that IgE expression in $\mu^+\varepsilon^+$ B cells does not involve the S_μ-S_ε rearrangement.

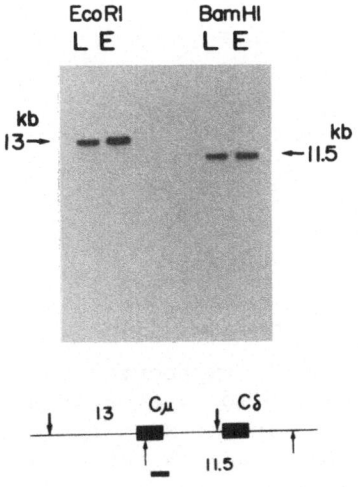

Fig. 13. Analysis of EcoRI and BamHI fragments of ε-bearing cell and SJA/9 liver DNAs using cloned mouse C_μ gene as probe. The fragments produced by EcoRI and BamHI digestion of ε-bearing cell DNA (E) and SJA/9 liver DNA (L) were electrophoresed and blotted to nitro cellulose filters. The restriction map surrounding probe used is shown below. Each lane contains about 1µg DNA. ↓ , EcoRI; ↑ , BamH1.

3) Class Switching Proceeds by Two Biochemical Steps

Given these results we propose that differentiation of IgM-bearing B lymphocytes to IgE-secreting plasma cells may proceed by at least two biochemical steps as shown in Fig. 14. The first step (step I) promotes differentiation of IgM-bearing B lymphocytes into IgM-IgE-bearing B lymphocytes, which involves the activation of differential RNA processing of a single large RNA transcript containing V_H, C_μ, C_δ, C_γ and C_ε gene sequences. The large transcript may be spliced into μ or ε mRNA by specific enzymes and/or specific assisting molecules such as low molecular weight RNA (Lerner et al., 1980 ; Roger and Wall, 1980). The size of the primary transcript is estimated to be about 180 kb from the C_H gene organization (Shimizu et al., 1982a). Naturally, the μ and ε mRNAs share an identical V_H region sequence. Since we handled a mixed population of $\mu^+\varepsilon^+$ lymphocytes, we were unable to obtain the evidence that the same V_H sequence was associated with the C_μ and C_ε sequences in a single cell. However, IgD and IgM molecules were shown to bear the identical V_H region in a $\mu^+\delta^+$ lymphoma (Maki et al., 1981). We presume that the step I does not involve any major DNA rearrangement.

IgM-IgE-bearing B lymphocytes differentiate into IgE-secreting B cells or plasma cells by the step II which involves the S_μ-S_ε recombination and the simultaneous DNA deletion as established before (Nishida et al., 1981). Needless to say, similar mechanism should apply to the switch from IgM-bearing B

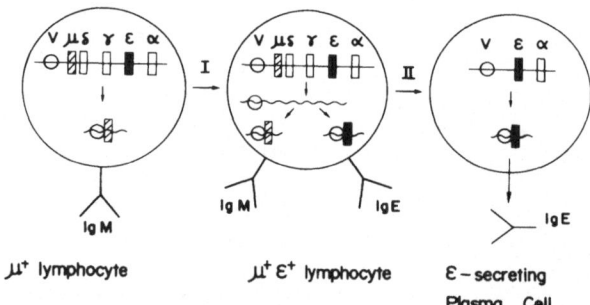

Fig. 14. Two steps of differentiation from μ^+ lymphocytes to ε-secreting plasma cells. Step I involves the activation of differential splicing. Alternate splicing of a long transcript containing V_H, C_μ, C_γ and C_ε sequences will produce mRNA encoding either μ or ε chain with the same V region sequence. Step II involves DNA deletion. Taken from Yaoita et al., (1982).

cells to IgD-, IgG-or IgA-secreting plasma cells. It is not clear whether DNA rearrangement accompanies the differentiation from IgM-bearing B cells to IgM-secreting plasma cells. It is worth noting that most of the IgM-secreting myelomas and hybridomas seem to have deletion in the S_μ region (Coleclough et al., 1980; Hurwitz et al., 1980 ; Yaoita and Honjo, 1980). We think it reasonable that deletion of the S_μ region facilitates the transcription of the C_μ gene and promotes the secretion of IgM since the extremely GC-rich S_μ region (Nikaido et al., 1981) may hinder the efficient transcription.

There are no data as to how long the primary transcript of μ mRNA is in IgM-bearing B cells. They may transcribe the whole C_H gene locus from the beginning. If so, the step I is mediated by the activation of a new differential splicing system. Alternatively, the primary transcript in IgM-bearing B cells may contain only the V_H and C_μ sequences. In this case the step I requires at least two new biochemical events, i.e. the transcription of a much larger RNA and the activation of a new differential splicing system. To avoid the premature termination of transcription lymphocytes may have to introduce some biochemichal changes in the C_H gene loci such as demethylation (Razin and Riggs, 1980). In fact the C_δ gene is demethylated in $\mu^+\delta^+$ hybridoma but not in μ^+ lymphoma (Rogers and Wall, 1981).

This model favors that the splicing as well as recombination mechanism is class-specific. Otherwise, the isotype expression in B cells should be transient and multiple (more than three isotypes per cell) untill they become plasma cells. Several lines of evidence suggest that the expression of a certain V_H sequence is closely associated with a specific C_H isotype. CBA/N mice have genetic defects which make them incapable of producing anti-phosphorylcholine antibody of any classes other than IgE whereas anti-phosphorylcholine antibody of IgM and IgG is very common in most mouse strains (Sher et al., 1975 ; Kishimoto et al., 1979). A lymphoma cell line I.29 was shown to switch always from μ to α (Sitia et al., 1981). Such results appear to indicate that the S-S recombination is catalyzed by the class-specific enzyme(s).

IgM-IgE-bearing lymphocytes accumulated in spleens of N. brasiliens-infected SJA/9 mice are capable of differentiating into IgE-secreting plasma cells when T cells of SJL are provided (K. Okumura, unpublished data). Since SJA/9 mice can synthesize normal amounts of IgM, IgG and IgA, the defect of SJA/9 seems to reside in IgE-specific regulatory T cells (Kishimoto, 1982). Furthermore, the step II is a likely step at which the T cells affect the B cell differentiation.

Perlmutter and Gilbert (1982) found the existence of the

C_μ gene in γ_1-bearing B cells purified from normal spleen using antibody-coated petri dishes. Alt et al. (1982) reported that the C_μ and $C_{\gamma 2b}$ genes remain intact in a γ2b chain-producing variant of the Abelson virus-transformed cell line 18-81.

IV. MOLECULAR MECHANISM OF THE S-S RECOMBINATION

1) Nucleotide Sequences of S Regions

In order to elucidate molecular mechanism for the S-S recombination we have determined the nucleotide sequences of the S regions (Takahashi et al., 1980a ; Kataoka et al., 1981 ; Nikaido et al., 1981, 1982). The results indicate that the 5' flanking regions of all the C_H genes except for the C_δ gene contain the S regions which comprise tandem repetition of short unit sequences. The nucleotide sequences of the repeat units of the S reigons are summerized in Fig. 15. Comparison of the nucleotide sequences of all the S regions revealed that length as well as nucleotide sequences of the S region sequences vary among different classes of the C_H gene but share short common sequences, (G)AGCT and TGGG(G). The nucleotide sequence of the S_μ region is homologous to those of the other S regions in the decreasing order of the S_ε, S_α, $S_{\gamma 3}$, and ($S_{\gamma 1}$, $S_{\gamma 2b}$, $S_{\gamma 2a}$) regions.

S_μ*	GAGCTGAGCTGGGGTGAGCT
$S_{\gamma 3}$	PGGACCAGGCTGGGACAGCTCTGGGGAGCTGGGGTGGGTGGGAGTGTGG
$S_{\gamma 1}$	GPPTCCAGGCTGAGCAGCTACAGGGGAGCTGGGGYAPPTGGGAPTPTPG
$S_{\gamma 2b}$	GGGACCAG$^{T}_{A}$CCTAGCAGCTPTGGGGGAGCTGGGGA$^{A}_{T}$GGTPGGAPTPTGA
$S_{\gamma 2a}$	GGGACCAGGCAGTACAGCTCTGGGTPGGGPNCAGGCAGTACAGCTCTGNGTG
S_ε*	GGGCTGGGCTGAGCTGPGCTGAGCTGPGCTGAGCTGPPNT
S_α	ATGAGCTGGGATGAGCTGAGCTAGGCTGGAATAGGCTGGGCTGGGCTGGT GTGAGCTGGGTTAGGCTGAGCTGAGCTGGA
common sequences	(G)AGCT(G), TGGG(G)

*, variable unit length

Fig. 15. Nucleotide sequences of repeat units of S regions. The consensus sequence of the repeat unit of each S region is shown. Common short sequences are underlined. P, purine ; Y, pyrimidine. Taken from Nikaido et al. (1982).

The order of the S region homology mentioned above does not seem to correlate with the relative contents of the immunoglobulin classes in mouse serum. In contrast, the order of the S region lengths appears to bear some correlation with the relative contents of the immunoglobulin classes in the mouse serum. In BALB/c IgG1 is the most abundant immunoglobulin class, followed by IgG2a, IgG2b and IgA in decreasing order (Kalpaktsoglou et al., 1973). This observation is consistent with the fact that the $S_{\gamma 1}$ region is the longest among the S reigons of BALB/c (Fig. 16). In C57BL/6 serum IgG2b is the highest in the concentration, followed by IgG1, IgG2a and IgA in that order (Barth et al., 1965), which is in general agreemnt with the order of the S reigon length in this strain, namely the $S_{\gamma 2b}$, $S_{\gamma 1}$, $S_{\gamma 2a}$, $S_{\gamma 3}$ and S_{α} regions (Fig. 2). In both strains the S_{ϵ} is the shortest and IgE is the least abundant.

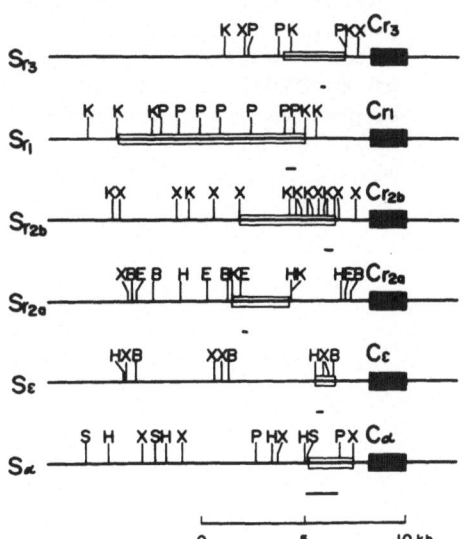

Fig. 16. Locations and ranges of the S regions. Schematic representation of the locations and sizes of the $S_{\gamma 3}$, $S_{\gamma 1}$, $S_{\gamma 2b}$, $S_{\gamma 2a}$, S_{ϵ} and S_{μ} regions is shown. Open boxes indicate the location of restriction DNA fragment containing the S region. Structural genes are shown as closed boxes with direction of transcription from left to right. Taken from Nikaido et al. (1982).

It is hard to believe that the length of the S reigon and the S reigon homology with the S_{μ} region directly determine the relative concentration of the immunoglobulin class as the latter depends on many other regulatory steps such as the B-lymphocyte proliferation and the half life of immunoglobulins. However, it is conceivable that the C_H gene organization may affect the relative abundance of the immunoglobulin class to some extent because the longer the S region, the higher the chance of the class switch recombination.

We have compared the nucleotide sequences immediately adjacent to the recombination sites of seven rearranged genes as shown
in Fig. 17.   Note that tetranucleotides TGAG and/or TGGG are
always found except for one case.   Such tetranucleotides may
constitute a part of the recognition sequence of a putative
recombinase.   These results provide a support to our previous proposal that the S-S recombination may be facilitated by short common sequences dispersed in all the S regions.

Clones		S regions
Igε-1	GA<u>TGGG</u>T<u>GGG</u>CTTCTCT<u>GAG</u>	Sμ
	TGTAGGGGAGĊAGGGATAGG	Sγ2b
Igε-1	AGGGAGC<u>TGGG</u>GCAGG<u>TGGG</u>	Sγ2b
	CTAAGCTTAGTTTAGC<u>TGAG</u>	Sε
J606	C<u>TGAG</u>C<u>TGGG</u>G<u>T</u>GAGC<u>TGAG</u>	Sμ
	GGGAGTG<u>TGGG</u>GACGGGTTG	Sγ3
MOPC141	TGTTAAAGAAṪGGTATCAAA	Sμ
	GCCAGGAGAGTTGTCCGATT	Sγ2b
MC101	<u>TGAG</u>GTGATTAĊTC<u>TGAG</u>GT	Sμ
	C<u>TGAG</u>CTGGAA<u>TGAG</u>C<u>TGGG</u>	Sα
MC101	GCTAGGTTGGṪC<u>TGAG</u>CTGA	Sα
	CTGGAGCTGA<u>TGGG</u>TATAAA	Sγ1
TEPC15	TGGTATCAAAĠGACAGTGCT	Sμ
	TGGAA<u>TGAG</u>Ċ<u>TGGG</u>TT<u>GAG</u>C	Sα
M603	<u>TGGG</u>GC<u>TGAG</u>Ċ<u>TGAG</u>C<u>TGAG</u>	Sμ(deleted)
	ATAGGT<u>TGGG</u>Ċ<u>TGGG</u>C<u>TGGT</u>	Sα
MPC11	TAGAGCTGAĊ	Sγ3
	GCGGGGATAGG<u>TGGG</u>AGTAT	Sγ2b

Fig. 17. Nucleotide sequences around S-S recombination
sites. TGGG and TGAG are
underlined. Dots indicate
putative recombination
sites. Nucleotide sequences
of MOPC141, TEPC15 and M603
sequences are taken from
Davis et al., (1980).

2) Sister Chromatid Exchange Model

The basic mechanism for the S-S recombination may be a sort
of a homologous recombination mediated by short reiterated common
sequences.   It is now established that the S-S recombination is
accompanied by deletion of C_H genes.   Two alternative models can
be proposed to explain the mechanism of the C_H gene deletion in B-
lymphocytes as shown in Fig. 18.   The first model postulates that
the S-S recombination takes place on a single chromosome by mutual

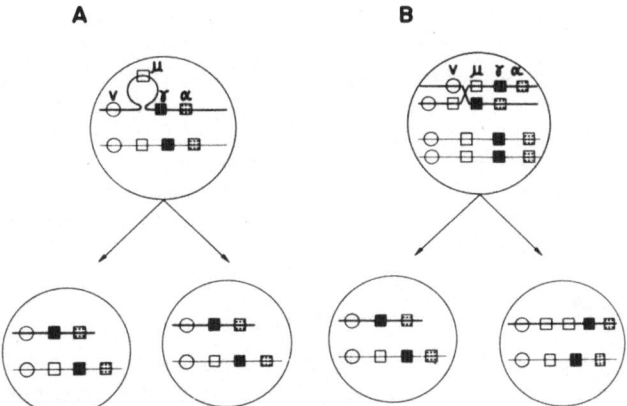

Fig. 18 Possible models for deletion of C_H genes in class switch recombination. A, looping-out model. B, sister chromatid exchange model. Taken from Obata et al. (1981).

recognition of two S regions. The intervening DNA segment is looped out and lost from the chromosome. This model is referred to as a looping-out model. Such recombination can occur at any stage of the cell cycle in principle. The other model, called a sister chromatid exchange model, explains the deletion of DNA segment by an unequal crossing-over event between sister chromatids (Honjo et al., 1981a ; Obata et al., 1981). According to this model one of the daughter cells contains an additional copy of the C_H gene that is lost in the other daughter cell. Sister chromatid exchange is unlikely to occur at any other stage of the cell cycle except for the mitotic phase.

I will describe observations which lead us to conclude that the sister chromatid exchange model is more favorable than the looping-out model. First, the expressed $\gamma 1$ gene from MC101 myeloma contains the S_α segment between the S_μ and $S_{\gamma 1}$ regions (Obata et al., 1981). It appears as if the presence of the S_α segment between the S_μ and $S_{\gamma 1}$ segments contradicted the linear arrangement of C_H genes ($5'-C_\mu-C_{\gamma 3}-C_{\gamma 1}-C_{\gamma 2b}-C_{\gamma 2a}-C_\varepsilon-C_\alpha-3'$) and the deletion mechanism for the class switch. It is too complicated to explain such rearrangement by recombination events within a chromosome. The generation of such $\gamma 1$ gene, however, can be explained by two or three successive unequal crossing-over events. There are various possible pathways to create the MC101 $\gamma 1$ gene.

Secondly, inhibition of the cell division leads to an increase in the frequency of binucleated cells able to direct synthesis of both IgM and IgG under the conditions that a single lymphocyte can give rise to progeny cells synthesizing IgM, IgG or IgA (Lawton et

al., 1977; van der Loo et al., 1979). The results suggest that
the class switch from IgM to IgG may involve an asymmetric cell
division, which is consistent with the sister chromatid exchange
model although they do not necessarily exclude the looping-out
model. Since the percentage of cells containing both IgM and IgG
relative to cells containing only IgG was rather high (10-20%) and
increased 2 to 3 fold by inhibition of cell division, switching
process appears to take place during cell division, probably
during or after replication of DNA.

3) S-S Recombination in E. coli Extracts

    Assay system   The molecular mechanism of the S-S recom-
bination including the possibility of the sister chromatid
exchange can be directly tested by the in vitro recombination
system. For this purpose it is important to set up an assay
system that allows us to detect an extremely small number of
recombinants like one recombinant out of 10^7 molecules (Kataoka et
al., 1982). The basic idea of this assay system is illustrated in
Fig. 19. We made two kinds of λ phage derivatives, each carrying
an immunoglobulin S region as well as a coding sequence. In this
case μ and α phages are shown. The two phages have different

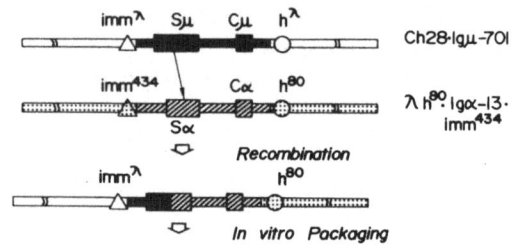

Fig. 19. In vitro assay system for the S-S recombination.
Ch28·Igμ-701 was constructed by a simple transfer of the insert
EcoRI fragment of λgtWES·IgH 701 (Kawakami et al., 1980).
λhϕ80·Igα-13·imm434 was constructed by recombination between
Ch28·Igα-13 and a recombinant phage λhϕ80·Imm434·pgal, followed by
the second recombination between the recombinant obtained
(Ch28·Igα-13·hϕ80) and a λ phage (hλ·imm434). Two phages were
incubated with lymphocyte extracts and DNAs were extracted. DNAs
were packaged in vitro into coat proteins and the recombinants
produced by recombination within two genetic markers were recovered by infection to E.coli K993 [ϕ80S·λR (imm434)].

genetic markers on each arms.   The μ phage has immunity to λ and
the tail protein (host restriction) of λ phage whereas the α phage
has immunity to λ434 and the tail protein of φ80. After in vitro
reaction with lymphocyte extracts, we can extract phage DNAs,
package them into coat proteins and have them infect E.coli to
recover recombinant phages. If we choose a proper host bacteria
like K993 which is φ80-sensitive, λ-resistant and immune to λ434,
we can detect a recombinant very efficiently.

Recombination in vitro To our surprise, however, we soon
found that this assay system has very high back ground. Many
recombinants were produced without lymphocyte extracts.   So we
decided to characterize the recombinational system in E.coli or λ
phage which seem to catalize the S-S recombination of the immunoglobulin gene. To exclude the recombination which took place

Table 2   Recombination of Immunoglobulin Genes in E.coli and
             in vito Packaging System

Experimental System	Recombination frequency	Recombination site[a] (%)	
	(x10^{-4})	insert	vector
Expt I (in vitro packaging)			
Complete	3.5	30	70
With inversely inserted μ gene	1.6	1.6	98
Mixed after separate packaging	2.0	2	98
Expt II (double infection)			
Complete	43	0	100
With inversely inserted μ gene	37	0	100

a, recombinat phages were screened by in situ hybridization using
the DNA fragment 5' to the S_μ region and that 3' to the C_α gene
as probes.   Recombinants that hybridized to both probes were
classified into those which recombined within the inserts.

48   T. HONJO ET AL.

within phage arms between two genetic markers, putative recombinants grown on K993 were screened by hybridization with μ and α
probes. We determined the number of clones which hybridized to
both μ and α probes. As shown in Table 2 the recombination frequency is in the order of 10^{-4}. The reaction requires that two S
regions are in the same orientation because the S-S recombination
was not detected when one of the insert is inverted. The recombination reaction seems to take place or initiate during the in
vitro packaging reaction because the S-S recombination was not
observed when two phages were packaged separately. Also double
infection at 100 times higher moi did not induce the S-S recombination although the recombination in the vector arms took place
at 100 times higher frequency.

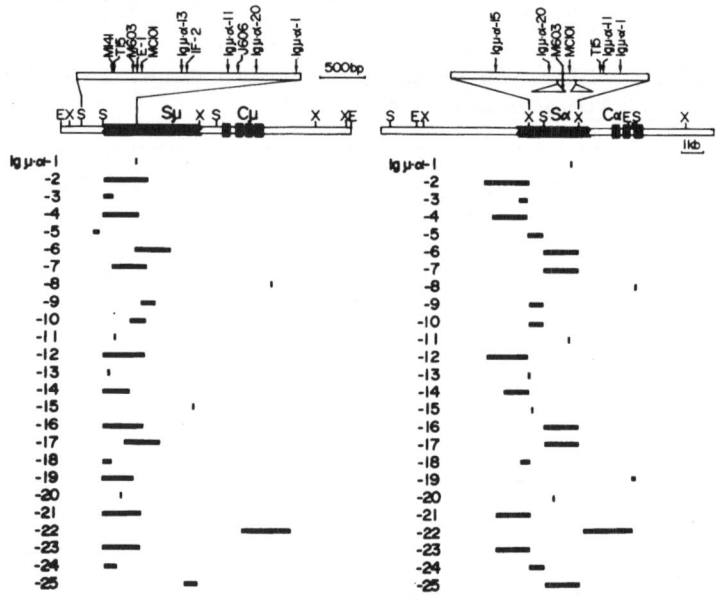

Fig. 20. Distribution of the recombination sites on μ and α chain
genes. The left and right horizontal rectangles represent the
restriction cleavage sites of the Igμ-701 and Igα-13 inserts,
respectively. Horizontal bars below the restriction maps of the
parental clones indicate the estimated ranges of the recombination
sites. In the clones, the recombination sites of which are definitely assigned, the sites are shown as the vertical lines. Top
rectangles above Igμ-701 and Igα-13 represent enlargements of portions of the S_μ and S_α regions which include the class switch
recombination sites of various myelomas or hybridomas as well as
those of the several in vitro recombinant clones. Triangles below
the top bar of Igα-13 indicate the locations of deletions intro-
duced upon cloning of $\lambda h^{\phi}80 \cdot Ig\alpha-13 \cdot imm^{434}$. S, SacI; X, XbaI;
E, EcoRI.

Nucleotide sequences surrounding recombination sites We have
determined locations of recombination sites of randomly-chosen 25
recombinant phages by restriction site mapping. The majority of
recombination (about 90%) occurred within the S_μ and S_α regions.
Some took place in the coding regions (Fig. 20). Then, we have
arbitrarily chosen 4 recombinants and determined the nucleotide
sequences surrounding recombination sites. As shown in Fig. 21
the recombinations must have taken place somewhere within the
boxed regions. These regions always contain TGAG or TGGG which is
also found around the class switch recombination site in mouse
myelomas. These results taken together, the λ phage-E.coli system
may have the recombinational system that can recognize short
sequences similar to those used in the class switch recombination
of the immunoglobulin gene.

Note that the Chi sequence (TCTGGTGG), which enhances the
generalized recombination in E.coli (Smith et al., 1981), bears
striking homology with the S_μ sequence and short sequences found
around the recombination sites in E.coli as well as in myelomas.
We have recently shown that the nucleotide sequences almost identical to the mouse S_μ region are represented in variety of organisms such as yeast, sea urchin and Drosophila (Sakoyama et al.,
1982). Although the biological function of these sequences is not
known, one may speculate that these sequences have been conserved
in variety of organisms because they serve as recognition signals
for DNA recombination of other genes.

```
Recombinant 1    GAGCTGAGCTGAGCTGGGCTAGGCTGAGTTAGTCT
Germline Sα      GGAATGAATTAGTCTGGGCTAGGCTGAGTTAGTCT

Recombinant 11   AGCTGAGCTGGAGTGAGCTGAGCTAGACTTAGGGT
Germline Sα      GGCTACAATGGATTGAGCTGAGCTAGACTTAGGGT

Germline Sμ      CCGGATGTTTTGAGTTGAGCTGGGGTAAGATGAGC
Recombinant 15   CCGGATGTTTTGAGTTGAGCTAGGTTGAGATGGGC
Germline Sα      TGGGCTGAGTTGTGTTGAGCTAGGTTGAGATGGGC

Recombinant 20   GAGCTGAGCTGGGGTGAGCTGGGTTGAGCTGAGCT
Germline Sα      AGGCTGGGCTGGTGTGAGCTGGGTTGAGCTGAGCT

Myeloma Sμ       TGAGGTGATTACTCTGAGGT
        Sα       CTGAGCTGGAATGAGCTGGG
```

Fig. 21. Nucleotide sequences of recombination sites in S-S
recombinants isolated from E.coli. Nucleotide sequences of recombination sites in four independent S-S recombinants were
determined. The germline S_μ sequence was not available except for
the recombinant 15 but the nucleotide sequence of the S_μ region
where these recombination took place is shown to be represented by
$[(GAGCT)_3 GGGGT]_n$ (Nikaido et al., 1981). Myeloma sequence (MC101)
is taken from Obata et al. (1981). Possible recombination sites
are boxed. TGGG or TGAG closest to the recombination sites is
underlined.

ACKNOWLEGMENT

    We are grateful to Ms. S. Nishida and Y. Nakayama for their
expert technical assistance and to Ms. F. Oguni for her exellent
secretarial assistance. We appreciate collaborations with Drs. K.
Okumura and Y. Kumagai (Tokyo Univ.), Dr. T. Miyata (Kyushu Univ.)
and Dr. K. Moriwaki (Genetic Inst.). This investigation was supported by grants from the Ministry of Education, Science and
Culture of Japan.

REFERENCES

Alt, F.W., Rosenberg, N., Casanova, R.J., Thomas, E. and
        Baltimore, D. (1982) Nature 296, 325-331.
Baltimore, D. (1981) Cell 24, 592-594.
Barth, W.F., Mclaughlin, C.L. and Fahey, J.L. (1965) J. Immunol.
        95, 781-790.
Borges, M.S., Kumagai, Y., Okumura , K., Hirayama, N., Ovary, Z.
        and Tada, T. (1981) Immunogenetics 13, 499-507.
Cheng, H,-L., Blattner, F.R., Fitzmanrice, L., Mushinski, J.F. and
        Tucker, P.W. (1982) Nature 296, 410-415
Coleclough, C., Cooper, C. and Perry, R.P. (1980) Proc. Natl.
        Acad. Sci. USA 77, 1422-1426.
Cory, S. and Adams, J.M. (1980) Cell 19, 37-51.
Cory, S., Jackson, J. and Adams, J.M. (1980) Nature 285, 450-456.
Darnell, J.E. Jr, (1978) Science 202, 1257-1260.
Davis, M.M., Calame, K., Early, P.W., Livant, D.L., Joho, R.,
        Weissman, I.L. and Hood, L. (1980a) Nature 283, 733-739.
Davis, M.M., Kim, S.K. and Hood, L. (1980b) Science 209,
        1360-1365.
Dunnick, W., Rabbitts, T.H. and Milstein, C. (1980) Nature 286,
        669-675.
Early, P., Rogers, J., Davis, M., Calame, K., Bond, M., Wall, R.,
        and Hood, L. (1980) Cell 20, 313-319.
Edelman, G.M., Cunningham, B.A., Gall, W.E., Gottlieb, P.D.,
        Rutishauser, U. and Waxdal, M.J. (1969) Proc. Natl. Acad.
        Sci. USA 63, 78-85.
Ellison, J., Buxbaum, J. and Hood, L. (1981) DNA 1, 11-18.
Ellison, J. and Hood, L. (1982) Proc. Natl. Acad. Sci. USA 79,
        1984-1988.
Gilbert, W. (1978) Nature 271, 501.
Hollis, G.F., Hieter, P.A., McBride, O.W., Swan, D. and Leder, P.
        (1982) Nature 296, 321-325.
Honjo, T. and Kataoka, T. (1978) Proc. Natl. Acad. Sci. USA 75,
        2140-2144.
Honjo, T., Obata, M., Yamawaki-Kataoka, Y., Kataoka, T., Kawakami,
        T., Takahashi, N. and Mano, Y. (1979) Cell 18, 559-568.
Honjo, T., Kataoka, T., Yaoita, Y., Shimizu, A., Takahashi, N.,
        Yamawaki-Kataoka, Y., Nikaido, T., Nakai, S., Obata, M.,

Kawakami, T. and Nishida, Y. (1981a) Cold Spring Harbor Symp. Quant. Biol. 45, 913-923.

Honjo, T., Nakai, S., Nishida, Y., Kataoka, T., Yamawaki-Kataoka, Y., Takahashi, N., Obata, M., Shimizu, A., Yaoita, Y., Nikaido, T. and Ishida, N. (1981b) Immunol. Review 59, 33-67.

Hurwitz, J.L., Coleclough, C. and Cebra, J.J. (1980) Cell 22, 349-359.

Kalpaktsoglou, P.K., Hong, R. and Good, R.A. (1973) Immunol. 24, 303-314.

Kataoka, T., Kawakami, T., Takahashi, N. and Honjo. T. (1980) Proc. Natl. Acad. Sci. USA 77, 919-923.

Kataoka, T., Miyata, T. and Honjo, T. (1981) Cell 23, 357-368.

Kataoka, T., Takeda, S. and Honjo, T. (1982) submitted.

Kawakami, T., Takahashi N. and Honjo, T. (1980) Nucl. Acids Res. 8, 3933-3945.

Kishimoto, T., Shigemoto, S., Watanabe, T. and Yamamura, Y. (1979) J. Immunol. 123, 1039-1043.

Kishimoto, T. (1982) Prog. Allergy (ed. P. Kallos, K. Ishizaka and B. Waksman) Kalger Pub. Inc., Basel, in press (1982).

Lalanne, J.L., Bregegere, F., Abastado, J.P., Gachelin, G. and Kourilsky, P. (1982) Nucl. Acids Res. 10, 1039-1049.

Lefranc, G., Rivat, L., Sulier, J.P., van Loghem, E., Aydenian, H., Zalzal, P., Chakhachiro, L., Loiselet, K. and Ropartz, C. (1977) Am. J. Hum. Genet. 29, 523-536.

Lawton, A.R., Kearney, J.F. and Cooper, M.D. (1977) Progress in Immunology 3, 171-182.

Lerner, M.R., Boyk, J.A., Mount, S.M., Wolin, S.L. and Steitz, J.A. (1980) Nature 283, 220-224.

Liebhaber, S.A., Goossens, M. and Kan, Y.W. (1981) Nature 290, 26-29.

Liu, C.-P., Tucker, P.W., Mushinski, G.F. and Blattner, F.R. (1980) Science 209, 1348-1353.

Maki, R., Roeder, W., Traunecker, A., Sidman, C., Wabl, M., Raschke, W. and Tonegawa, S. (1981) Cell 24, 353-365.

Michaelsen, T.E., Frangione, B. and Franklin, E.D., (1977) J. Biol. Chem. 252, 883-399.

Miyata, T., Yasunaga, T., Yamawaki-Kataoka, Y., Obata, M. and Honjo, T. (1980) Proc. Natl. Acad. Sci. USA 77, 2143-2147.

Moore, K.W., Rogers, J., Hunkapiller, T., Early, P., Nottenburg, C., Weissman, T., Bazin, H., Wall, R. and Hood, L.E. (1981) Proc. Natl. Acad. Sci. USA 78, 1800-1804.

Nakai, S., Vernon, O., Herzenberg, L.A., Yamagishi, H., and Honjo, T. (1982) Biomed. Res. 3, 37-45.

Natvig, J.B., Kunkel, H.G. and Litwin, S.D. (1967) Cold Spring Harbor Symp. on Quant. Biol. 32, 173-180.

Nikaido, T., Nakai, S. and Honjo, T. (1981) Nature 292, 845-848.

Nikaido, T., Yamawaki-Kataoka, Y. and Honjo, T. (1982) J. Biol. Chem. 257, 7322-7329.

Nilsson, K. (1971) Int. J. Cancer 7, 380-396.

Nishida, Y., Kataoka, T., Ishida, N., Nakai, S., Kishimoto, T., Böttcher, I. and Honjo, T. (1981) Proc. Natl. Acad. Sci. USA 78, 1581-1585.

Nishida, Y., Miki, T., Hisajima, H. and Honjo, T. (1982) Proc. Natl. Acad. Sci. USA 79, 3833-3837.

Nishioka, Y., Leder, A. and Leder, P. (1980) Proc. Natl. Acad. Sci. USA 77, 2806-2809.

Nottenberg, C. and Weisman, I.L. (1981) Proc. Natl. Acad. Sci. USA 78, 484-488 (1981).

Obata, M., Kataoka, T., Nakai, S., Yamagishi, H., Takahashi, N., Yamawaki-Kataoka, Y., Nikaido, T., Shimizu, A. and Honjo, T. (1981) Proc. Natl. Acad. Sci. USA 78, 2437-2441.

Ollo, R. and Rougeon, F. (1982) Nature 296, 761-763.

Perlmutter, A. P. and Gilbert, W. (1982) Proc. Natl. Acad. Sci. USA, in press.

Pink, J.R.L., Buttery, S.H., deVries, G.M. and Milstein, C. (1970) Biochem. J. 117, 33-47.

Rabbitts, T.H., Forster, A., Dunnick, W. and Bentley, D.L. (1980) Nature 283, 351-356.

Rabbitts, T.H., Forster, A. and Milstein, C. (1981) Nucl. Acids Res. 9 4509-4524.

Ravetch, J.V., Kirsch, I.R. and Leder, P. (1980) Proc. Natl. Acad. Sci. USA 77, 6734-6738.

Razin, A. and Riggs, A.D. Science 210, 604-610 (1980).

Roeder, W., Maki, R., Traunecker, A. and Tonegawa, S. (1981) Proc. Natl. Acad. Sci. USA 78, 474-478.

Rogers, J., Early, P., Carter, C., Calame, K., Bond, M., Hood, L. and Wall, R. (1980) Cell 20, 303-312.

Rogers, J. and Wall, R. (1980) Proc. Natl. Acad. Sci. USA 77, 1877-1879.

Rogers, J., Choi, E., Souza, L., Carter, C., Word, C., Kuehl, M., Eisenberg, D. and Wall, R. (1981) Cell 26, 19-27.

Rogers, J. and Wall, R. (1981) Proc. Natl. Acad. Sci. USA 78, 7497-7501.

Sakano, H., Maki, R., Kurosawa, Y., Roeder, W. and Tonegawa, S. (1980) Nature 286, 676-683.

Sakoyama, Y., Yaoita, Y. and Honjo, T. (1982) Nucl. Acids Res. in press.

Schrier, P.H., Bothwell, A.L.M., Mueller-Hill, B. and Baltimore, D. (1981) Proc. Natl. Acad. Sci. USA 78, 4495-4497.

Sher, I., Ahmed, A., Strong, D.M., Steinberg, A.D. and Paul, W.E. (1975) J. Exp. Med. 141, 788-803.

Shimizu, A., Takahashi, N., Yamawaki-Kataoka, Y., Nishida, Y., Kataoka, T. and Honjo, T. (1981) Nature 289, 149-153.

Shimizu, A., Takahashi, N., Yaoita, Y. and Honjo, T. (1982a) Cell 28, 499-506.

Shimizu, A., Hamaguchi, Y., Yaoita, Y., Moriwaki, K., Kondo, K. and Honjo, T. (1982b) Nature 298, 82-84.

Sitia, R., Rubartelli, A. and Hammerling, U. (1981) J. Immunol. 127, 1388-1394.

Slightom, J.L., Blechl, A.E. and Smithies, O. (1980) Cell 21,
        627-638.
Smith, G.R., Kunes, S.M., Schultz, D.W., Taylor, A. and Trinan,
        K.L. (1981) Cell 24 429-436.
Takahashi, N., Kataoka, T. and Honjo, T. (1980a) Gene 11,
        117-127.
Takahashi, N., Nakai, S. and Honjo, T. (1980b) Nucl. Acids Res. 8,
        5983-5991.
Takahashi, N., Shimizu, A., Obata, M., Nishida, Y., Nakai, S.,
        Nikaido, T., Kataoka, T., Yamawaki-Kataoka, Y., Yaoita,
        Y., Ishida, N. and Honjo, T. (1981) C. Janeway, E.E.
        Sercarz and H. Wigzell, eds. (New York : Academic Press),
        pp 123-134.
Takahashi, N., Ueda, S., Obata, M., Nikaido, T. and Honjo, T.
        (1982) Cell 29, 671-679.
Tucker, P.W., Liu, C.-P., Mushinski, J.F. and Blattner, F.R. (1980)
        Science 209, 1353-1360.
Tucker, P.W., Slighton, J.L. and Blattner, F.R. (1981) Proc. Natl.
        Acad. Sci. USA 78, 7684-7688.
Tyler, B.M., Cowman, A.F., Gerondakis, S.D., Adams, J.M. and
        Bernard, O. (1982) Proc. Natl. Acad. Sci. USA 79,
        2008-2012.
van der Loo, W., Gronowicz, E.S., Strober, S. and Herzenberg, L.A.
        (1979) J. Immunology 122, 1203-1208.
Wang, An-Chuan, Tung, E. and Fudenberg, H. (1980) J. Immunol. 125,
        1048-1054.
Wilde, C.D., Crowther, C.E., Cripe, T.P., Lee, M. G.-S. and Cowan,
        N.J. (1982) Nature 297, 83-84.
Yamawaki-Kataoka, Y., Kataoka, T., Takahashi, N., Obata, M. and
        Honjo, T. (1980) Nature 283, 786-789.
Yamawaki-Kataoka, Y., Miyata, T. and Honjo, T. (1981) Nucl. Acids
        Res. 9, 1365-1381.
Yamawaki-Kataoka, Y., Nakai, S., Miyata, T. and Honjo, T. (1982)
        Proc. Natl. Acad. Sci. USA 79, 2623-2627.
Yaoita, Y. and Honjo, T. (1980a) Biomed. Res. 1, 164-175.
Yaoita, Y. and Honjo, T. (1980b) Nature 286, 850-853.
Yaoita, Y., Kumagai, Y., Okumura, K. and Honjo, T. (1982) Nature
        297, 697-699.

DISCUSSION

Leder: Indirect evidence from a human IgE-producing cell line suggests that the E pseudogene (called E2 by Honjo) is 5' to the active gene - that is, the pseudogene is deleted in this line.

Milstein: Dr. Honjo, did you say most of the C_H has been left intact, but that some may be deleted?

Honjo: No, it is identical to the germ line sequence.

Vitetta: Have you tried activating the epsilon positive cells with LPS to see if they will be activated to secretion? That is, can you induce a DNA rearrangement?

Honjo: This has not been done.

Jones: What is the role of antigen in expanding the number of cells with a particular combination of C_H on the surface? Do you think that the decision of which second C_H will be expressed (through long transcript) along with C_u is random, with a role for antigen in selecting B cells expressing a certain C_H?

Honjo: T cells may recognize the surface Ig and may prefer a certain V region associated with a particular C_H region. If T cells give a special signal to begin the class-specific S-S recombination, this will result in a tight coupling of RNA splicing (step I) and DNA recombination (step II).

Leder: Are these epsilon positive cells normal B cells?

Honjo: Yes.

Leder: How do you know that you are not looking at both chromosomes?

Honjo: Because the analysis is quantitative.

Cohn: What happens in E. coli that lack Rec. A?

Honjo: Switch recombination in the E.coli system does not depend on Rec. A.

Hood: Expression of immunoglobulin IgA by plasmacytomas occurs as a result of DNA rearrangement that brings the variable gene, (V_H), a few kilobases 5' to the constant region gene, C_{alpha}. We have demonstrated that the allelic or nonexpressed C_{alpha} gene also is rearranged in virtually all plasmacytomas. Cloning, restriction mapping, heteroduplex analyses, and sequence analyses of the nonproductively rearranged C_{alpha} genes from two plasmacytomas, M603 and M167, have demonstrated that the nonproductive rearrangement occurs within the alpha switch region, S_{alpha}. In each case, the same DNA sequence has been joined to the 5' side of the C gene and we have termed this DNA NIRD (for nonimmunoglobulin rearranged DNA). Southern blotting analysis of genomic DNAs from a variety of IgG-, IgM-, or IgA-producing plasmacytomas suggests that NIRD is rearranged in almost all plasmacytomas. However, NIRD rearranges to the S_{alpha} regions only in IgA-producing cells and not in IgM or IgG producers.

Cytogenetic evidence has shown than translocations between chromosones 12 and 15 are common in murine plasmacytomas. Immunoglobulin heavy genes are located on chromosome 12 and the translocation breakpoint in plasmacytomas occurs near the immunoglobulin genes. NIRD has been mapped to chromosome 15 by Southern blotting analysis of mouse or hamster cell lines, suggesting that the nonproductively rearranged C_{alpha} gene clones represent the 12-15 chromosomal translocations identified cytogenetically. Therefore, we have identified a region of DNA on chromosome 15 that is commonly rearranged in transformed mouse lymphocytes. Obviously one can speculate on the possible significance of the NIRD sequence in the neoplastic transformation of mouse lymphocytes, particularly with regard to the possibility that it is a cellular oncogene that has been activated through chromosomal rearrangement.

Leder: We have also seen this rearrangement (Kirsch et al., Nature, 1981) and find that it has occurred in all the non-u myelomas we have looked at.

Cohn: What happens in the abberrantly rearranged chromosome when the expressed chromosome switches to another class?

Weigert: In what B cells do you find the rearranged x sequence?

Hood: We find that it is rearranged in every IgA producer and in some B cells expressing other classes of immunoglobulins. In these latter case we do not know where x rearranges to.

Cohn: The switch from IgM to other Ig classes is driven by the effective level of T helper activity

There are two views possible on the regulation of this class switch. Either the switch is random in which case any disproportionate expression of an isotype must involve an isotype recognizing mechanism, or the switch is directed (non-random), in which case any disproportionate expression of an isotype must involve a set of isotype inducing hormones.

The argument used by Lee Hood that the switch is non-random is based on studies with C_{alpha}. It is not strong because C_{alpha} is the

3' ultimate C-gene and successive random switches in both chromo-somes would have to end up at C alpha, deleting everything in between. Besides, I believe that there exist data showing that the chromosome pair does not switch in parallel to the same C-gene.

In any case, the randomness or non-randomness of the switch is the key question to settle before discussions of mechanism can become meaningful. It is the reason I asked the question "What happens to the aberrantly rearranged chromosome during class switching of the functionally rearranged chromosome?"

Leder: I simply wish to point out that this is one of two poorly understood genetic rearrangements that occur in immunoglobulin producing cells. The other is the disappearance or inevitable re-arrangement of kappa genes in lambda producing B-cells.

Nabholz: Carlo Croce has claimed that the Burkitt lymphoma specific rearrangements involve the "non-expressing" Ig-chromosome. Is this true?

Leder: I think both models are valid even if the translocation is to the "inactive" chromosome. For example, both kappa alleles are transcribed, though only one makes a "normal" transcript.

Mäkelä: How low is actually the production of circulating IgE in the SJA mouse? It is probably increased by the nematode infection, is it still low enough to exclude the problem of cytophilic antibodies?

Hood: Dr. Honjo has demonstrated that one may strip IgE from these B cells and in five hours they regain (presumably resynthesize) surface IgE.

Vitetta: One could answer this more definitely by looking at the size of the H chains on the cell surface IgE. Cell surface IgE should be larger than secreted IgE.

Uhr: I want to clarify Dr. Honjo's speculation concerning the coordination of RNA splicing and DNA rearrangements, which is necessary for a B cell to differentiate into a plasma cell that secretes the same isotype as was expressed by the B cell. Your last figure suggested that a T cell was responsible. The implication, therefore, is that the non-IgM isotype is a receptor for an isotype specific T helper cell or T cell derived lymphokine that signals the B cell to undergo the DNA rearrangements resulting in synthesis of the isotype in question. Is this your viewpoint?

Honjo: T cells may recognize the surface Ig and may prefer a certain V region associated with a particular C_H region. If T cells give a special signal to begin the class-specific S-S combination, this will result in a tight coupling of RNA splicing (step I) and DNA recombination (step II).

Coutinho: If we come back to Dr. Honjo's model, I would like to ask him about the "rigidity" of the relationship he postulates between the specificities of the splicing and recombination steps. The model postulates that such specificities are related, in order to "use" surface expression in the regulation of the secreted isotypes (e.g. by isotype-specific helper cells or factors). In contrast, however, we have evidence pointing out that the relationship between membrane and secreted isotypes is not absolute in the case of IgG subclasses. Together with Luciana Forni at the Basel Institute for Immunology we have analysed the production of membrane and secreted forms of all isotypes (except IgD) in single clones of normal B cells and at single cell level. We detected a sizeable fraction of all cells bearing any given IgG which also express a second IgG isotype on the membrane. Furthermore, and here the data have direct implications to the model, a proportion of all cells carrying a given membrane IgG are secreting a different IgG subclass, indicating that the specificity of splicing (membrane expression) is often different from the specificity of recombination (secreted forms).

Honjo: It is possible that the IgM-IgE-bearing lymphocytes are in a transient stage and they can shift to express the different isotypes. In that case there is no solid linkage between the steps I and II.

Session III

MHC Genes

Chairman: J. Strominger

MOLECULAR ANALYSES OF MHC ANTIGENS

O.Kämpe, D.Larhammar, K.Wiman, L.Schenning, L.Claesson, K.Gustafsson, S.Pääbo, J.J.Hyldig-Nielsen, L.Rask, and P.A.Peterson

Dept. of Cell Research, The Wallenberg Laboratory, Box 562, S-751 22 Uppsala, Sweden

The major histocompatibility complex (MHC) has an essential role in the immune system. In a direct manner some of the MHC antigens, the class I molecules, seem to be involved in combatting virus-infections inasmuch as MHC antigens on virus-infected cells are part of the target for T-killer cells. Such T-cell killing is generally restricted to the virus and one or more of the class I molecules of the infected cell (see ref. 1). Whether one T-cell receptor jointly recognizes a virus product in association with a class I antigen or whether separate T-cell receptors independently recognize the virus product and the class I antigen, respectively, is not yet resolved (for a recent review see ref. 2). In this paper we will discuss our approach to analyze this issue.

The class II antigens of the MHC are directly or indirectly involved in several immunological events. Thus, antigen-presenting cells seem to display class II molecules in an obligatory manner. T-helper cells responding to the antigen-presenting cell recognize a given class II antigen presented together with a foreign substance. At subsequent antigen challenge the T-helper cell seems to recognize the same foreign substance only when it is presented together with the initially recognized class II molecule (see ref. 3). The class II antigens also seem to serve as controling elements in the interactions between T-helper cells and B-cells (4) and between T-suppressor cells and other T-cells (5). Furthermore, delayed-type hypersensitivity is to a great extent controled by the class II antigens (6).

Detailed knowledge of the structure of class II antigens has largely been lacking, which, of course, preclude attempts to

61

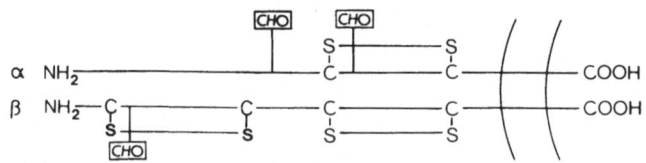

Figure 1. Schematic picture of a class II antigen. Both α and ß
          chains contain disulfide loops and carbohydrate moieties
          (CHO). The most NH$_2$-terminal CHO moiety of the α-chain is
          of the high-mannose type (L. Claesson, unpublished
          observations).

describe the immunological phenomena of class II antigens in molecular detail. As a first step towards approaching the molecular
function of the class II antigens several laboratories including
our own, have begun to elucidate their structure.

General Structure of Human Class II Antigens

     Using recombinant DNA technology we have isolated several cDNA
clones corresponding to human class II α (7) and ß chains (8). The
nucleotide sequences of some of these clones have been reported
(9-11). The amino acid sequences predicted from the sequences of
the cDNA clones confirm that class II antigens are composed of
heterodimers, as shown in Fig. 1. The two polypeptide chains appear
to be of about equal length. Both chains contain hydrophobic
stretches of amino acids close to their COOH-termini followed by 10
to 15 mostly hydrophilic amino acids. In agreement with previous
indirect data (12, 13) this suggests that both chains are integral
membrane proteins and that their COOH-terminal regions reside on
the cytoplasmic side of the plasma membrane.

     The extracellular portions of the human class II antigen α
chains are composed of two domains, each containing an Asn-linked
carbohydrate unit. An immunoglobulin-like disulfide loop occurs in
the domain closest to the membrane-integrated portion of the chain
(for further details see ref. 11).

     The ß chains of the human class II antigens are also composed
of two extracellular domains. In contrast to the α chain both ß
chain domains contain disulfide loops of the immunoglobulin type. A
single carbohydrate unit is attached to the first Asn in position
18 (see ref.10).

Class II Antigen α Chains

     The predicted amino acid sequence of the human HLA-DR antigen

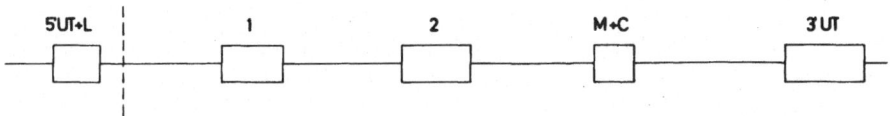

Figure 2. Outline of the murine E   gene. Exons are denoted by the
boxes. Information to the left of the broken line is
tentative.

α chain was recently elucidated (11). Using probes derived from a
cDNA clone corresponding to this chain, Southern blot analyses of
EcoRI-digested human genomic DNA derived from HLA-DR homozygous
individuals revealed a single band. Thus, no evidence for
polymorphism at the genomic level was obtained. However, repeating
the analyses with Bgl II-digested DNA gave a pattern that was
allotype-specific (not shown). Since the sequenced cDNA α chain
clones do not contain any Bgl II restriction sites it seems reasonable to conclude that the HLA-DR antigen α chain genes contain
variable Bgl II sites in the intron sequences and/or in the flanking sequences.

Recently, at least two, new putative α chain cDNA clones have
been isolated whose restriction maps differ markedly from that of
the analyzed HLA-DR antigen α chain cDNA clones. It is assumed that
at least one of these clones should correspond to the human gene
product equivalent to the murine α chain of the I-A region.

The HLA-DR antigen α chain cDNA clones hybridize specifically
to genomic clones containing the murine E_α gene (T. Lund and R.
Flavell, unpublished). From a cosmid library containing approximately 40 kb fragments of genomic DNA of mice of the $H-2^d$
haplotype, two F_α gene-containing clones were isolated. Restriction
mapping and Southern blot hybridizations suggested that the two
clones contained the same gene. This gene has been sequenced in its
entirety apart from the region to the left of the broken line in
Fig. 2. We have determined the leader sequence of a human α chain,
which codes for 25 amino acid residues, so it seems reasonable to
conclude that the fine structure of the murine E_α gene is that of
Fig. 2, although the size of the first intron is presently unknown.
Following the first intron the exon coding for the first domain of
the α chain appears (Fig. 2). It contains information for amino acid
residues 3 to 85 (numbering is according to the sequence of the
human α chain). The second extracellular domain of the E_α chain
corresponds to residues 86 to 178 and is encoded in the third exon.
The fourth exon contains contiguous information both for the membrane-embedded and the intracellular sequences, respectively, of the

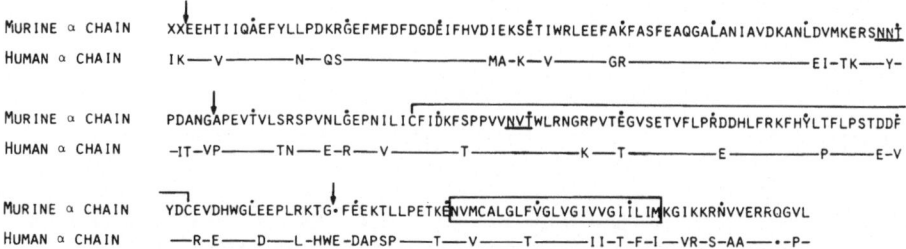

Figure 3. Predicted amino acid sequences of a murine $E_\alpha{}^d$ and a human HLA-DR α chain. <u>Arrows</u> denote exon-intron boundaries. Underlined residues represent putative carbohydrate attachment sites. Residues within the box are probably embedded in the lipid matrix of the plasma membrane. The dots above the residues mark every 10 residue. Dots within the sequences denote gaps introduced to maximize the homology.

E_α chain. The 3'-untranslated portion of the mRNA is encoded in the fifth exon. In contrast to class I antigens (14, 15), whose cytoplasmatic region appears to be encoded in two or three separate exons, the E_α gene does not seem to have the potential for alternative splice events in the corresponding region (for discussion, see ref. 16).

The amino acid sequence predicted from the nucleotide sequence of the E_α gene is compared to that of the HLA-DR antigen αchain in Fig. 3. It can be seen that the two sequences have several features in common. The Asn-linked carbohydrates and the single disulfide loop seem to occur in analogous positions. The membrane-embedded portions of the two chains are apparently identical in size. The overall homology between the two sequences is 74%. However, both the first domains (second exon) and the second domains (third exon) display 80% homology while the membrane-integrated and cytoplasmic stretches of the chains (fourth exon) only share identical residues in 59% of the positions. Consequently, the evolutionary pressure appears to be greater on the extracellular portions of the α chain than on the membrane-integrated and intracellular portions. It is particularly interesting to note that serine-219 in the human sequence is replaced by an arginine in the murine E_α chain since this serine has been implicated in phosphorylation events (see ref. 13). Recent data in our laboratory suggest that the major portion of the phosphorylation occurs on a human α chain distinct from the HLA-DR antigen α chain (O. Kämpe, unpublished information).

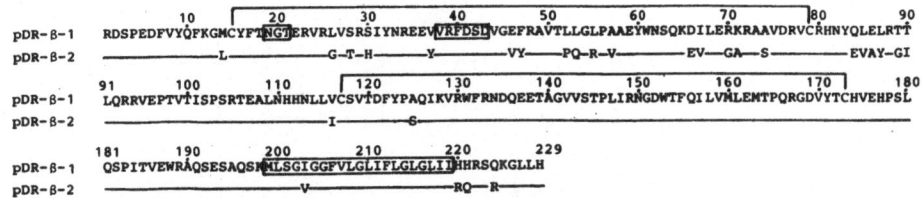

Figure 4. Predicted amino acid sequences of two human class II antigen ß chain cDNA clones. The boxes denote, in order of appearance, the carbohydrate binding site, the invariant hexapeptide (see Fig. 9) and the membrane-embedded portion of the chain, respectively.

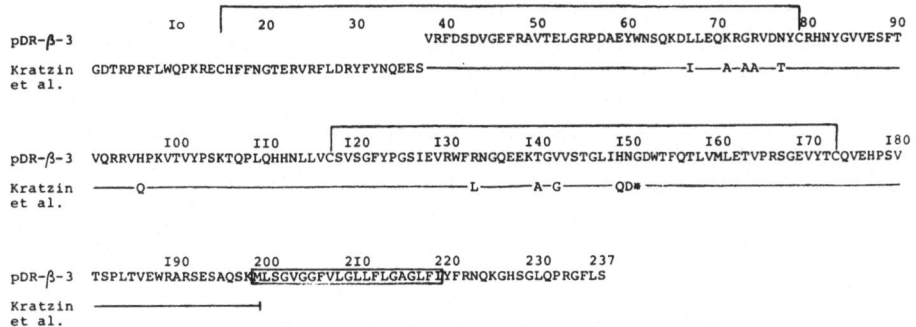

Figure 5. Amino acid sequence comparison between two human class II antigen ß-chains. The upper sequence was predicted from the pDR-ß-3 nucleotide sequence. The lower sequence was taken from ref. 21.

Class II Antigen ß Chains

The initially isolated cDNA clone displays a translated amino acid sequence that does not correspond to HLA-DR antigen ß chain sequences (see ref. 9 and 10). Instead, its amino acid sequence is more similar to chains of the murine A_β type than to the E_β type (17). This substantiate previous investigations claiming that at least two and possibly more loci in or near the HLA-D region code for class II antigen ß chains (18-20). Therefore, we continued to isolate several more class II antigen ß chain cDNA clones, three of which have been sequenced. Fig. 4 shows the predicted amino acid sequence of two clones which may represent alleles at a single locus. The amino acid sequences of these clones are more homologous to A_β than E_β chains of the mouse (see ref. 17). The two human sequences are identical apart from 28 amino acid replacements. This high degree of homology (88%) is, however, regionally distributed. The first domain exhibits about 77% homology while the second domain exhibits as much as 98% homology.

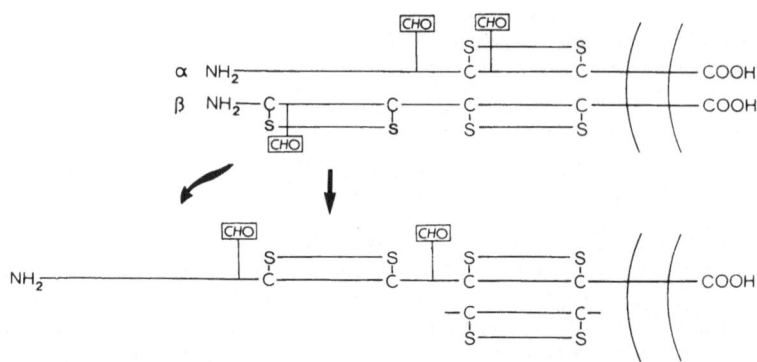

Figure 6. Schematic picture of class II (top) and I (bottom)
          antigens. The second carbohydrate moiety in the class I
          antigen heavy chain has been found in H-2 but not in HLA
          molecules. The second class II antigen α and β chain
          domains, and the class I antigen heavy chain domain
          closest to the membrane and β_2-microglobulin are homolo-
          gous to Ig constant domains and to the NH_2-terminal
          domain of the α chain. The latter is also homologous to
          the NH_2-terminal β chain domain. The first and second
          domains of the class I antigen heavy chain are homologous
          to each other and to the NH_2-terminal β-chain domain.

        The third β chain cDNA clone does not contain the 5'-end of
the translated region, so information is only available from amino
acid 38 and onwards (Fig. 5).The predicted amino acid sequence of
this cDNA clone, pDR-β-3, overlapped with the previously determined
NH_2-terminal amino acid sequence of HLA-DR β chains (8). This
information combined strongly suggests that the pDR-β-3 clone
corresponds to an HLA-DR antigen β chain and, thus, is more similar
to murine E_β than to A_β chains. In fact, the 3'-untranslated region
of pDR-β-3 encompasses a stretch of nucleotides that is very dissi-
milar to that of the pDR-β-1 and β-2 clones (not shown). These
particular nucleotide sequences hybridize to unique human genomic
DNA fragments on blot analyses clearly demonstrating that pDR-β-3
is derived from another locus than are the pDR-β-1 and β-2 cDNA
clones.

        The amino acid sequence predicted for the pDR-β-3 cDNA was
compared to the protein sequence of a recently published β-chain
(21). Fig. 5 shows that the homology between the two sequences is
93% for the 163 residues available for comparison. However, when
the protein sequence corresponding to the pDR-β-3 clone is used to
include the 37 NH_2-terminal residues (8) the homology drops to 89%.

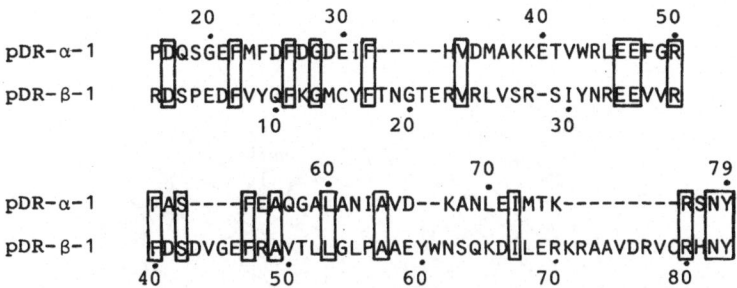

Figure 7. Alignment of the predicted NH$_2$-terminal amino acid sequences of the pDR-α-1 and pDR-ß-1 cDNA clones. The amino acid sequence comparison was carried out using the program ALIGN. The score, A=5.03, is statistically highly significant (see ref. 22).

Interestingly, the NH$_2$-terminal domains display a homology of 84% while the second domains are more alike, i.e. the homology is 94%.

Although data on the number of human class II antigen loci and their allelic variation are limited, the present observations may suggest that for the two ß chain loci identified here the gene products display most of its polymorphism in the first domain, corresponding to the second exon of the genes (unpublished observations). However, more allelic forms have to be analyzed to confirm or refute this suggestion, particularly since the human HLA-D region seems to contain three or more ß chain loci (J. Böhme, unpublished observations).

Similarities in Structure Between Class I and II Antigens

Due to differences in their overall structure class I and II antigens were not generally believed to display sequence homology. This notion was reinforced by the observation that various types of serological reagents seemed specific for each class of molecules. However, using various types of statistical procedures (see ref. 22) we have found that class I and II antigens exhibit a substantial degree of homology (10, 11). Fig. 6 summarizes the data. The second domains of the class II antigen α and ß chains are homologous to the third domain of the class I antigen heavy chain and to ß$_2$-microglobulin. These four domains are also homologous to immunoglobulin constant regions (23-25). As noted previously the first and second domains of class I antigen heavy chains are homologous to each other (22, 23) and to the first domain of the ß-chain (10). Moreover, the first domain of the α chain is

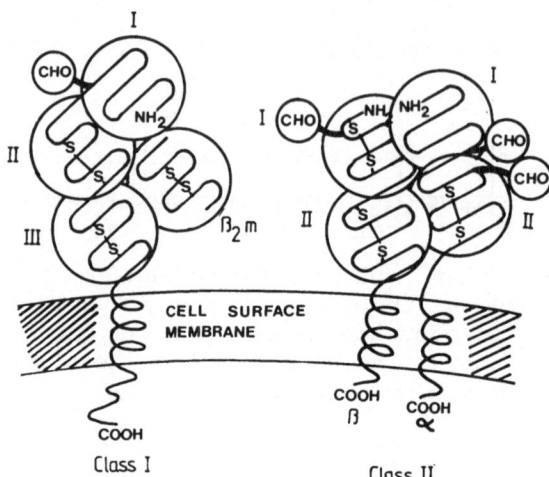

Figure 8. Arrangement of class I and II antigen domains which may yield similar overall structures. Roman numerals denote domains.

homologous to the first domain of the ß–chain (Fig. 7) and to the second domains of both α and ß chains (not shown). These data strongly suggest that immunoglobulins, class I and class II antigens have had an interrelated evolution.

Despite the homologies in primary structure between class I and II antigens X-ray crystallography is required to establish whether similarity exists also at the three-dimensional level. In the absence of such information it may be predicted that both types of molecules are composed of four extracellular domains (Fig. 8). In each molecule two of the domains are similar in primary structure to immunoglobulin constant regions. A third domain contains an immunoglobulin-like disulfide loop and one domain is devoid of cysteines. Since both class I and II antigens contain a large amount of ß-structure (26-28), a feature consistent with the basic immunoglobulin fold (29), the models of the two types of molecules displayed in Fig. 8 may not be entirely without foundation. Regardless of how class I and II antigens will turn out to be folded Fig. 8 highlights an important issue: May antigen receptors on T-killer and T-helper cells, which preferentially react with class I and II antigens, respectively, be recognizing very similar structures?

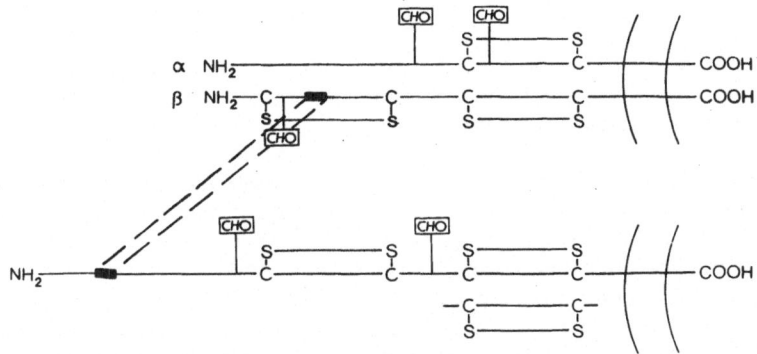

Figure 9. Schematic outline of class I and II antigens indicating
the position of the hexapeptide -Val-Arg-Phe-Asp-Ser-Asp

Occurrence of an Invariant Hexapeptide in Class I and II Antigens

For several receptor-ligand pairs it is well established that
structures which are in direct physical contact accumulate mutations at a significantly slower rate than structures not involved
in interactions. Thus, the region of the insulin molecule interacting with the insulin receptor has been under stricter evolutionary
constraints than other portions of the molecule (30). With this
notion in mind it is very intriguing to note that all class I
antigen heavy chains and all class II antigen ß-chains sequenced so
far contain an invariant hexapeptide (Fig. 9). Arguments that go
beyond this presentation make it conceivable that T-cells do not
only recognize whatever is foreign on the cell surface but also
whatever is invariant among the MHC antigens. Whether the hexapeptide represents such an invariant structure is under investigation.

Assembly of Class II Antigens

The data above provide evidence for the existence of at least
two human ß chain loci. In the murine system it is known that two
types of class II molecules exist. They are composed of $A_\beta A_\alpha$ and E_β
E_α chains, respectively (17). There does not seem to exist any
reports demonstrating the occurrence of hybrid molecules, i.e. $A_\beta F_\alpha$
etc. The two human ß chain loci may correspond to the murine A_β and
E_β loci, respectively, and, the ß chains will therefore most
probably associate with different types of α chains. In view of the
high degree of homology between the two types of ß chains it is not
obvious how the assembly of the class II antigens occur in view of
the fact that the same cell may produce class II molecules derived
from different loci. However, the existence of an intracellular,

invariant chain (termed γ chain) associated with murine (31) and human (32) class II antigens may provide an answer to this problem. It has been reported that the γ chain can only leave the endoplasmic reticulum while protein synthesis occurs (33). Thus, the γ chain is transported to the Golgi complex associated with α and ß chains. Recently, we have shown that the γ chain dissociates from the class II antigens concomitant with terminal glycosylation of α, ß and γ chains. The chain and the class II antigens are then separately transported and integrated into the plasma membrane (L. Claesson, unpublished observations). The γ chain may fullfil a role in the sorting of the various class II antigen chains provided it binds to both chains of only one type of the class II antigens. Should that be the case class II antigens of one type may assemble in the endoplasmic reticulum while those of another type, associated with the γ chain, may assemble only after transport to the Golgi complex.

Association of Virus Proteins with Class I Antigens.

Since we presently favour the view that T-killer cells recognize MHC and foreign antigens by a process more compatible with the altered self concept than with the dual recognition hypothesis (see ref. 1) we have searched for a class I antigen-virus protein complex that is stable enough to withstand molecular analyses. So far the association of an adenovirus protein with rat class I antigens seem to be the only virus protein-MHC antigen complex that has been described in some detail (34). Several authors have demonstrated that various virus proteins on the surface of cells co-cap with class I antigens. However, such analyses have been subject to criticism since in most cases the serological reagents used may have contained extraneous antibodies. In view of the scarce evidence for complex formation between class I antigens and virus proteins it is highly relevant to ask whether the adenovirus protein is just an odd virus protein? Thus, the adenovirus protein may bind to class I antigens like Staphylococcus aureus protein A binds to IgG.

However, part of the difficulty in establishing the existence of a physical association between class I antigens and virus protein is inherent in the experimental system itself. Assuming that x molecules of a class I antigen (C) may bind y copies of a virus protein (V) the following situation exists:

$$xC + yV \Leftrightarrow C_x V_y$$

This equilibrium is, of course, subject to change when the concentration of any one of the components changes. Thus, using antibodies reacting better with free than with complexed molecules will diminish complex formation. It should also be pointed out that complex formation may depend on the high local concentration of the reactants, which is brought about by both molecules being anchored in the lipid bilayer of the plasma membrane. Solubilization of the membranes will drastically lower the effective concentration of the class I antigens and the virus proteins, thereby promoting dissociation of the complex.

According to the altered self concept the protein complex $C_x V_y$ is being recognized by T-killer cells (1). As yet no information is available as to whether 1%, 10% or 100% of the relevant molecules may have to exist in the complexed form to serve as targets for the T-killer cells. Thus, should only 10% of the molecules occur in complexes the large amount of free molecules would probably render the detection of the complexed molecules impossible.

With these conceptual and technical obstacles in mind it is surprising that the adenovirus protein E19 forms complexes with class I antigens that can be detected. However, E19 seems to occur as a dimer (O. Kämpe, unpublished observations). Should class I antigens be able to bind to several determinants on the virus protein, complex formation would be enhanced. Having multiple determinants may be the particular "oddity" of this adenovirus protein.

Association of the E19 Adenovirus Protein with Human Class I Antigens

We have previously described that the adenovirus-2 early glycoprotein E19 from the E3 region (35) associates with class I antigens in a transformed rat fibroblast line (34). To extend this observation we examined whether the E19 protein would also associate with human class I antigens in productively infected HeLa cells. After radioactive labeling of the cells and solubilization of their membranes class I antigens were isolated by indirect immunoprecipitation and analyzed by SDS-polyacrylamide gel electrophoresis (PAGE). Fig. 10 demonstrates that an antiserum against the class I antigen heavy chain co-precipitated the E19 protein and that the antiserum did not co-precipitate the E19 molecule in mock-infected cells. An interesting and reproducible difference between the two lanes of Fig. 10 is the amount of β_2-microglobulin co-precipitated. From the virus-infected cells much less β_2-microglobulin was recovered than from the mock-infected cells. This does not seem to idicate that β_2-microglobulin is dissociated from the class I antigen heavy chain on its forming a complex with the E19 protein since monoclonal antibodies directed against β_2-microglobulin co-precipitated the virus protein (not shown). A more likely explanation is that the association between the heavy chain and β_2-microglobulin is diminished due to conformational changes induced in the heavy chain upon binding of the E19 protein.

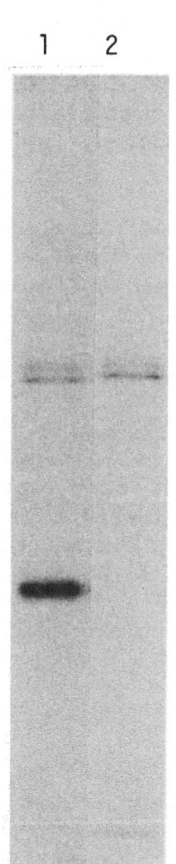

Figure 10. SDS-PAGE of ^{35}S-Methionine-labeled, adenovirus- (lane 1) and mock-infected (lane 2) molecules precipitated by an antiserum against class I antigen heavy chains. The class I antigen heavy chains occur as a doublet while E19 (lane 1) gives a single band. β_2-Microglobulin is hardly visible in lane 1.

The association between human class I antigens and E19 may be due to many factors. To exclude that other virus proteins promoted complex formation we isolated the coding region for E19 (36) and inserted it into a eucaryotic expression vector (S. Pääbo, F. Weber, W. Schaffner et al., unpublished observations). This vector only produces E19 mRNA and cells transfected with the vector expressed E19, which formed complexes with class I antigens. Thus, the interaction between E19 and class I antigens does not seem to depend on other virus proteins.

Biogenesis of the Class I Antigen - E19 Protein Complexes.

To identify the cellular localization where class I antigens and E19 formed complexes extensive studies on the biosynthesis and intracellular transport of the two proteins were carried out. The class I antigens were synthesized and transported as in mock-infected cells (see ref.37). The E19, which contains two Asn-linked carbohydrate moieties, is core-glycosylated in the endoplasmic reticulum. Trimming of the glucose residues, accompanied by an apparent decrease in molecular weight, is followed by the removal of most of the mannoses, again accompanied by a decrease in the apparent molecular weight. No terminal glycosylation seems to occur on either one of the two carbohydrate moieties. Approximately 60 min after synthesis E19 appears on the cell surface. It is then, and only then, that complex formation with class I antigens occur. Thus, class I antigens and E19 are transported separately to the cell surface (O. Kämpe, unpublished observations).

Size Determination of the Protein Complexes Consisting of Class I Antigens and the E19 Protein.

Since our data show that E19 may exist as a homodimer we attempted to estimate the approximate size range of the E19-class I antigen complexes by using cleavable cross-linkers.

Radioactively labeled glycoproteins from the adenovirus-transformed rat cell line and from adenovirus-infected HeLa cells, respectively, were treated with the crosslinker dithiobis(succinimidyl)propionate (DTSP) prior to the immunoprecipitations. Antibodies directed against class I antigen heavy chains precipitated complexes from both cell types that were so large that they hardly entered the running gel (Fig. 11, B and E). De-crosslinking of the isolated complexes released three types of molecules; namely, class I antigen heavy chains, β_2-microglobulin and E19 (Fig. 11, C and F). This experiment demonstrated that about equal amounts of radioactivity were present in the three types of chains. This contrasts with the data obtained when the immunoprecipitations were carried out prior to the crosslinking. Fig. 11 A and D display little if any β_2-microglobulin. Fig. 11A displays more radioactivity in the heavy chain than in E19 while the converse is true in Fig. 11D. These data demonstrate that the protein complexes found are large and that their stoichiometry is easily influenced by the reactivity of the antibodies.

Do Class I Antigens have the Role of Defense Molecules at the Single Cell Level?

In view of the large size of the complexes formed between class I antigens and E19 the question arose whether such complexes were removed from the cell surface by endocytosis. It is well established that a number of cell surface receptors are taken up by endocytosis following their interaction with the ligand (see ref. 38). Some of the receptors end up in the lysosomes and become

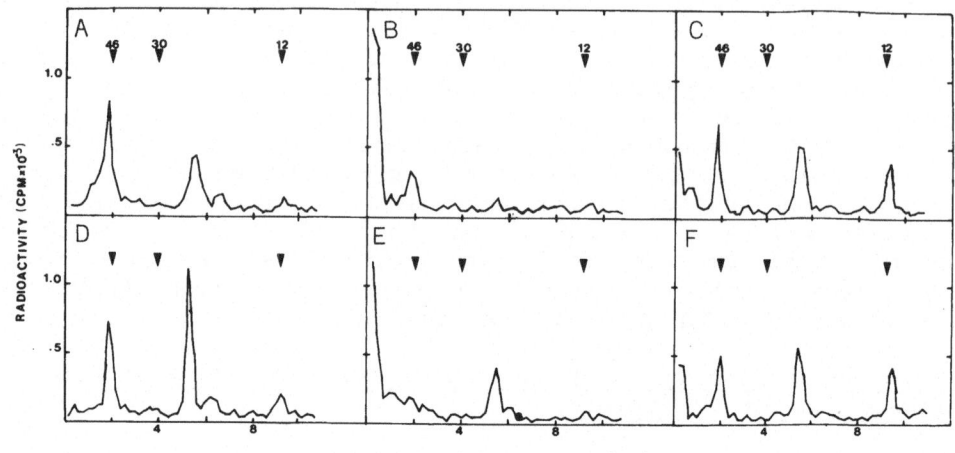

Figure 11. SDS-PAGE of cross-linked class I antigen-E19 complexes. The glycoprotein fraction of ^{35}S-methionine-labeled adenovirus-transformed rat fibroblasts (A-C) and adenovirus-infected HeLa cells (D-F) were separately treated with the covalent crosslinker DTSP. Molecules reactive with antisera against class I antigen heavy chains were precipitated and analyzed by SDS-PAGE. A and D show immunoprecipitates obtained prior to the crosslinking. B and E display the immunoprecipitates recovered after crosslinking. C and F exhibit the polypeptide patterns of the crosslinked complexes after de-crosslinking. The arrows denote apparent mol.wts. in k-daltons.

degraded (39) while others leave their ligands in the lysosomes and recirculate back to the plasma membrane (40).

     To examine the fate of the class I antigen – E19 protein complexes we investigated the half-life of the individual molecules in the transformed rat cell line. Despite the fact that the great majority of the two types of molecules occurred in complexed form (see Fig. 11) the class I antigens had a half-life more than 10-fold longer than that of E19. The half-life of E19 increased to that of the class I antigens on blocking the lysosomal degradation by treating the cells with chloroquine. Identical results were obtained in monensin-treated cells (41) while neither drug affected the half-life of the class I antigens.

     These data in conjunction with current knowledge about receptor-mediated endocytosis suggest the scheme depicted in Fig. 12. The protein complexes get trapped in coated pits (or in regions of the plasma membrane similar in function) and are taken up by the

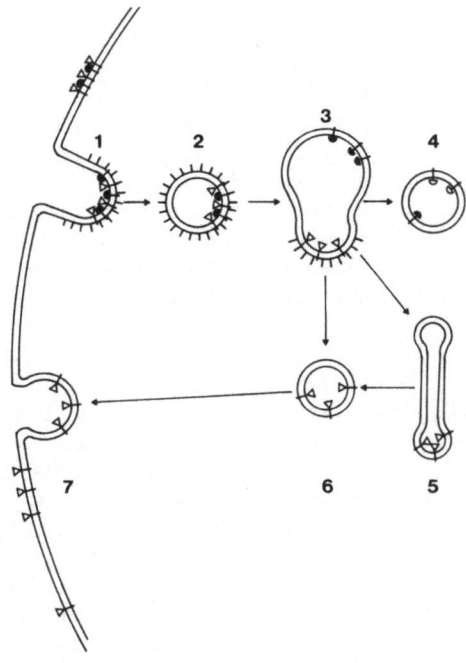

Figure 12. Schematic outline of the putative fate of class I
           antigen-E19 complexes. The class I antigens (open
           triangles) are bound to the E19 protein (filled half-
           circles) and may get trapped in coated pits (1). Coated
           vesicles are formed (2) which, after divesting the
           clathrin-coat, turn into endosomes (3). Due to the
           decreasing pH class I antigens and the E19 protein may
           become sequestered so that the E19 protein ends up in a
           lysosome (4) while the class I antigens return to the
           cell surface (7), either with a distinct type of vesicle
           (6) or via the exocytotic route of the Golgi complex
           (5).

cell through the formation of coated vesicles. After removal of the
clathrin the pH of the endosome drops. This may trigger the
segregation of class I antigens and E19. While E19 becomes degraded
in the lysosome the class I antigens return to the cell surface,
either by a specific transport vesicle or, less likely, by passage
through part of the Golgi complex.

The data briefly reported here may, if generalized, suggest
that class I antigens serve as defense molecules at the level of
the single cell. Thus, whatever binds to the class I antigens will
be removed and degraded in the lysosomes. Should this route of
degradation be insufficient T-killer cells may become agressive.

The endocytosis and recirculation concept is in a sense contradictory to the notion that T-killer cells recognize MHC antigens and foreign substances. However, is complex formation restricted to the cell surface, as is the case for E19, the endocytotic process will only diminish, not abolish, the occurrence of complexes exposed on the cell surface. Thus, T-killer cells will react with fewer molecules if the rate of endocytosis is significant. This may in fact ascertain that T-killer cells do not encounter too much antigen should receptor crosslinking in T-cells, like in B-cells, be required for activation.

Conclusions

The present article demonstrates that class I and II antigens are more similar in structure, and thereby possibly in mechanism of action, than hitherto known. However, three-dimensional structure analyses are needed to evaluate the evolutionary relationship between the two types of molecules. Should the MHC antigens turn out to be similar in structure to immunoglobulins it is tempting to suggest that the virus protein-class I antigen interaction described here have features in common with antigen-antibody complexes. However, also in this case it is obvious that the type of interaction should be unravelled at the three-dimensional level. Such analyses will undoubtedly reveal whether "allotypic" residues in the class I antigens are engaged in the complex formation.

The endocytosis and recirculation of class I antigens associated with the virus protein suggest that class I antigens may have a function at the single cell level. Should this behaviour of the class I antigens (and class II antigens during antigen presentation) be general in other types of cells and for other virus proteins, it may afford an excellent example on how evolution has selected a molecule with a "primitive" function to participate in a more sophisticated system serving the same function. However, other virus proteins must be examined to generalize these findings.

ACKNOWLEDGEMENTS

We are grateful to our collegues who allowed us to cite their unpublished results. Expert assistance in preparing this manuscript was provided by Ms C. Plöen. This work was supported by grants from the Swedish Cancer Society, King Gustaf the V:s 80-years fund, Centrala Försöksdjursnämnden and the Swedish Board of Technical Development.

REFERENCES

1. P.C. Doherty, R.V. Blanden, and R.M. Zinkernagel, Specificity of virus-immune effector T-cells for H-2K or H-2D. Compatible

interactions: Implications for H-antigen diversity. Transpl.
Rev. 29:89-123 (1976)

2. P. Matzinger, A one-receptor view of T-cell behaviour, Nature
292:497-501 (1981)

3. R.W. Thomas, L. Clement, E.M. Shevach, T lymphocyte stimulation
by hapten-conjugated macrophages. Immunol. Rev. 40:181-204
(1978)

4. D.H. Katz, B. Benacerraf, Genetic control of lymphocyte interactions and differentiation. In: "The role of products of the
histocompatibility gene complex in immune responses". D.H. Katz,
and B. Benacerraf (eds.) Academic Press, London, pp. 355-385
(1976)

5. T.Tada and J. Taniguchi, In: "The role of products of the
histocompatibility gene complex in immune responses". D.H. Katz,
and B. Benacerraf (eds.) Academic Press, New York p. 531-
(1976)

6. J.F.A.P. Miller, M.A. Vadas, A. Whitelaw, A., and J. Gamble, H-2
gene complex restricts transfer of delayed-type hypersensitivity
in mice Proc. Natl.Acad. Sci. USA. 72:5095 (1975)

7. K. Gustafsson, P. Bill, D. Larhammar, K. Wiman, L. Claesson, L.
Schenning, B. Servenius, J. Sundelin, L. Rask, and P.A.
Peterson, Isolation and identification of a cDNA clone coding
for an HLA-DR transplantation antigen chain. Scand J. Immunol.
(in press)

8. K. Wiman, D .Larhammar, L.Claesson, K. Gustafsson, L. Schenning,
P. Bill, J. Böhme, M. Denaro, B. Dobberstein, U. Hammerling, S.
Kvist, B. Servenius, J. Sundelin, P.A. Peterson, and L. Rask,
Isolation and identification of a cDNA clone corresponding to an
HLA-DR antigen ß-chain, Proc. Natl. Acad. Sci. USA 79:1703-1707
(1982)

9. D.Larhammar, K. Wiman, L. Schenning, L. Claesson, K. Gustafsson,
P.A. Peterson, and L. Rask, Evolutionary relationship between
HLA-DR antigen ß chains, HLA-A, B, C antigen subunits and
immunoglobulin chains. Scand J. Immunol. 14:617-622 (1981)

10.D. Larhammar, L. Schenning, K. Gustafsson, K. Wiman, L.
Claesson, L. Rask, and P.A. Peterson. The complete amino acid
sequence of an HLA-DR antigen-like ß chain as predicted from the
nucleotide sequence: Similarities with immunoglobulins and
HLA-A, B, C antigens. Proc. Natl. Acad. Sci. USA 79:3687-3691
(1982)

11.D. Larhammar, K. Gustafsson, L. Claesson, P. Bill. K. Wiman, L.
Schenning, J. Sundelin. E. Widmark. P.A. Peterson, and L. Rask,
HLA-DR transplantation antigen chain is a member of the same
protein superfamily as the immunoglobulins. Cell 30:153-161
(1982)

12.F.S. Walsh, and M.,J. Crumpton, Orientation of cell-surface
antigens in the lipid bilayer of lymphocyte plasma membrane.
Nature 269:307-311

13.J.F. Kaufman, and J.L. Strominger, Both chains of HLA-DR bind to
the membrane with a penultimate hydrophobic region and the heavy

chain is phosphorylated at its hydrophilic carboxyl terminus. Proc. Natl. Acad. Sci. USA 76:6304-6308 (1979)

14. K.W. Moore, B.T. Sher, Y.H. Sun, K.A. Eahle, and L. Hood, DNA sequence of a gene encoding a BALB/C mouse L^d transplantation antigen, Science 215:679-683 (1982)

15. M. Malissen, B. Malissen, and B.R. Jordan, Exon/intron organization and complete nucleotide sequence of an HLA gene. Proc. Natl. Acad. Sci. USA 79:893-897 (1982)

16. M. Steinmetz, K.W. Moore, J.G. Frelinger, B. Taylor Sher, F.W. Shen, E.A. Boyse, and L. Hood, A pseudogene homologous to mouse transplantation antigens: Transplantation antigens are encoded by eight exons that correlate with protein domains. Cell 25:683-692 (1981)

17. J.W. Uhr, J.D. Capra, E.S. Vitetta, and R.G. Cook, Organization of the immune response genes. Both subunits of I-A and I-E/C molecules are encoded within the I region, Science 206:292-297 (1979)

18. R.S. Accolla, N. Gross, S. Carrel, and G. Corte, Distinct forms of both   and ß subunits are present in the human Ia molecular pool. Proc. Natl. Acad. Sci USA 78:4549-4551 (1981)

19. L.M. Nadler, P. Stashenko, R. Hardy, K.J. Tomaselli, E.J. Yunis, S.F. Schlossman, and J.M. Peao, Monoclonal antibody identifies a new Ia-like (p29, 34) polymorphic system linked to the HLA-D/DR region. Nature 290:591-593

20. S. Shaw, P. Kavathas, M.S. Pollack, D. Charmot, and C. Mawas, Family studies define a new histocompatibility locus, SB, between HLA-DR and GLO. Nature, 293:745-747 (1981)

21. H. Kratzin, C.-Y. Yang, H. Götz, E. Pauly, S. Kölbel, G. Egert, F.P. Thinnes, P. Wernet, P. Altevogt, and N. Hilschmann, Primary structure of class II human histocompatibility antigens. Hoppe-Seyler´s Z. Physiol. Chem. 362:1665-1669 (1982)

22. L. Trägårdh, L. Rask, K. Wiman, J. Fohlman, and P.A. Peterson, Complete amino acid sequence of pooled papain-solubilized HLA-A, B, C antigens: Relatedness to immunoglobulins and internal homologies. Proc. Natl. Acad. Sci. USA 77:1129-1133 (1980)

23. L. Trägårdh, O. Kämpe, U. Hammerling, J. Böhme, L. Claesson, L. Rask, and P.A. Peterson, $ß_2$-microglobulin and transplantation antigens. Scand. J. clin. Lab. Invest. 40, Suppl. 154 (1980)

24. H.T. Orr, D. Lancet, R.J. Robb, J.A. Lopez de Castro, and J.L. Strominger, The heavy chain of human histocompatibility antigen HLA-B7 contains an immunoglobulin-like region. Nature 282:266-270, (1979).

25. L. Trägårdh, L. Rask, K. Wiman, J. Fohlman, and P.A. Peterson, Amino acid sequence of an immunoglobulin-like HLA antigen heavy chain domain. Proc. Natl. Acad. Sci. USA 76:5839-5842 (1979)

26. L. Trägårdh, B. Curman, K. Wiman, L. Rask, and P.A. Peterson, Chemical, physical-chemical, and immunological properties of papain-solubilized human transplantation antigens. Biochemistry 18:2218-2226

27. D. Lancet, P. Parham, and J.L. Strominger, Heavy chain of HLA-A and HLA-B antigens is conformationally labile. A possible role for ß$_2$-microglobulin, Proc. Natl. Acad. Sci. USA 76:3844-3848 (1979)

28. K. Wiman, L. Claesson, L. Rask, L. Trägårdh, and P.A. Peterson, Purification and partial amino acid sequence of papain-solubilized HLA-DR transplantation antigens, Biochemistry (in press)

29. R.J. Poljak, Three-dimensional structure, function and genetic control of immunoglobulins, Nature 256:373-376 (1975)

30. P. De Meyts, E. van Obberghen, J. Roth, A. Wollmer, and D. Brandenburg, Mapping of the residues responsible for the negative cooperativity of the receptor-binding region of insulin, Nature 273:504-509 (1978)

31. P.P. Jones, D.B. Murphy, D. Hewgill, and H.O. McDevitt, Detection of a common polypeptide chain in I-A and I-E subregion immunoprecipitates. Mol. Immunol. 16:51-60 (1979)

32. D.J. Charron, and H.O. McDevitt, Analysis of HLA-D region-associated molecules with monoclonal antibody. Proc. Natl. Acad. Sci. USA, 76:6567-6571 (1979)

33. S. Kvist, K. Wiman, L. Claesson, P.A. Peterson, and B. Dobberstein, Membrane insertion and oligomeric assembly of HLA-DR histocompatibility antigens. Cell 29:61-69 (1982)

34. S. Kvist, L. Östberg, H. Persson, L. Philipsson, and P.A. Peterson, Molecular association between transplantation antigens and a cell surface antigen in an adenovirus-transformed cell line. Proc. Natl. Acad. Sci. USA 75:5674-5678 (1978)

35. S.R. Ross, S.J. Flint, and A.J. Levine, Identification of the adenovirus early proteins and their genomic map positions. Virology 100:419-432 (1980)

36. J. Hérissé, G. Courtois, and F. Galivert, Nucleotide sequence of the EcoRI D fragment of adenovirus 2-genome. Nucleic Acids Res. 8:2173-2192 (1980)

37. H.L. Ploegh, H.T. Orr, and J.L. Strominger, Major histocompatibility antigens: The human (HLA-A, -B, -C) and murine (H-2K, H-2D) class I molecules. Cell 24, 287-299 (1981)

38. J.L. Goldstein, G.W.E. Anderson, and M.S. Brown, Coated pits, coated vesicles, and receptormediated endocytosis. Nature 279, 679-685 (1979)

39. F.R. Maxfield, J. Schlessinger, Y.L. Shechter, I. Pastan, and M.C. Willingham, Collection of insulin, EGF and $_2$-macroglobulin in the same patches on the surface of cultured fibroblasts and common internalization. Cell, 14:805-810 (1978)

40. R.G.W. Anderson, E. Vasile, R.J. Mello, M.S. Brown, and J.L. Goldstein, Immunocytochemical visualization of coated pits and vesicles in human fibroblasts: Relation to low density lipoprotein receptor distribution. Cell 15:919-933 (1978)

41. S.K. Basu, J.L. Goldstein, R.G.W. Anderson, and M.S. Brown, Monensin interrupts the recycling of low density lipoprotein receptors in human fibroblasts. Cell 24:493-502 (1981).

DISCUSSION

Strominger: Per, what is the conserved hexapeptide and where exactly is it located?

Peterson: The hexapeptide has the sequence -V-R-F-D-S-D- (see Fig. 9) and occurs in all class I antigen heavy chains and class II antigen beta -chains sequenced so far.

G. Möller: Since the MHC antigens have much less variability than antibodies you should expect the binding of MHC antigens to viral proteins to differ much from an antigen-antibody interaction?

Peterson: Our knowledge is too limited to answer this question. However, conceptually I cannot see that the binding between class I antigens and a virus protein has to be qualitatively different from that between antigens and antibodies. In other words, the prediction is that a given class I antigen may bind many different molecules but with low binding constants. So one may ask, how many structurally different molecules will bind to a given monoclonal antibody with a binding constant that is equal to or greater than say 5×10^3?

Nabholtz: What is the function of the adenovirus protein?

Peterson: This is not known, but it is clear that the E19 protein is not needed for transformation or assembly of the virus particle.

Coutinho: The number of minor antigens that Jim (Forman) is talking about is so large that Per Peterson's model is suicidal. Since anti-minor responses occur between MHC-identical strains, you would postulate that all minors against which a T cell response can be induced are "recognized" by self MHC, as for example, a viral protein. This not only means that MHC cannot be ascribed the function of self non-self discrimination, but it would also result in the complete and continuous "clogging up" of all MHC molecules on cell surfaces, I would think.

I think it is questionable to draw conclusions from such homologies and to assume functions of antigen "recognition" and ultimate consequences in MHC restriction, since we know that also Thy-l shows the same homologies and neither "recognizes" antigen (in your model) nor does it function as a restricting element, and this we know. If those homologies could be recognized by antibodies, then antibodies could "confuse" MHC and Ig.

Strominger: The model of interaction of viral antigen and class I antigen implies some kind of specificity in binding. It seems likely that the polymorphic region of the class I molecule is somehow involved in that interaction.

Peterson: This is, of course, what we would like to believe but presently we do not have data neither for nor against this notion. As you know, model building of class I antigens based on the immuno-globulin structure suggest that a substantial portion of the polymorphic residues may form a cluster similar to the antigen-combining site of antibodies, However, it is yet too early to decide whether there is any similarity between class I and II antigens at the three-dimensional model. Finally, I would just like to add that the extensive genetic polymorphism of the class I antigens is, of course, explained by making the polymorphism functional.

Jones: Several laboratories have used monoclonal antibodies in cross-blocking studies to define different, independent alloantigenic sites. Are all these distinct sites independent antigen-recognition sites?

Peterson: Again, I do not have an answer to your question. In analogy with antibodies, where both idiotypes and paratopes can be distinguished, I would guess that all allo-antigenic sites are not directly related to antigen recognition. Indeed, are any of these sites involved?

Benacerraf: Are all polymorphic areas of variability exposed on the surface of the molecule?

Strominger: We still do not know much about which residues are actually exposed, but that information should come out of the x-ray analysis of the crystal structure.

Peterson: In the absence of a true three-dimensional structure for the class I and II antigens a correct answer to your question cannot be given. However, by making the reasonable assumption that charged residues occur on the surfaces of the molecules it is possible to predict that a sizeable portion of the allotypic residues do occur on the surfaces.

Cohn: I question two of Per Peterson's arguments which lead to an "altered self" or new antigenic determinant (NAD) view of restrictive recognition of antigen.

First, the fact that the C-region of the immunoglobulin heavy chain and the heavy chain of class I restricting elements have a common evolutionary precursor, does not permit the conclusion that their functions are identical, namely to bind a vast number of unrelated antigens. The Thy-1 surface component is also derived from this same precursor. Would you conclude that it too functions by binding vast number of unrelated antigens? Further, binding antigen is

not a property of the C-region of immunoglobulin but of the V-region and, unlike restricting elements, there are many of them in each animal in at least a one to one relationship with antigenic determinants. As a general case, given the altered self view, **each** Class I or II restricting element (RI or RII) must interact with roughly the same vast array of antigens. Each is effectively a universal glue. In fact, in any one homozygous mouse there must be at least ten sets of (RX) interactions leading to non-overlapping NADs. In the RI class, there are at least three distinguishable elements (K,D,L); in the RII class, there are at least two (A,E); and in the world of antigens there are self and nonself determinants. In the heterozygous animal there are at least 20 non-overlapping NAD sets. Is this not a rather rococco justification for your arbitrary requirement that the language of antigen Xs be translated into the language of NADs before T cells can recognize them? What in your formulation is special about R that permits recognition of (RX)NAD and not X? In addition, even were I to accept that the "altered self" formulation had merit, nothing could be said about the T-cell receptor. It could be a single receptor (one triggering signal) as proposed by Bevan or a double receptor (two triggering signals as proposed by Janeway/Wigzell/Binz).

This leads to a second point, your assumption that there is evolutionary selection to make the self-nonself discrimination at the level of the interaction between a restricting element (R) and the antigen-X, self (X_S) or nonself (X_F). R does not interact with X_S but it does with X_F. The first argument you have made and this assumption are clearly incompatible. However, let me illustrate why this assumption is untenable.   A given mother (Mo) has a set of R^{Mo} which reacts with foreign antigens $X_F(R^{Mo}X_F)$ but **not** with her self antigens (X_{MoS}); $R^{Mo}X^{Mo}_S$ is excluded by evolutionary selection. A given father has a set of R^{Fa} which react with foreign antigens X_F ($R_F^{Fa}X_F$), but not with his self antigens (X^{Fa}_S); $R^{Fa}X^{Fa}_S$ is excluded by evolutionary selection. The children would die of autoimmune disease since X^{Mo}_S is X_F for the father and X^{Fa}_S is X_F for the mother. It is **absolutely** required that the self-nonself discrimination be **learned** by each individual during ontogeny. It cannot be determined by a germline evolutionary process. I do not understand why these self-marker theories of the self/nonself discrimination can never be laid to rest.

My last comment is one of principle. There is no properly developed "altered self" model: there are only bits and pieces of a model. The problem is not whether R can bind to X. Any protein can be postulated to bind to any other substance at some level of affinity. A thoughtful model of restriction must account for the following facts:

Although I would venture that there is no chance that, as a general case, the origin of restrictive recognition could be due to an **obligatory** R+X to RX interaction, the assumption is testable by determining whether establishing of tolerance is **obligatorily** restricted (R-dependent) as predicted by "altered-self" or can behave unrestricted (R-independent) as predicted by the dual recognition model we have proposed.

Strominger: The HLA-B locus gene is located at some distance from the HLA-A locus, about 1 centimorgan. Perhaps gene conversion or reciprocal recombination events can occur after unequal pairing of genes located at that distance, but in any event it is also possible that some "HLA-B7 like" polymorphic sequence is carried by some pseudogene with which the postulated "gene conversion" events may have occurred.

Cohn: The arguments that polymorphism of MHC is driven by pathogen mimicry are incomplete until one answers "Why mimic MHC?". Jerne proposed that the germline V-gene pool encodes anti-R, because the somatically generated repertoire is derived by mutational escape from self-tolerance. His proposal that the repertoire is derived from but a small fraction of the germline V-gene pool is disproven for the B cell and certain to be wrong on many grounds for the T cell. In any case, Jerne's proposal does not account for either allele-specific recognition or the violating of the effector function/class of R relationship when R_F (allo-R) is the target. Further, it does not explain either why the gaps in the repertoire of each animal should drive polymorphism and not polygeneism or how the polymorphic set of R-genes and V-genes are selected upon to evolve in tandem.

If one argues that
1) the germline V_T-locus encodes anti-allele-specific determinants on R, and
2) the total V_T-gene pool is used as a starting point for somatic diversification then we can understand polymorphism.

The selection pressure is at two levels:
1) Any animal which cannot recognize its own restriction elements will have a defective immune system and this tends to eliminate that individual favouring those which do.
2) While the recognition of determinants common to all or many R alleles would permit perfectly functional restrictive recognition, the V_T-genes encoding anti-common determinants cannot be used as starting points for somatic diversification, because cells expressing them would be eliminated by tolerance. Only those V_T-genes encoding allele-specific recognition could function as sources of somatic variants because they are **not** prevented in a given individual from being expressed due to tolerance. This is strictly anti-Jernerian. The polymorphism is driven by the need to disperse the initial V_T-gene pool from which somatic variants derive. It is a consequence of the vicissitudes of evolution that the V_T-gene pool from which the antigen-specific repertoire is derived somatically. The two selection

pressures, i.e. the requirement for restrictive recognition and for dispersion in the germline of the V_T-genes from which the repertoire is somatically derived, drive polymorphism (not polygeneism) of the MHC encoded R elements.

Strominger: It appears to us that the changes which distinguish HLA-A28 from HLA-A2 did **not** come about by random mutational changes, but we cannot entirely rule out an effect of structural constraints in influencing these non-random changes. A full discussion can be found in our recent publication (PNAS, June 1982). What we mean to say is that "gene conversion" is a process which needs to be seriously considered as a mechanism for generation of HLA poly- morphism and that our data have led us to think in that direction.

Hood: The major histocompatibility complex of mouse encodes several families of molecules including the class II or Ia antigens. These antigens are present on B cells, macrophages, and some T cells. They regulate the recognition of foreign antigens on the surfaces of these immune-related cells in the afferent portion of the immune response. These interactions lead to high or low immune responses to antigenic determinants controlled by the so-called Ir (immune response) genes. The Ia antigens appear to be equivalent to the Ir gene products.

The I region has been divided by recombinational analysis into five subregions: I-A, I-B, I-J, I-E, and I-C. The I-A and I-E subregions contain at least four genes encoding the Ia antigens. Two biochemi- cally well-characterized Ia antigens, I-A and I-E, are heterodimers composed of a 33-35,000-dalton alpha chain and a 28-31,000-dalton beta chain and are expressed primarily on B cells and macrophages. The A_{alpha}, A_{beta}, and E_{beta} chains are encoded in the I-A subregion, whereas the E peptide is encoded in the I-E subregion. The I-J subregion appears to encode one or more soluble T-cell factors in cell- surface antigens on T cells and macrophage which suppress immune responses. Our laboratory has employed cDNAs complementary to human alpha and beta messenger RNAs encoding class II chains which were obtained from the laboratory of Bernard Mach at Geneva. We have employed two of these human cDNA clones, (DR_{alpha}) (homo- logous to mouse E_{alpha}) and DC1beta (homologous to class II beta chains), and chromosomal walking procedures to isolate about 200 kilobases (kb) of contiguous DNA from the' I region of the inbred BALB/c mouse. This 200 kb of I region DNA includes 18 overlapping cosmid clones. This cloned I region contains four class II genes. We have demonstrated by cross-hybridization to human probes and, more recently, by DNA sequence analysis that the order of these genes is centromere-A_{beta} -E_{beta} -E_{beta2} E_{alpa}. Three of these genes appa- rently encode serologic products that have been previously defined whereas the fourth, E_{beta2}, may or may not be a pseudogene. It will require DNA analysis to determine whether the E_{beta2} gene is actually functional. We have employed DNA blot analyses with appropriate probes to demonstrate that it is likely the BALB/c genome only contains two alpha-like genes and four to six beta-type genes. Thus, the number of class II genes is remarkably small for the complex phenotypic functions that they appear to carry out-most strikingly that of the exquisitely specific control of immune responses.

Immunogeneticists have divided the I region into five subregions by recombinational analysis of various immune responsiveness traits. Restriction site polymorphisms have permitted us to correlate our molecular map with the genetic map of the I region. Thus, we have subcloned ten single-copy probes from various regions throughout the 200 kb of I region DNA and we have used the single-copy probes to probe the DNAs from a variety of different inbred strains of mice to map these probe positions by restriction enzyme site polymorphisms to particular subregions of the I region. From these types of analyses we can make several interesting points. First, the E_{alpha} gene maps to the I-E subregion. The A_{beta} gene and E_{beta} and the 5' portion of the E_{beta} gene maps to the I-A subregion. Second, our restriction enzyme site polymorphism analyses demonstrate the the I-B and I-J subregions must be combined to a region of DNA that is less than 3.4 kb in length. There has in the past been controversy as to whether the I-B subregion really in fact exists. However, there seems to be no controversy about the fact serologically-defined gene products have been identified which apparently are encoded in the I-J subregion. What is striking about our mapping results is that the 3.4-kb region to which these two subregions must be confined is centered about the 3' end of the E_{beta} gene.

Several models may explain how a gene in this region might encode I-J products. First, the I-J gene may be encoded outside of the I region. This possibility cannot be excluded since the generation of the recombinant congenic strains to use define the I-J subregion also involved recombinational events outside the I region on chromosome 17. However, this possibility seems unlikely because the I-J subregion appears to segregate with the I region and not with any other region of the H-2 complex. Second, expression of the I-J gene product may be controlled by a regulatory element which is encoded in this 3.4-kb region. Again, this possibility seems unlikely because of the poly- morphism observed in the congenic mice with identical backgrounds (i.e., non-I region genes). Third, the I-J product may arise from alternative RNA splicing patterns of the E_{beta} gene so that some coding sequences overlap the E_{beta} gene and other coding sequences are distinct, for example, due to the splicing of alternative down- stream exons. Finally, the I-J and E_{beta} polypeptides may be identical. The I-J chain, however, may differ in its antigenic properties from the E_{beta} chain because of post-translational modifications, such as glycosylation or because of conformational differences if it is associated with a polypeptide different from E_{alpha} or, alternatively, if it is expressed as a single polypeptide chain on the surface of T-suppressor cells. Studies in progress should allow us to differentiate between these two different alternative possibilities.

I region recombination is localized in and around the E_{beta} gene. Indeed, the nine independently generated recombinant congenic mice that we have studied all map to this 3.4-kb region. Indeed, all of these recombinational events could have occurred at precisely the same position. Thus, it is clear that recombinational events in the I region are not randomly scattered but rather that they are highly localized in a very small region. Obviously this has important implications for any attempt to correlate recombinational map distances generated by classic genetics and molecular map distance generated by chromosomal walking. Obviously in the future one is going to have to be very carefully about attempting to correlate these two types of data.

The cloning of the I region will permit precise identification of the genes involved in immune responsiveness and other phenotypic traits encoded by this region. We will be able to use the techniques of gene transfer and in vitro mutagenesis to determine which genes control specific traits and how they function to regulate these traits. Finally, it is clear the genetic map of the I region can now start to be replaced with a molecular map which localizes precisely genes encoding various types of class II polypeptides.

Leder: How did you define the boundaries of the class II genes?

Hood: We used synthesized DNA probes and human cDNA clones to the alpha and beta class II genes obtained from Bernard Mach at Geneva.

Sachs: Can you tell us anything more about the E_{beta}-like gene? Is it found in other haplotypes than H-2^d? In particular, we have found a second I-E molecule in H-2^d but not in H-2^k using the same reagents and I wonder whether there might be a correlation?

Hood: We have used clear restriction enzyme polymorphism to move within 3 kb of one another the right hand boundery of the I-A region and the left hand boundary of the I-E region. The J gene, if it is in the I region, must reside in this 3 kb region.

Sachs: What is the E_{beta}-like gene?

Hood: It is a gene that hybridizes with the human beta cDNA clone, but not with a synthesized 15 mer DNA probe. This DNA probe was synthesized from an amino acid sequence obtained from the N-terminus of the E_{beta} molecule. This molecule was purified by Drs. Ken Sung and Pat Jones at Stanford.

Milstein: Some‧ years ago we prepared a monoclonal antibody NAI/34 which was a putative homologue in man of the TLa antigen in mouse (McMichael et al., Eur. J. Immunol. 9, 205-210, 1979). This antibody precipitated from human T cell line Molt4 a molecule containing two chains of similar size to Class I antigens. However, on close examination we were able to demonstrate that its light chain was different from beta$_2$microglubin and we called it beta-t (Ziegbo, A. and Milstein, C. Nature, 279, 243-244, 1979). Molt4 cells express moderate amounts of the antigen HTA-1 recognized by NA1/34 and also HLA,A,B,C as recognized by another monoclonal antibody derived by us - WG/32 (Barnstable et al., Cell, 14, 9-20, 1978). This combination of reactivities is unexpected in that cortical thymocytes which recognize NAI/34 do not recognize in our hands WG/32.

We were interested in the correlation between those two antigens and prompted by reports that alpha-interferon affected the level of HLA expression in human cells (e.g. Heron et al., Proc. Natl. Acad. Sci. USA, 75, 6215-6219, 1978; Fellous et al., Eur. J. Immunol., 11, 524-526, 1981) decided to test its effect on Molt4 cells using this time highly purified alpha-interferon prepared in my laboratory by D. Secher (Secher, D.S. and Burke, D.C., Nature, 285, 446-450, 1980). This work was done in collaboration with O. Burrone and also with B. Wright and D. Gilmore in later stages.

Alpha-IFN increased the expression of HLA,A,B,C antigens as detected by WG/32 but of neither NAI/34 or WG/34 another monoclonal antibody which reacts with Molt4 cells or indeed others I will not list. A time course of IFN treatment showed that after a lag period of about 10 h the amount of WG/32 bound increases dramatically over a period of days to reach a maximum at about 6 days which is about 10 fold higher than untreated controls. The effect is reversible and due to an increase in the rate of both HLA,A,B,C and beta$_2$microglobulin molecules as demonstrated by analysis of ^{35}S-methionine incorporation into specific proteins. Using a cDNA clone as a probe (kindly provided by Good et al., Proc. Natl. Acad. Sci. USA, 78, 616-620) we have also demonstrated that IFN stimulates a high level of specific HLA mRNA. The increase has been measured to be of the order 10-20 fold and correlates with the increase in the synthesis and membrane expression of the HLA molecules. We have described these results recently (Burrone and Milstein, EMBO Journal, 1982) and since then we have prepared a subline of Molt4 which is capable of an even higher level of IFN action. This has been cloned and the clone M4WH5 after treatment with IFN for several days expressed 20-fold increase in surface HLA (about twice better than Molt4). Iodination of IFN treated Molt4 cells, showed increased HLA,A,B,C and beta$_2$microglobulin levels as well as of another component MW 16.000 which we call P16. This component not observed with IFN not treated cells, is also observed following IFN treatment of Raji and DAUDI cells. We are now trying to further characterize P16.

Session IV

MHC Antigens and T Cell Function

Chairman: J. Klein

IMMUNOLOGICAL SURVEILLANCE: T CELL REPERTOIRE AND THE BIOLOGICAL FUNCTION OF MHC ANTIGENS

Peter C. Doherty

Department of Experimental Pathology
The John Curtin School of Medical Research
Canberra A.C.T. 2601, Australia

INTRODUCTION

Ten years ago we had no clear idea of the biological role of the major histocompatibility complex (MHC), though many people were trying to deal with the issue intellectually.[1-4] The phenomenon of alloreactivity dominated both experiments and concepts. Considerable effort had been put into the study of graft rejection and the strong transplantation antigens. Could it be that these extremely potent immune responses, and the glycoproteins at which they were directed, had no physiological function other than the elimination of transplanted tissues? Was alloreactivity a phylogenetic remnant of the need to avoid mutual parasitism in primitive life forms, now used in complex vertebrates to limit the emergence of spontaneous tumors? Such thinking led to Burnet's formulation of the immunological surveillance concept.[5]

The discovery of immune response (Ir) genes[6] mapping to the MHC[7] had no discernable influence on speculations concerning the nature of alloreactivity, though the idea that the Ir gene products were involved in cell-cell interactions for T-B help was considered.[2,7] However most attention was focused on the possibility that the Ir genes might encode all, or part of, the T cell receptor.[8-10]. This proposal still dominated thinking about T cell-macrophage and T-cell-B cell collaboration as late as 1975[11] but has since been de-emphasized by most of the groups working in the area.[12,13]

This change in thinking reflected the influence of models proposed in 1974-75 to explain the MHC restriction of virus and hapten-

specific cytotoxic T cells.[14-17] The nature of these experimental
systems, and the fact that effector function mapped to the strong
transplantation antigens instead of the then somewhat vaguely defined Ir genes, led logically to the concept that T cells were recognizing 'altered self' or 'self + x'.[18-20] Attention was thus focused
onto the target/stimulator cell and the idea that the MHC glycoprotein themselves were being recognized by the self-monitoring T cell,
rather than functioning as lymphocyte receptors. The debate continues whether self + x reflects an actual physical association between the two molecules, or the fact that they simply need to be presented close together in the plasma membrane of the same cell. This
will probably only be resolved when we understand more about the
nature of the T cell receptor(s).

The present article considers the biology of the MHC in two
ways. The first part (Section II) is a general discussion of the
role of MHC glycoproteins, argued in the context of a contemporary
immunological surveillance hypothesis. The latter part (Section III)
deals specifically with the virus immune cytotoxic T cell response
associated with H-2^k, H-2^b and the H-2K^b mutant (K^{bm}) glycoproteins.
The idea here is to provide specific instances of many of the points
raised in Section II. A brief discussion of T cell receptors serves
as a conclusion.

II.   IMMUNOLOGICAL SURVEILLANCE 1982

We need first to differentiate between immunological surveillance,[5] which shows the characteristics of an adaptive immune response (fine specificity, clonal expansion, memory), and natural
surveillance. Natural killer (NK) cells may show a degree of specificity but at this stage, they cannot be regarded as conventionally
'immune'.[21,22] This is not in any way to decry the importance of
natural surveillance, mediated by NK cells, monocyte-macrophages
and so forth. The narrower definition of immunological surveillance
that now seems appropriate is that, "immunological surveillance
is the process of specific monitoring for abnormal cell-surface
phenotype". This can be stated, with emerging clarity, in the context of the biological mechanisms underlying self-non-self discrimination at the level of the plasma membrane of somatic cells.

II. (1) The Nature of Self

Self is defined for the immune system by the antigens encoded
by the MHC, and by the molecular entities that constitute the receptors on T cells and B cells. There are thus at least two,[20,23] and
possibly three (at time of writing), genetic systems concerned with
specifically monitoring the integrity of self and maintaining a
stable milieu interior.

II. (2) Cytotoxic T Cells: Effectors of Cell-Surface Surveillance

Cytotoxic T cells recognize neoantigens (virus, TASA) presented on cell-surface in the context of class I MHC antigens (H-2KD, HLA-AB).[20] These class I MHC glycoproteins are present on all cells throughout the body, so there is thus the potential for effector function in any anatomical site. Inflammatory exudates induced by both viruses and tumors may contain numerous cytotoxic T cells,[24,25] and it is reasonably established that these lymphocytes are involved in the specific elimination of cells expressing abnormal surface phenotypes.[20]

II. (3) Helper-Inducer T Cells: The Promoters of Immune Response

Helper T cells recognize neoantigens presented in the context of class II MHC antigens (Ia, HLA-D), which are expressed principally on the surface of cells (T and B lymphocytes, macrophages, dendritic cells, Langerhans cells) that are involved in the development of the immune response.[11,13,26] Most of these cell types are present in, or pass through, lymphoid tissue. The restriction pattern of the helper-inducer thus focuses them into the anatomical sites (lymph node and spleen) where all components of the immune response come together, and can be influenced by secreted factors which operate at short range (Il-1, Il-2).[28] Cells of the helper class may also be recruited to sites of inflammatory process where Ia+ cells (monocytes→activated macrophages) are already present, and operate to promote the level of delayed type hypersensitivity (DTH). However, the concurrent involvement of cytotoxic T lymphocytes also seems to be essential if (for instance) virus-infected cells are to be eliminated.[29,30]

II. (4) Adaptive Immune Response Versus Autoimmunity

Effective immunological surveillance against virus-infected cells and tumors may require that both arms of an immune response, cytotoxic-effector and helper-inducer-DTH T cell, are involved.[31] This is readily achieved in virus diseases, where the immune system is exposed to large, complex antigens and the viruses may actually grow in the stimulator cells. However, antigenic changes on the surface of spontaneously transformed cells may be both less likely to engage a variety of cytotoxic T cell clones, and to be presented in an appropriate way on Ia+ stimulators. This need for a two-component response may operate to minimize the possibility of auto-immunity, while tending to work against effective immunological surveillance for tumors. The practical challenge in the latter case may be to develop ways to circumvent, or provide a replacement for, T cell help.

II. (5) Immune Response Genes

Immune response gene effects may reflect the frequency of T cell precursors capable of recognizing a particular association between class I or class II MHC gene products and a given neoantigen.[18-20] It is now reasonably established that the Ir gene product is the MHC antigen itself[32,33] The more complex the invading virus, the greater than chance that an antigenically appropriate interaction will occur. Lack of response to self + x could also result from an absence of lymphocytes expressing suitable receptor configurations, perhaps reflecting 'preclusion' rules[34] and differentiation events occurring in bone marrow, thymus and periphery.[35, 36] The limits of cell-surface surveillance by T lymphocytes may be largely determined by the need to balance the maintenance of self-tolerance with the capacity to mount an effective immune response.

II. (6) MHC Polymorphism and the Role of Multiple Loci

The existence of many different forms of class I and class II MHC molecules presumably ensures that the species as a whole will not be eliminated by a novel pathogen, or transforming agent.[18,20] The Qa antigens, which are structurally similar to H-2KD glycoproteins but do not have a known T cell-restricting function, are not highly polymorphic.[37] Also, the existence of two loci concerned with cytotoxic effector function (K and D, A and B) tends to ensure that any individual will be a responder. Furthermore, as most free-living vertebrates are heterozygous at the MHC, the gene products of 4 loci can potentially be involved in the cytotoxic response. In addition, the heterozygote possesses at least two loci concerned with stimulation of helper T cells, and hybrid Ia molecules (which act as restricting elements[32,33] are also found.[38] There are thus reasonable grounds for arguing some immunological component in heterozygote advantage.[18]

The fact that there are very few non-responders to viruses at the cytotoxic T cell level[39,40] could reflect either that viruses have not been as important as we originally argued in selecting for MHC polymorphism, or that the MHC genes associated with defective cell-mediated immunity to major pathogens have been eliminated. The standard laboratory mouse strains, which all originate from the more temperate zones of the world, are mostly non-responders to mosquito-borne, tropical togaviruses.[42]

II. (7) Alloreactivity

Alloreactivity is, in birds and mammals, probably an epiphenomnon of the need to see self + x,[43,44] a logical prediction of the altered self hypothesis.[18] Many cloned cytotoxic and helper T cell lines are both self-restricted and alloreactive.[45-47] This does not preclude the possibility that the contemporary T cell surveillance mechanism may have evolved from a much older biological system which, in more primitive life forms such as sponges[47] and cyclostomes,[5] was concerned with preventing mutual parasitism. The answer to this question, and the search for 'V genes' specific for alloantigens,[48] rests with the development and use of suitable probes by molecular archeologists.

II. (8)   The Law of Conservation of T Cell   Function

The cytotoxic T cell response involves a one-on-one interaction between effector and target, though the lymphocytes may go on to kill more than once. The success, or otherwise, of the response is thus determined by the number of effectors that can be recruited to a particular tissue site of pathology. The magnitude of response is therefore a direct, quantitative expression of both the precursor frequency and the doubling-time of the cells involved: T cell memory is, so far as we know, simply a function of expanded precursor frequency.

On the other hand, an individual B cell may differentiate to a plasma cell, which secretes immense amounts of immunoglobulin. A considerable excess of antibody in serum can usually be detected by day 6 or 7 after priming, when T cell responses are first apparent. Thus, if cell mediated immunity is to operate, there must be no blocking of either T cell proliferation or effector function by antibody. Also, it would obviously be detrimental if T cells were to bind antigen directly. This makes sense in hindsight, and fits the facts concerning T cell specificity. It is generally impossible to block virus-immune T cells with anti-viral antibody, though some success may be achieved with selected monoclonal immunoglobulins used at very high titer. The recently described antibodies that are considered to bind virus + H-2 have yet to be examined in this context.[49] Cytotoxic and helper T cells (though not suppressors) are not readily shown to bind antigen.

The immune system has thus evolved in such a way that the possibility of blocking of effector T cell function with antibody or antigen is minimized. Perhaps T cells and antibodies interact with the same viral molecules, but recognize different determinants.[50,51] Antibody to MHC components, which is not (of course) found in a normal immune response in self, readily blocks T cell function.[52,54] The divergence in T and B lymphocyte specificity patterns thus reflects the need to conserve the T cell for its major biological function, surveillance of cell-surface phenotype and the elimination of abnormal cells.

II. (9) Towards an Immunological Surveillance Hypothesis

There has been a revolution in our understanding of T cell function since 1970, when Burnet stated the immunological surveillance
concept.[5] It now seems appropriate to update the idea in the light
of subsequent advances concerned with the function of T cell subsets
and the role of the MHC. None of this could have been foreseen in
1970. Also, Burnet stated quite clearly that he did not wish to propose a rigid dogma, or even an hypothesis. Immunological surveillance is a very good term to describe what T cells actually do.
However there is a need for some change of emphasis in interpretation.
We should also distinguish immunological surveillance from natural
surveillance, mediated by NK cells and other relatively non-specific
mechanisms.

The original form of the immunological surveillance concept
stated that the central role of T cells is the monitoring of cell-
surface for the expression of transformed phenotype, and the elimination of potentially malignant cells. We now know that cytotoxic T
cells are focused onto the surface of other somatic cells by the concurrent presence of self class I MHC antigens and changes induced
by conventional lytic viruses, tumor viruses and haptens. Furthermore, these lymphocytes kill cells expressing such modifications of
plasma membrane.

The historical reasons for the obsession with malignancy in the
original immunological surveillance concept are thus no longer particularly compelling: we now have a biological function for the MHC
and know that T cells are of major importance in the host response
to pathogens.[18,20] Immunological surveillance can be re-stated very
simply as the monitoring of cell surface with resultant elimination
of cells expressing modifications of self phenotype. Self is defined
by the MHC, and non-self by the combination of MHC and foreign anti-
gen(s). We do not yet know whether the latter involves actual physical association, or simple presentation of both components in reasonable proximity on the same membrane.[55]

The question still exists whether the initial lymphocyte-target
interactions that characterize immunological surveillance can occur
in other than lymphoid foci, or in tissue sites (around Langerhans'
cells in skin?) where stimulators, helper-inducers and cytotoxic
effectors can be brought in close proximity.[56] Such conditions might
also occur in, for instance, sites of inflammation induced by lytic
viruses, where monocyte and NK cell recruitment may precede T cell
invasion.[57] It seems that, for the expression of immunological surveillance function, both cytotoxic and helper-inducer subsets may be
involved. This is probably a mechanism to minimize the possibility
of autoimmunity. However, the need to involve the helper set may
work against the elimination of transformed cells that express little
in the way of surface change, and may not present determinants that

can be recognized by helper cells (associated with class II MHC glycoproteins) after antigen processing. Alternatively, involvement
of helper-inducers alone in a tumor could promote growth of that
tumor by secretion of Il-2, which could explain results of Prehn[58]
and others. There is thus a need for rigorous experimental studies
before the iniation of treatment protocols designed to promote helper
function.

III. VIRUS-IMMUNE CYTOTOXIC T CELL RESPONSES ASSOCIATED WITH H-2^k

AND H-2^b

We have examined the virus-immune cytotoxic T cell responses
associated with H-2^k and H-2^b for two different virus systems, vaccinia virus and the influenza A viruses. The first is a large DNA
virus which is assembled in cytoplasmic factories, the second is an
RNA virus that buds from cell membrane. Vaccinia virus has proved
particularly useful for situations where we need to develop a potent,
primary CTL response in vivo. The influenza model has the advantage
of sophisticated viral genetics,[59] and is thus the virus of choice
for the analysis of fine specificity patterns.

III. (1) Divergence Between CTL and Antibody Specificity Patterns

The influenza A viruses are subdivided into various serotypes
on the basis of determinants expressed on the haemagglutinin (H)
and Neuraminidase (N), which are the main viral constituents found
on the surface of both the virion and the virus infected cell.
There is no serological cross-reactivity at all between the surface
antigens of (for instance) an H1N1 and an H3N2 influenza virus,
though internal components such as the matrix (M) and nucleoprotein
(NP) are antigenically very similar for all influenza A viruses.

Limit dilution analysis has shown that approximately 90% of the
CTL clones generated by priming with an H1N1 virus are completely
cross-reactive for MHC-compatible cells infected with an H3N2
virus.[60,61] Such cross-reactivity could be directed at the NP antigen, which is present as a minority component on the surface of infected cells:[62] we need to look at normal targets modified by exposure to liposomes incorporating NP. However, such cells that have
been incubated with liposomes containing isolated viral haemmagglu-
tinin are also seen by at least some of the cross-reactive CTL.[63]
The inference is thus that, for the haemagglutinin, antibodies and
T cells may see different determinants on the same molecule. Further
complexity was encountered when the reactivity patterns of one of
the relatively rare[64] haemagglutinin-subtype-specific (for H1) CTL
clones was examined using a range of recombinant viruses.[65] It was
found that,[66] for optimal lysis, the infecting virus needed to con-

tain a particular combination of genes encoding the haemagglutinin,
the nucleoprotein and a viral polymerase!

Two important points are thus made for the understanding of
immunological surveillance and T cell repertoire. The first is
that serological markers may be useful for identifying a particular
molecule recognized during a T cell response, but concurrently provide no hint as to the nature of the determinants seen by the cytotoxic lymphocyte.[50] The second is that gene products that are not
normally thought of as being expressed on cell surface[66] may contribute to the antigenic entities seen by self-monitoring lymphocytes. This may, in particular, have implications for tumor immunology.

III. (2) Hierarchies and Immune Response Genes

The term I-region, encompassing genes encoding class II antigens in the mouse, is particularly unfortunate as class I MHC glycoproteins also operate to mediate Ir gene function.[67,68] Mice primed
with influenza and vaccinia viruses show evidence of potent CTL generation associated with $H-2K^k$, and a concurrently low level of response at $H-2D^b$. However, if $H-2K^k$ is not present, the level of CTL
activity mapping to $H-2D^b$ is greatly increased. The basis of this
interaction between $H-2K^k$ and $H-2D^b$ is not understood, and has so
far defied analysis using a variety of cell-mixture and negative
selection procedures.[69] The problem does not seem to be at the level
of the target, as virus-infected $H-2K^kD^b$ cells are readily lysed by
$H-2K^bD^b$ CTL. Also, virus-infected $H-2K^kD^b$ stimulators cause the
generation of potent $H-2D^b$-restricted virus-immune CTL from $H-2K^bD^b$
T cell populations that have first seen depleted of alloreactivity
for $H-2K^k$. The converse ($H-2K^kD^b$ lymphocyte, K^bD^b stimulator) is
also true. Thus, there does not seem to be a major defect at the
level of either T cell repertoire or stimulator presentation. Interactions occurring during development, on the surface of the virus-
infected stimulator and between different lymphocytes subsets in the
immune response, may be involved.

A somewhat different type of Ir gene effect is found for influenza virus associated with $H-2K^b$. No CTL activity specific for $H-2K^b$-
influenza virus is seen following either primary or secondary stimulation in vivo.[67] Similarly, when such virus-primed memory T cells
are exposed to virus for 6 days under limit-dilution conditions
in vitro, no response is recognized for cultures that do not incorporate an exogenous source of Il-2. Generally, for $H-2^k$ and $H-2^d$,
addition of Il-2 does not increase influenza specific T cell frequency by more than 20%, if at all.[61] However, the concurrent presence
of Il-2 throughout stimulation allows the emergence (in some individuals) of $H-2K^b$-restricted, influenza-immune CTL.[41]

We are thus able to define a heirarchy of CTL responsiveness in another way: the weaker and more variable the response, the more Il-2-dependent it will be.[41] It should also be recognized that such in vitro culture conditions may define the absolute extent of the T cell repertoire, rather than indicating the T cell specificity patterns that will be engaged under normal conditions of host response in vivo.

III. (3) Cross-Reactivities for Some MHC-Restricted Responses

Experimental evidence emerged in 1977-78 that T cells from $\{(AxB)F_1 \to A\}$ bone marrow radiation chimeras, when A and B are different H-2 haplotypes, were restricted to recognition of virus presented in the context of A.[70,71] In addition, the MHC phenotype of the thymus was shown to be central to determining the subsequent restriction patterns of peripheral T cells. We found for $\{(H-2^{kxb})F_1 \to H-2^k\}$ and $\{(H-2^{kxb})F_1 \to H-2^b\}$ radiation chimeras that the above was true for thymocytes taken more than 4 weeks after bone marrow reconstitution and stimulation with vaccinia virus for 6 days in irradiated, virus-infected recipients.[72] However, a divergence was observed in spleen: $\{(H-2^{kxb})F_1 \to H-2^k\}$ chimeras remained tightly restricted to H-2^k, while the $\{(H-2^{kxb})F_1 \to H-2^b\}$ show a progressive increase in the level of CTL function for H-2$^{k\cdot}$ + virus. It thus seemed that the thymus was imposing an absolute MHC restriction pattern, which was being gradually lost in the periphery in one case but not the other.

These results followed earlier findings from acute negative selection experiments, where alloreactive T cells were first removed from mature lymphocyte populations by acute filtration through irradiated, virus-infected recipients. The H-2^b T cells were able to generate CTL specific for H-2^k + virus, but the converse could not be shown.[73] The conclusion that may be drawn is that the MHC restricted repertoire for H-2^b is able to allow the emergence of CTL specific for H-2^k + vaccinia virus, while the opposite is not true for H-2^k T cells.

The debate continues about the relative roles of bone-marrow (pre-thymic), thymus and peripheral lymphoid tissue (post-thymic) in the determination of the MHC-restricted T cell repertoire.[35,36,70,71] It seems obvious that physiological events involving negative selection of some reactivity patterns must occur, in order to ensure self-tolerance. There is also reasonable evidence for the idea of a positively-selected, self MHC-restricted repertoire. It is now known that T cells specific for A + x may also recognize B + y[74] or alloantigen C.[44-46] There are numerous cloned, cell lines that demonstrate such characteristics. Some of us consider that such results support a "one receptor-self + x" (or "altered-self") model, but alternatives can be argued. Again we await the deliberations of the protein and DNA chemists.

III. (4) Analysis with H-2K[b]-Mutant Mice

The H-2K[b] and H-2K[bm1] molecules differ for only two amino acids[75] and are not readily distinguished by conventional antisera.[76,77] However, less than 30% of clones generated in a third-party allo-reactive response are cross-reactive for these two MHC types.[78] Also, for bulk populations of virus-immune spleen cells, absolute MHC restriction is seen between H-2K[b] and H-2K[bm1].[79-81]

Other H-2K[b] mutants recognize virus-infected wild-type (K[b]D[d]) targets to a varying extent. However, the virus-specific cross-reactivity patterns between the mutants have not previously been examined, because all mutants share a common H-2D[b]-restricted response. We thus established limit-dilution cultures, and excluded all clones that recognized the wild-type (K[b]D[b]) virus-infected or normal target.[82] Cultures that were positive for the homologous, virus-infected mutant cell line were expanded, and tested on a variety of targets. The results are summarized in Table 1. Considerable cross-reactivity was seen for mutants that differed by as many as four amino acids[75] (e.g. bm1 and bm3), though the likelihood of detecting shared specificity patterns was increased when the mutations specified close amino acid changes. In general, the degree of MHC-restricted cross-reactivity was inversely related to the capacity to generate alloreactive CTL on cross-stimulation.[83]

Table 1. Cross Reactivity Patterns for Vaccinia-Specific Limit Dilution
         Cultures From bm1 and bm3 Mutants After Removal of Effector
         Populations Lytic for Virus-Infected and Normal K[b]D[b] Targets[82]

Vaccinia-infected mutant target	Position of amino acid substitution[75]	% Of Cross-reactive Cultures bm1 effectors	bm3 effectors
bm11	77	10	94
bm3	77,89	32	100
bm9	116,121	76	80
bm1	155,156	100	30
bm10	165	67	23

These findings cannot readily be interpreted as favouring the old idea that T cells are specific solely for short, linear sequences of amino acids (reviewed in 13). Topographic influences must also be involved. This also seems to be true for non-MHC antigens, such as cytochrome, myoglobin and insulin.[84-87] The most reasonable conclusion may be that T cells are very much concerned with three dimensionally-defined determinants on both self and x, or self + x.[18,80]

IV. RECEPTORS AND REPERTOIRE

We may now have a sound operational knowledge of the biology of MHC restriction.[18,20] However, the problem with defining the T cell repertoire is that we have been attempting to answer questions concerning molecules by extrapolating from findings generated from the analysis of cell-cell interactions. This is obviously inappropriate, though it has served to pose questions. It is difficult to see how further speculation will be of much value until we gain at least a minimal understanding the nature of the T cell receptor(s), or of the DNA encoding the receptor(s).[88] At the moment, most evidence[23] can be considered to favor the idea of a one or two component receptor[89] recognizing some complex of self + x (Fig. 1). Perhaps the receptor serves to bring self and x together, or vice versa. Our understanding of molecular clustering on cell surface seems very limited, though such events may be central to T cell function.[90]

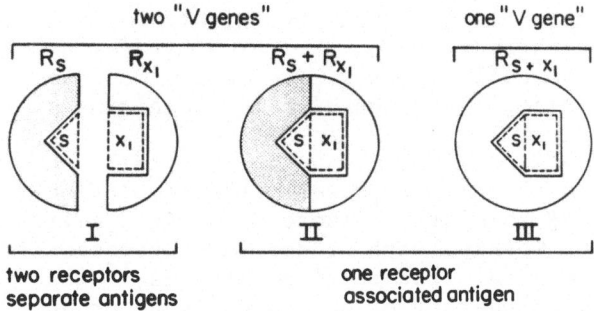

Fig. 1 Possible Organization of T Cell Receptor Binding Sites
        Encoded by One, or Two, Distinct Genetic Element(s).

The idea of two separate receptors, that act quite independently, seems untenable. Kappler, Marrack and colleagues[91] were unable to show reassortment of T cell specificity patterns (A + x and B + y did not give A + y) on cell fusion: this is currently disputed,[92] and needs to be repeated. Also, it has always been difficult to understand why two, different "low-affinity" receptors would not (if each is present in multiple copies) act independently to promote cell-cell binding.[93] Proposals requiring 'two signals' (each acting through one receptor to mediate function) may be advanced,[34] but why should this be needed for binding?[17] The retreat position for protagonists of two receptors has thus been to say that one is normally hidden, or that the first 'receptor' acts to change the functional (or binding) characteristics of the second.

It is also difficult to accomodate the two receptor idea with the fact that some T cell clones recognize both A + x and alloantigen (C): this is even more problematic for a clone that sees A + x and B + y. In the first case, the conventional escape has been to say that the alloantigen is bound via Rx[34] (Fig. 1): alloreactivity thus needs only one receptor, self monitoring requires two. However, if this were the case it should be possible to compete for alloreactive recognition of C by the A + x reactive clone by incorporating x alone, or cells expressing D + x. The one receptor model, in either the one or two chain form (Fig. 1), readily accomodates such cross-reactivity by proposing that the complex binding site can fit different antigenic configurations with varying degrees of affinity.[73]

We would also, if there are two distinct receptors, expect to identify clones that have low affinity for self MHC[36] (as a result of selection in bone marrow and/or thymus) but high affinity for x. The only point at which cells with high affinity for x could reasonably be expected to be subject to negative selection is during the process of antigenic stimulation. One possibility that could be argued is that such cells exist and are either deleted, or driven along a suppressor pathway by being blocked by free antigen prior to encountering x on cell surface. The latter could result in failure to receive a 'signal' via concurrent recognition of the MHC glycoproteins.

Anything is possible. At present, the resolution[23] seems likely to rest with the DNA chemists,[88] those studying T cell 'idiotypes' and[94,95] and groups working with helper and suppressor factors.[96,97] The prediction of the 'altered-self' hypothesis,[18] that recognition depends ultimately on whether or not an MHC gene product can form an appropriate association with a particular nominal antigen, still seems to be of value, and is generally supported by clear structural evidence that the Ia antigens are the Ir gene products[32] and functional indications that the same is true for class I MHC glycoproteins.[67,68,98] Once the basic question about the nature of T cell receptors is resolved, there will be a great need to understand how physiological exposure to particular MHC gene products can skew the emerging repertoire.[70,72] The central questions of the nature of differentiation and self-non-self discrimination remain, though events over the past 10 years have greatly modified both our technical and conceptual approaches to these problems.

ACKNOWLEDGEMENT

Some of the work summarized here was supported by grants AI-14162 and AI-15412 from the National Institutes of Health.

REFERENCES

1.   Snell, G.D.   The H-2 locus of the mouse: Observations and
     speculations concerning its comparative genetics and its poly-
     morphism. Folia.Biologica (Praha) 14: 335 (1968).
2.   Amos, D.B., W.F. Bodmer, R. Ceppellini, P.G. Condliffe, J. Daus-
     set, J.L. Fahey, H.C. Goodman, G. Klein, J. Klein, F. Lilly,
     D.L. Mann, H. McDevitt, S. Nathenson, J. Palm., R.A. Reisfeld,
     N.G. Rogentime, A.R. Sanderson, D.C. Shreffler, M. Simonsen,
     and J.J. Van Rood. Biological significance of histocompatibility
     antigens. Fed. Proc. 31: 1087 (1971).
3.   Bodmer, W.F. Evolutionary significance of the HLA System.
     Nature (Lond.) 237: 139 (1972).
4.   Burnet , F.M. Multiple polymorphism in relation to histocompati-
     bility antigens. Nature (Lond.) 245: 359 (1973).
5.   Burnet , F.M. "Immunological Surveillance", Pergamon Press,
     Sydney (1970).
6.   McDevitt, H.O. and B. Benacerraf. Genetic control of specific
     immune responses. Advan. Immunol. 11: 31 (1969).
7.   McDevitt, H.O., B.D. Deak, D.C. Shreffler, J. Klein, J.H. Stimp-
     fling, and G.D. Snell. Genetic control of the immune response.
     Mapping of the Ir-1 locus. J. Exp. Med. 135: 1259 (1972).
8.   Benacerraf, B. and H.O. McDevitt. Histocompatibility-linked
     immune response genes. Science 175: 273 (1972).
9.   Benacerraf, B. "Genetic Control of Immune Responsiveness: Rela-
     tionship to Disease Susceptibility." H.O. McDevitt and M. Landy,
     eds., Academic Press, New York, pp. 716-718 (1972).
10. Shevach, E.M. and A.S. Rosenthal. Function of macrophages in
     antigen recognition by guinea pig T lymphocytes. II. Role of
     the macrophage in the regulation of genetic control of the immune
     response. J. Exp. Med. 138: 1213 (1973).
11. Benacerraf, B. and D.H. Katz. The histocompatibility-linked
     immune response genes. Advances in Cancer Research 21: 121 (1975).
12. Greineder, D.K., E.M. Shevach and A.S. Rosenthal. Macrophage-
     lymphocyte interaction. III. Site of alloantiserum inhibition
     of T lymphocyte proliferation induced by allogeneic or aldehyde-
     bearing cells. J. Immunol. 117: 1261 (1976).
13. Benacerraf,B. A hypothesis to relate the specificity of T lympho-
     cytes and the activity of I-region-specific Ir genes in macro-
     phages and B lymphocytes. J. Immunol. 120: 1809 (1978).
14. Zinkernagel, R.M. and P.C. Doherty. Immunological surveillance
     against altered self components by sensitized T lymphocytes in
     lymphocytic choriomeningitis. Nature (Lond.) 251: 547 (1974).
15. Shearer, G.M. Cell-mediated cytotoxicity to trinitrophenyl-
     modified syngeneic lymphocytes. Eur. J. Immunol. 4: 527 (1974).
16. Doherty, P.C. and R.M. Zinkernagel. H-2 compatibility is re-
     quired for maximal T cell-mediated lysis of target cells in-
     fected with lymphocytic choriomeningitis virus. J. Exp. Med.
     141: 502 (1975).

17. Zinkernagel, R.M. and P.C. Doherty. H-2 compatibility require-
     ment for T cell-mediated lysis of target cells infected with
     lymphocytic choriomeningitis virus. Different cytotoxic T cell
     specificities are associated with structures coded for in H-2K
     or H-2D. J. Exp. Med. 141: 1427 (1975).
18. Doherty, P.C. and R.M. Zinkernagel. A biological role for the
     major histocompatibility antigens. Lancet i: 1406 (1975).
19. Shearer, G.M. and A. Schmitt-Verhulst. Major histocompatibility
     complex restricted cell mediated immunity. Adv. Immunol. 25:
     55 (1977).
20. Zinkernagel, R.M. and P.C. Doherty. MHC-restricted cytotoxic T
     cells: Studies on the biological role of polymorphic major
     transplantation antigens determining T cell restriction-specifi-
     city function and responsiveness. Adv. Immunol. 27: 51 (1979).
21. Roder, J.C. and T. Haliotis. Do NK cells play a role in anti-
     tumor surveillance? Immunology Today 1: 96 (1980).
22. Herberman, R.B. and J.R. Ortaldo. Natural killer cells: Their
     role in defense against disease. Science 214: 24 (1981).
23. Janeway, C.A., Jr., R.E. Cone and R.W. Rosenstein. T cell recep-
     tors: through a glass darkly... Immunology Today 3: 83 (1982).
24. Cerottini, J.C. and K.T. Brunner. Cell-mediated cytotoxicity,
     allograft rejection and tumor immunity. Adv. Immunol. 18: 67
     (1974).
25. Brunner, K.T., H.R. MacDonald, and J.C. Cerottini. Quantitation
     and clonal isolation of cytolytic T lymphocyte precursors selec-
     tively infiltrating murine sarcoma virus-induced tumors. J. Exp.
     Med. 154: 362 (1981).
26. Hurwitz, J.L., R. Korngold, and P.C. Doherty. Specific and non-
     specific T cell recruitment in viral meningitis: Implications
     for multiple sclerosis. Submitted for publication.
27. Sprent, J. Role of H-2 gene products in the function of helper
     cells from normal and chimeric mice measured in vivo. Immunol.
     Rev. 42: 108 (1978).
28. Farrar, J.J., W.R. Benjamin, M.L. Hilfiker, M. Howard, W.L.
     Farrar and J. Fuller-Farrar. The biochemistry, biology and role
     of interleukin 2 in the induction of cytotoxic T cell and anti-
     body-forming B cell responses. Immunol. Rev. 63: 129 (1982).
29. Ada, G.L., K.N. Leung, and H. Ertl. An analysis of effector T
     cell generation and function in mice exposed to influenza A or
     Sendai viruses. Immunol. Rev. 58: 5 (1981).
30. Lu, Y.L. and B.A. Askonas. Biological properties of an influ-
     enza A virus-specific T cell clone. Inhibition of virus repli-
     cation in vivo and induction of delayed-type hypersensitivity
     reactions. J. Exp. Med. 154: 225 (1981).
31. Reiss, C.S. and S.J. Burakoff. Specificity of the helper T cell
     for the cytolytic T lymphocyte response to influenza A viruses.
     J. Exp. Med. 154: 541 (1981).

32. Matis, L.A., P.P. Jones, D.B. Murphy, S.M. Hedrick, E.A. Lerner, C.A. Janeway, Jr., J.M. McNicholas, and R.H. Schwartz. Immune response gene function correlates with the expression of an Ia antigen. II. A quantitative deficiency in Ae:Eα complex expression causes a corresponding defect in antigen-presenting cell function. J. Exp. Med. 155: 508 (1982).

33. Alpert, B. and J. Sprent. Role of the H-2 complex in induction of T helper cells in vivo. III. Contribution of I-E subregion to restriction sites recognized by I-A/E restricted T cells. J. Exp. Med. 155: 548 (1982).

34. Langman, R.E. The role of the major H complex in immunity: a new concept in the functioning of a cell-mediated immune system. Rev. Physiol. Biochem. Pharmacol. 81: 1 (1978).

35. Schwartz, R.H. A clonal deletion model for Ir gene control of the immune response. Scand. J. Immunol. 7: 3 (1978).

36. Doherty, P.C. and J.R. Bennink. An examination of MHC restriction in the context of a minimal clonal abortion model for self tolerance. Scand. J. Immunol. 12: 271 (1980).

37. Forman, J., J. Trial, S. Tonkonogy, and L. Flaherty. The Qa 2 subregion controls the expression of two antigens recognized by H-2-unrestricted cytotoxic T cells. J. Exp. Med. 155: 749 (1982).

38. Jones, P.P., D.B. Murphy and H.O. McDevitt. Two gene control of the expression of a murine Ia antigen. J. Exp. Med. 148: 295 (1978).

39. Doherty, P.C. Surveillance of self: Cell-mediated immunity to virally modified cell surface is defined operationally by the major histocompatibility complex. Proceedings of the Fourth International Congress of Immunology, Paris, Academic Press, New York, p. 563 (1980).

40. Zinkernagel, R.M. and K.L. Rosenthal. Experiments and speculations on antiviral specificity of T and B cells. Immunol. Rev. 58: 131 (1981).

41. Allouche, M., J.A. Owen and P.C. Doherty. Limiting-dilution analysis of weak influenza-immune T cell responses associated with H-2K^b and H-2D^b. J. Immunol., in press.

42. Mullbacher, A and R.V. Blanden. Murine cytotoxic T cell response to alphavirus is associated mainly with H-2D^k. Immunogenetics 7: 551 (1978).

43. Burakoff, S.J., R. Finberg, L. Glimcher, F. Lemonnier, B. Benacerraf, and H. Cantor. The biologic significance of alloreactivity. The ontogeny of T cell sets specific for alloantigens or modified self antigens. J. Exp. Med. 148: 1414 (1978).

44. Bevan, M.J. Killer cells reactive to altered self antigens can also be alloreactive. Proc. Natl. Acad. Sci. USA 74: 2094 (1977).

45. von Boehmer, H., H. Hengartner, M. Nabholz, W. Lenhardt, M. Schreier, and W. Haas. Fine specificity of a continuously growing killer cell clone specific for H-Y antigen. Eur. J. Immunol. 9: 592 (1979).

46. Braciale, T.J., M.E. Andrew and V.L. Braciale. Simultaneous expression of H-2 restricted and alloreactive recognition by a cloned line of influenza virus-specific cytotoxic T lymphocytes. J. Exp. Med. 153: 1371 (1981).

47. Hildemann, W.H. and D.S. Linthicum. Transplantation immunity in the Palaun sponge, Xestospongia exigua. Transplantation 32: 77 (1981).

48. Jerne, N.K. The somatic generation of immune recognition. Eur. J. Immunol. 1: 1 (1971).

49. Wylie, D.E., L.A. Sherman and N. Klinman. Participation of the major histocompatibility complex in antibody recognition of viral antigens expressed on infected cells. J. Exp. Med. 155: 403 (1982).

50. Doherty, P.C., R.B. Effros and J.R. Bennink. Heterogeneity of the cytotoxic T cell response following immunization with influenza viruses. Proc. Natl. Acad. Sci. 74: 1209 (1977).

51. Maizels, R.M., J.A. Clarke, M.A. Harvey, A. Miller, and E.E. Sercarz. Epitope specificity of T cell proliferative response to lysozyme. T proliferative cells react predominately to different determinants from those recognized by B cells. Eur. J. Immunol. 10: 509 (1980).

52. Fischer Lindahl, K. and H. Lemke. Inhibition of killer target cell interactions by monoclonal anti-H-2 antibodies. Eur. J. Immunol. 9: 526 (1979).

53. Blanden, R.V., A. Mullbacher, and R.B. Ashman. Different D-end dependent antigenic determinants are recognized by H-2 restricted cytotoxic T cells specific for influenza and Bebaru viruses. J. Exp. Med. 150: 166 (1979).

54. Allouche, M., J.R. Bennink, T.J. McKearn, and P.C. Doherty. A monoclonal antibody to an interspecies major histocompatibility determinant inhibits a virus-specific T cell clone. Cell. Immunol. 68: 1 (1982).

55. Ciavarra, R. and J. Forman. Cell-membrane antigens recognized by anti-viral and anti-trinitrophenyl cytotoxic T lymphocytes. Immunol. Rev. 58: 73 (1981).

56. Wagner, H., C. Hardt, K. Heeg, K. Pfizenmaier, W. Solbach, R. Bartlett, H. Stockinger, and M. Rollinghoff. T-T cell interactions during cytotoxic T lymphocyte (CTL) responses. T cell derived helper factor (Interleukin 2) as a probe to analyze CTL responsiveness and thymic maturation of CTL progenitors. Immunol. Rev. 51: 215 (1980).

57. Doherty, P.C. and R. Korngold. Characteristics of viral meningoencephalitis: Distribution of natural killer cells and cytotoxic T lymphocytes in a pox-virus-induced inflammatory exudate. Submitted for publication.

58. Prehn, R.T. Do tumors grow because of the immune response of the host? Transplantation Rev. 28: 34 (1976).

59. Webster, R.G. and W.J. Bean, Jr. Genetics of influenza virus. Ann. Rev. Genet. 12: 415 (1978).

60. Askonas, B.A., A. Mullbacher and R.B. Ashman. Cytotoxic T memory cells in virus infection and the specificity of helper T cells. Immunol. 45: 79 (1982).

61. Owen, J.A., M. Allouche and P.C. Doherty. Limiting dilution analysis of the specificity of influenza immune cytotoxic T cells. Cell. Immunol. 67: 49 (1982).

62. Yewdell, J.W., E. Frank and W. Gerhard. Expression of influenza A virus internal antigens on the surface of infected P815 cells. J. Immunol. 126: 1814 (1981).

63. Koszinowski, U.H., H. Allen, W.J. Gething, M.D. Waterfield, and H.D. Klenk. Recognition of viral glycoproteins by influenza A specific cross-reactive cytolytic T lymphocytes. J. Exp. Med. 151: 945 (1980).

64. Braciale, T.J., M.E. Andrew and V.L. Braciale. Heterogeneity and specificity of cloned lines of influenza-virus-specific cytotoxic T lymphocytes. J. Exp. Med. 153: 910 (1981).

65. Palese, P. The genes of influenza virus. Cell. 10: 1 (1977).

66. Bennink, J.R., J.W. Yewdell and W. Gerhard. A viral polymerase involved in recognition of influenza virus-infected cells by a cytotoxic T cell clone. Nature (Lond.) 296: (1982).

67. Doherty, P.C. W.E. Biddison, J.R. Bennink, and B.B. Knowles. Cytotoxic T cell responses in mice infected with influenza and vaccinia viruses vary in magnitude with H-2 genotype. J. Exp. Med. 148: 534 (1978).

68. Zinkernagel, R.M., A. Althage, S. Cooper, G. Kreeb, P.A. Klein, B. Sefton, L. Flaherty, J. Stimpfling, D. Shreffler, and J. Klein. Ir genes in H-2 regulate generation of antiviral cytotoxic T cells. Mapping to K or D and dominance of unresponsiveness. J. Exp. Med. 148: 592 (1978).

69. Bennink, J.R. and P.C. Doherty. Reciprocal stimulation of negatively selected high responder and low responder T cells in virus-infected recipients. Proc. Natl. Acad. Sci. USA 76: 3482 (1979).

70. Bevan, M.J. and P.J. Fink. The influence of thymus H-2 antigens on the specificity of maturing killer and helper cells. Immunol. Rev. 42: 4 (1978).

71. Zinkernagel, R.M. Thymus and lymphohemopoietic cells: Their role in T cell maturation, in selection of T cells' H-2 restriction specificity, and in H-2 linked Ir gene control. Immunol. Rev. 42: 202 (1978).

72. Doherty, P.C., R. Korngold, D.H. Schwartz, and J.R. Bennink. The development and loss of virus-specific thymic competence in bone marrow radiation chimeras and normal mice. Immunol. Rev. 58: 38 (1981).

73. Doherty, P.C. and J.R. Bennink. Vaccinia-specific cytotoxic T cell responses in the context of H-2 antigens not encountered in thymus may reflect aberrant recognition of a virus H-2 complex. J. Exp. Med. 149: 150 (1979).

74. Hunig, T.R. and M.J. Bevan. Antigen recognition by cloned
     cytotoxic T lymphocytes follows rules predicted by the altered-
     self hypothesis. J. Exp. Med. 155: 111 (1982).
75. Nairn, R., K. Yamaga and S.G. Nathenson. Biochemistry of the
     gene productivity from murine MHC mutants. Ann. Rev. Genet.
     14: 241 (1980).
76. Melvold, R.W. and H.I. Kohn. Eight new histocompatibility mu-
     tants associated with the H-2 complex. Immunogenet. 3: 185 (1976)
77. Klein, J. H-2 mutations: Their genetics and effects on immune
     functions. Adv. Immunol. 26: 55 (1978).
78. Sherman, L.A. Dissection of the B10.D2 anti H-2K^b cytolytic T
     lymphocyte receptor repertoire. J. Exp. Med. 151: 1386 (1980).
79. Zinkernagel, R.M. H-2 compatibility requirement for virus-
     specific T cell-mediated cytolysis. The H-2K structure in-
     volved is coded by a single cistron defined by H-2K^b mutant
     mice. J. Exp. Med. 143: 437 (1976).
80. Blanden, R.V., M.B.C. Dunlop, P.C. Doherty, H.I. Kohn, and
     I.F.C. McKenzie. Effects of four H-2K mutations on virus-
     induced antigens recognized by cytotoxic T cells. Immunogenet.
     3: 541 (1976).
81. Doherty, P.C., J.R. Bennink, and P.J. Wettstein. Negatively-
     selected H-2^{bml} and H-2^b T cells stimulated with vaccinia virus
     completely discriminate between mutant and wild-type H-2K
     alleles. J. Immunol. 126: 131 (1981).
82. Hurwitz, J.L., S. Pan, P.J. Wettstein, and P.C. Doherty. Cross-
     reactivity patterns for vaccinia-specific cytotoxic T lymphocytes
     from H-2K^{bml} and H-2K^{bm3} mutant mice. Submitted for publication.
83. Melief, C.J.M., L.P. DeWaal, M.Y. Van Der Meulen, R.W. Melvold,
     and H.I. Kohn. Fine specificity of alloimmune cytotoxic T
     lymphocytes directed against H-2K. A study with K^b mutants.
     J. Exp. Med. 151: 993 (1980).
84. Barcinski, M.A. and A.S. Rosenthal. Immune response gene con-
     trol of determinant selection. I. Intramolecular mapping of
     the immunogenic sites on insulin recognized by guinea pig T and
     B cells. J. Exp. Med. 145: 726 (1977).
85. Corradin, G and J.M. Chiller. Lymphocyte specificity to protein
     antigens. II. Fine specificity of T cell activation with cyto-
     chrome C and derived peptides as antigenic probes. J. Exp. Med.
     149: 439 (1979).
86. Solinger, A.M., M.E. Ultee, E. Margoliash, and R.H. Schwartz.
     The T lymphocyte response to cytochome C. I. Demonstration of
     a T cell heteroclitic proliferative response and identification
     of a topographic antigenic determinant on pigeon cytochrome C
     whose immune recognition requires two complementing major histo-
     compatibility complex linked immune response genes. J. Exp. Med.
     150: 830 (1979).
87. Berkower, I., F.R.N. Gurd and J.A. Berzofsky. H-2 linked fine
     specificity of myoglobin primed T cells. Fed. Proc. 40: 998
     (1981).

88. Kurosawa, Y., H. von Boehmer, W. Haas, H. Sakono, A. Trauneker,
     and S. Tonegawa. Identification of D segments of immunoglobulin
     heavy chain genes and their rearrangement in T lymphocytes.
     Nature (Lond.) 290: 565 (1981).

89. Doherty, P.C., D. Gotze, G. Trinchieri, and R.M. Zinkernagel.
     Models for recognition of virally-modified cells by immune
     thymus-derived lymphocytes. Immunogenet. 3: 517 (1976).

90. Cohen, R.J. and H.N. Eisen. Interactions of macromolecules on
     cell membranes and restrictions of T cell specificity by pro-
     ducts of the major histocompatibility complex. Cell. Immunol.
     32: 1 (1977).

91. Kappler, J.W., B. Skidmore, J. White and P. Marrack. Antigen
     inducible, H-2 restricted, interleukin-2-producing T cell hybri-
     domas. Lack of independent antigen and H-2 recognition.
     J. Exp. Med. 153: 1198 (1981).

92. Lonai, P., S. Bitton, H.F.J. Savelkoul, J. Puri, and G.J. Ham-
     merling. Two separate genes regulate self-Ia and carrier recog-
     nition in H-2 restricted helper factors secreted by hybridoma
     cells. J. Exp. Med. 154: 1910 (1981).

93. Doherty, P.C., R.B. Effros, J.R. Bennink, and W. Gerhard. Cell-
     mediated immunity in influenza. Perspectives in Virology 10:
     73 (1977).

94. Infante, A.J., P.D. Infante, S. Gillis, and C.G. Fathman.
     Definition of T cell idiotypes using anti-idiotype sera pro-
     duced by immunization with T cell clones. J. Exp. Med. 155:
     1100 (1982).

95. Binz, H. and H. Wigzell. T cell receptors with allo-major
     histocompatibility complex specificity from rat and mouse.
     Similarity of size, plasmin susceptibility and localization of
     antigen-binding region. J. Exp. Med. 154: 1261 (1981).

96. Germain, R.N. and B. Benacerraf. Helper and suppressor T cell
     factors. Springer Sem. Immunopath. 3: 93 (1980).

97. Yamaguchi, K., N. Chao, D.B. Murphy, and R.K. Gershon. Molecular
     composition of an antigen specific Ly-1 T suppressor inducer
     factor. One molecule binds antigen and is I-J[+] another is I-J[−],
     does not bind antigen and imparts an Igh-variable region-linked
     restriction. J. Exp. Med. 155: 655 (1982).

98. Pan, S.H., P.J. Wettstein and B.B. Knowles. H-2K[b] mutations
     limit the CTL response to SV40 TASA. J. Immunol. 128: 243 (1982).

DISCUSSION

Paul: Peter (Doherty), I wish to bring up the issue you raised concerning the notion that the "self-reactivity" of T cells is greater in its precision of recognition than is the "antigen-reactivity" of such cells. I do not believe that the experiments you described adequately blots the issue. What you should determine is whether "self+X" specific cells, which do not recognize wild type "self+X", can recognize "alloantigens+X". Similarly, the fact that most influenza specific T cells do cross react among the existing mutant hemagglutinins does not imply any lack of precision in their recognition capacity, only that they do not recognize the sites which have been subject to mutation.

Doherty: You are quite correct, we cannot really make that comparison. The findings with influenza may simply reflect that the T cells are highly specific for an invariant region on the glycoprotein.

Benacerraf: I would like to ask Peter Doherty to comment on the weaker reactivity of T cells for xeno MHC antigens as compared to allo-MHC antigens which characterizes the specificity of T cells for MHC antigens. That is the specificity of T cells centers on MHC molecules very close to self.

Uhr: I want to pursue further Peter Doherty's conclusion concerning the limitation of the T cell repertoire for non-self antigens. There are examples in which T cells distingish minute chemical differences between antigens that are not detected readily at the antibody level. Thus, in the field of contact hypersensitivity, a rodent can distinguish dinitroflorobenzene from dinitrochlorobenzene whereas conventionally raised antibodies cannot; substitutions at different positions in the benzene ring are readily recognized, etc. In essence I believe the evidence in general supports the concept that the T cell repertoire for exogenous antigens may be just as large as the B cell repertoire for antigens.

Doherty: We know relatively little about the size of the T cell repertoire. It is obvious that there is extensive cross reactivity between self+X, alloantigen and even A+X and B+Y. This will only be resulved by analysis of the genes encoding the receptor(s).

Melchers: In response to your conclusion that T cells see determinants which are structurally different from those which B cell antibody see, and considering the same system you mentioned when talking about the experiments with cloned, virus-hemagglutinin-specific killer T cells I would like to remind you of experiments which we did in collaboration with Walter Gerhard at the Wistar Institute in Philadelphia. We cloned helper T cells specific for influenza virus hemagglutinin and found one clone which can distinguish hemagglutinins with a single amino acid exchange at position 122 (Lys to Gln). I would, therefore, say that it is possible that these helper T cells may see the same structural change in hemagglutinins as the corresponding monoclonal antibodies do, with which these mutant influenza strains were made. I would, however, also say that in part these helper T cells must also see it different from antibody, since they always also have to see Ia, being Ia-restricted. You, therefore, either believe in Norman Klinman's repertoir of B cell recognition of influenza virus, where he concludes that B cells also see the antigen in conjunction with Ia, or, if you do not believe that, that T cells have a different binding specificity from B cells, or, that T cells have one which is as good and therefore similar or identical in the binding site and additionally one which binds Ia.

Doherty: Walter Gerhard has an Ia restricted, influenza hemagglutinin-specific helper clone which discriminates between hemagglutinin glycoproteins changed by a single mutational event.

Klein: Are there non-restricted T cells in the periphery?

Doherty: There are such cells but they may or may not be in the minority. There are currently too many conflicting experiments to be sure. There is a need for careful analysis of frequency.

Cohn: What biological sense could there be to an immune system, which is full of gaps in recognition in the functional self-restricted repertoire, but is complete in any one of the any non-functional allo-restricted repertoires? What evolutionary or somatic process could maintain each member of the huge family of non-functional repertoires complete and the one functional repertoire incomplete? In fact, how could a significant allo-restricted repertoire exist and have the potential to function in an individual given that a self-learning process is required to establish the relationship between effector function and class of R (I or II)?

Sprent: One of the tenets of the thymus selection theory is that T cells from normal homozygous strain a mice should be unable to recognize non H-2 antigen (antigen X) in association with allo H-2 of strain b. The evidence here is conflicting. Testing this notion is complicated by the fact that before searching for strain **a** T cells with anti-**b** + X reactivity, one first has to remove cells with alloreactivity for strain **b**. Two approaches have been used to remove alloreactive cells. I have used an **in vivo** method in which Ta cells are filtered from blood to lymph through irradiated $(a \times b)F_1$ mice for 1 day. During this filtration, Ta cells with binding specificity for strain b become trapped in the spleen and fail to recirculate. The lymph-borne Ta_{-b} cells are transferred with antigen (sheep red cells) into irradiated $(a \times b)F_1$ mice for 5 days and then recovered. These

activated T helper cells collaborate effectively with strain **a** and
(**a** x **b**)F$_1$ B cells on further transfer but, significantly, do not provide
help for strain **b** B cells. Hence in this particular situation there is no
evidence that strain **a** T cells can show anti-**b** + X reactivity.

The second approach is to expose Ta cells to strain **b** cells **in
vitro** and then subject the cells to treatment with BUdR plus light, a
procedure which destroys proliferating cells. The key finding here is
that, in contrast to **in vivo** negative selection, **in vitro** selected Ta$_{-b}$
cells do show the capacity to respond to **b** + X.

In attempting to explain these diametrically opposite sets of
results I would like to suggest that **residual alloreactivity** may
account for the capacity of BUdR plus light-suicided Ta cells to
respond to **b** + X. My argument here rests on the assumption that
there are two categories of alloreactive T cells. One class of cells has
strong binding avidity for allo **b**. These are the cells which respond in
MLR and can be removed by negative selection **in vivo** and by
exposure to BUdR plus light plus **b** **in vitro**. The other category of
cells has a lower binding avidity for allo **b**. These cells bind to cells
expressing allo **b** but - and this is the crucial point - do not bind with
sufficiently high avidity to cause proliferation. Hence BUdR plus light
cannot delete these cells. These cells would be removed, however, by
filtration through irradiated strain **b** mice, where negative selection
reflects binding to allo **b**. In this respect Bill Ford observed several
years ago that although filtration of Ta cells through strain **b** rats
selectively removed about 10% of the cells; however only one half of
this 10% actually entered DNA synthesis after sequestration in the
lymphoid tissues of the host.

According to this line of reasoning, Ta cells exposed to strain **b**
cells and then BUdR plus light **in vitro** would contain a subset of
cells which, though unable to proliferate in response to strain **b**, would
be able to bind to strain **b** cells with significant avidity (higher than
the avidity of binding for self H-2). What then would happen if the
strain **b** cells were pulsed with antigen X? Here one could envisage
that some of the strain **a** cells would have anti-X receptors (assuming
that T cells have two receptors). The presence of antigen X on the
strain **b** cells would then allow high avidity binding as the result of
the combined actions of the anti-X and anti-H-2 receptors. The cells
would then be induced to proliferate. Such proliferation would not be
observed with **in vitro** selected cells, i.e. T cells lacking residual
alloreactivity.

If X-specific T cells with residual anti-**b** alloreactivity are part
of the anti-self **a** + X repertoire, these cells would be expected to
also respond to **a** + X, which they apparently do not. Here one can
invoke determinant selection and argue that the association of antigen
X with strain **a** vs. strain **b** determinants results in the display of

different X epitopes.

  Cohn: Since I am challenging the conclusion of Sprent's experiment, it is incumbent upon me to reinterpret it.

  I believe that an allo-restricted repertoire appears to exist and to be complete because the first experimental step involving elimination of cells proliferating to the allo-stimulus, by the use of BudR and light blocks their division but leaves intact their effector function as helpers, anti-allo R. In other words, castration is not synonymous with death.

  The consequence is that a low responder because of an insufficiency of antigen-specific T help becomes a responder in the second experimental step due to the presence of allo-T-help induced during the first experimental step designed to rid cells proliferating to the allo-stimulus. This makes the "allo-restricted" repertoire an artefact.

  We should remember that the antigens selected to reveal IR-gene differences are those with low avidity for the T cell receptor. The MHC haplotypes, which show a low response are those for which the germline encoded recognition of the restricting element is at the low end of the affinity distribution. Those haplotypes at the high end make up for the low affinity for antigen and are responders.

  In this particular system the low response in a proliferation assay is probably due to an insufficiency of interleukins. Antigen-sensitive T cells activated by associative recognition of antigen, but unable to proliferate because the allo-activated T helper interacting with the allo-APC results in the sufficiency of them. This "abnormal" source of help, i.e. a disassociative source of help, explains why an allo-restricted repertoire appears to exist and to be complete in each individual.

  The only reason that we get into polemics as to whether the IR-genes are expressed in T-cells or accessory cells (APC) is because we have been thinking in "altered-self or NAD" terms.

  Under the dual recognitive model, which we have proposed, this question is misleading because it takes two to tango. MHC (IR-1) genes encode restricting elements (R). It is the affinity of the R anti-R interaction (both germline encoded) which determines whether an X anti-X interaction at any given affinity will result in induction or not. It takes both the anti-R encoded in the non-MHC germline and the MHC encoded R to determine responsiveness to a given X. The T cell expresses anti-R and anti-X (non-MHC encoded); the APC expresses R (MHC encoded) and displays X. IR-1 genes encoding R, are expressed in the APC; non-IR-1 genes encoding the restrictively recognitive receptor are expressed in the T cell. The outcome of the T

helper/accessory cell (APC) interaction is the production of interleukins, which act in a second stage of induction on the T helper
activated T^*- or B^*-cell leading to division and differentiation.

The usual low responder results because the RII restricted T^H-
interactions via antigen X are of too low affinity to either activate T
or B cells or generate a sufficiency of interleukins from accessory
cells or both.

We can expect in the future many cases where the response to a
given antigen will be regulated by two sets of IR-genes one of which
is MHC encoded (R-elements expressed on antigen-sensitive and
accessory cells) and the other non-MHC encoded (the receptor
expressed on the effector T cell and its precursors).

Paul: I would like to continue the discussion as to the nature of
the expressed T cell repertoire in the periphery of an individual of
MHC type **a**. The issue that is raised is essentially whether this
repertoire is identical to the genotypic repertoire or whether it has
been skewed by a selection based upon recognition of self MHC
molecules of the a type, probably within the thymus. I would take the
view that it is and that the results which Thomas and Shevach and
that Nagy and you have obtained which show that such individals
contain cells which respond to antigen together with MHC restriction
elements of the **b** type can be accounted for by several of the
mechanisms described by the previous discussants. To restate this point
in a slightly different way I would argue that the cells of a and **b**
animals which recognize antigen +b restriction elements are very
different from one another and that few of the b-restricted cells
found in the **a** animal are actually used in the **b** animal. Indeed, the
finding that althogh **b** is a non-responder to a given antigen, **a** may
possess T cells which see that antigen together with **b** restriction
elements can probably be explained by this line of reasoning that is,
such cells display an individally high degree of "partial reactivity" to **b**
and are normally eliminated in b animals by the process of tolerance
induction.

Benacerraf: I think this discussion simply reflects the degeneracy
of the T cell system for MHC. It is the same receptor which reacts
with self+X and with alloantigens.

Sprent: It is true that the thymus selection theory is now viewed
with a certain amount of skepticism, largely because of the repeated
observation that T cells can show restriction to H-2 determinants not
encountered in the thymus. This evidence against the thymus selection
theory applies particularly to K/D-restricted T cells (CTL). In the case
of I-restricted T cells, by contrast, it is my impression that the vast
majority of the available data are consistent with this theory. This
might mean that the influence of the thymus in dictating T cell

specificity is crucial for I-restriction but rather loose for K/D-restriction.

E. Möller: Could we come to an agreement as to the available germ line repertoire in animals of different MHC genotypes? I would start off by claiming that the germ line repertoire is basically the same in different individals.

Forman: I agree.

Benacerraf: The main difficulty is that we do not have any idea of the mechanism whereby T cells become committed to MHC specificities and selected to react only with antigens presented in the context of MHC molecules.

Cohn: The diverse data showing a significant allo-restricted repertoire in a given animal must have an explanation as artefact. The argument cannot be made that there is nothing more to restrictive recognition than the immunogenic selection of T cells by (RX) interaction determinants or NADs (self or allo). Why?

The relationship between effector function ($T^{K/S}$ or $T^{H/DH}$) and restriction specificity (RI or RII) must be learned in the absence of foreign X. Independent of and distinct from tolerogenic or immunogenic selection by NADs, there must be a requirement for the learning of the RII_L-ness and RII_L-ness of a NAD by the $T^{K/S}$ and $T^{H/DH}$ cells, respectively. Even under an "altered-self" model a significant allo-restricted repertoire cannot exist.

This learning process cannot be placed at the level of immunogenic selection/induction by NADs because, as an example, the uncommitted T^o anti-(RII_F-X_S) NAD (i.e. alloreactive) would have to be induced to become a cytotoxic or killer T cell, T^K anti-(RII_F-X_S)NAD by presentation of the allo (RII_F-X_S)NAD via a second interaction with R_I, an obvious absurdity. Further, this process must explain the predilection for allele-specific recognition of the NADs. "Altered-self" or NAD models fail to do this.

Under "altered-self" models, the learning process whether it occurs in the thymus or the tail inevitably biases the repertoire toward (R_L-X_S)NAD recognition (no foreign X_F being present). The anti-(R_L-X_S)NAD repertoire is postulated to be low affinity (anti-self), but provides the functional anti-(R_L-X_F)NAD repertoire (anti-nonself) by high affinity heteroclitic cross reactivity. This position derived from Jerne was championed here by Benacerraf.

The assumption that low affinity anti-self NADs implies high affinity anti-nonself NADs is not a simple or adequate explanation for the origin of a functioning vailable T cell repertoire.

All "altered self" or "NAD" models that require self-selection in **the absence of foreign-X** to derive the repertoire which is heteroclitically anti-nonself, also require that the germline encode directly or indirectly the entire repertoire (i.e., an unselected or random repertoire must be presented for self-selection and learning) and that, once selected, somatic diversification play no role. This reinvents at the T cell level the so-called "germline theory" disproven at the B cell level.

First, somatic diversification is not permitted under this formulation, because the learning process which establishes the strict relationship between effector function and restriction specificity would be negated by somatic mutation, i.e. t^Kanti-(RI_L-X_S)NAD mutation to t^Kanti-$(RII_L-X_{S/F})$NAD. There is no way to prevent this if a random repertoire anti-NAD is further diversified somatically by random mutation.

Second, the assumption that out of a random germline encoded repertoire the learning process must select T cells anti-(R_L-X_S)NAD committed to a proper effector function/restriction specificity has many difficulties.

The selected T cells must have:
b) A heteroclitic high affinity for $(R_L-X_F)NAD_2$ with **strict** respect for the relationship between effector function and restriction specificity, i.e. $T^{K/S}$ are RI_L restricted and $T^{H/DH}$ are RII_L restricted. The T cells must know the RI_L-ness or RII_L-ness of the NAD.
c) A heteroclitic high affinity alloreactivity for $(R_F-X_S)NAD_3$ with **no** respect for the relationship between effector function and restriction specificity, i.e. both $T^{K/S}$ and $T^{H/DH}$ function perfectly well with either $(RI_F-X_S)NAD_3$ or $(RII_F-X_S)NAD_3$.
d) No reactivity toward $(R_F-X_F)NAD_4$ which is what defines restrictive recognition. The $(R_F-X_F)NAD_4$ must be "processed" to $(R_L-X_F)NAD_2$ and $(R_F-X_S)NAD_3$ the "true" immunogens.

The failure to recognize $(R_F-X_F)NAD_4$ requires that anti-NAD_4 be missing from the initial germline encoded repertoire since there can be no somatic selection to eliminate that specificity. Thus we face a nontrivial contradiction showing that the germline encoded repertoire cannot be random. Since every R haplotype selects a subset of t anti-(R_L-X_S)NADs $\cong$ anti-(R_L-X_F)NADs which lack anti-(R_F-X_F)NAD specificities, no repertoire can exist. Every subset anti-$(R_L-X_S)NAD_1$ $\cong$ anti-$(R_L-X_F)NAD_2$ is anti-$(R_F-X_F)NAD4$ in the eyes of another R haplotype. Thus the assumption of self-selection from a random repertoire in the absence of foreign-X is translatable into a **reductio ad absurdum.**

Coutinho: I agree with Mel Cohn's point that all what we know about restriction comes from effector stages and fractions. If you want to pursue this, however, you cannot make reasonable postulates about germ-line repertoires derived from such observations. If repertoires, as David Baltimore was saying, had no sense at all and contained all possibilities, the phenomenology we observe is a reflexion of the cellular expression and, particularly, of the function of the detectable restricting elements on the target cells for the effector T cells we study. For example, helper cells "restricted" to Thy-1 if they existed in the potential repertoire could never be detected or even function in antibody responses, because B cells do not express Thy-1.

Forman: Steve Clark in my laboratory has been studying cytotoxic T lymphocyte (CTL) H-2 restriction using H-2K^b mutant strains as the tool. Two parameters were being assayed, the ability of H-2K^b mutant molecules to crossreact in H-2 restriction with H-2K^b using the antigens vesiculostomatitis virus (VSV) and Sendai virus (SV), and the presence of H-2K^b CTL alloantigenic specificities on H-2K^b mutant molecules. We find that mutants can be divided into three groups. The first are mutants lacking most H-2K^b allodeterminants; these do not crossreact with H-2K^b in viral restriction. However, it should be noted that in many cases these mutant antigens convert to a nonresponder phenotype. A second group of strains with mutant molecules retain most of the H-2K^b allodeterminants and crossreact highly with H-2K^b in viral restriction. The most interesting is the third group which contains mutants that have lost allodeterminats but cross react in viral restriction and vice versa. If one analyses the ability to cross react with H-2K^b in CTL restricted responses using a very large panel of antigens by surveying published data, strains in the third group show a variable pattern of crossreactivity with H-2K^b depending on the antigen being tested. We interpret this as favouring an interaction antigen as the unit being recognized by CTL receptors. Finally, we have noted that anti-H-2K^b/VSV CTL crossreact with uninfected target cells from mutant strain H-2K^{bm8}. On the other hand, anti-H-2K^b SV CTL do not crossreact on noninfected H-2K^{bm8} cells or other H-2K^b mutant cells. This indicates that receptors that recognize a restricting determinant show unique crossreactions with particular H-2 alloantigens.

Simpson: The data shown in next page on Ir gene responsiveness to two antigens would appear to map the dominant H-2 linked Ir gene to I-B. If I-B is deemed no longer to exist, some explanation needs to be put forward to accommodate these data.

Strominger: Are the I-B data explainable on the basis of hybrid molecules, i.e. I-A, I E/C hybrids (e.g. A$_{alpha}$ E$_{beta}$) may be possible with some genes, but not with others?

Miller: In general, antibody production to related haptens, such as DNP and TNP is highly crossreactive (e.g. one uses TNP-red cells

Mouse strain	H-2 haplotype K A B E D	anti-H-Y DTH response	anti-oxazolone response
B10	b b b b b	+	-
B10.BR	k k k k k	-	+
B10.A(4R)	k k b b b	+	-
B10.A(2R)	k k k k b	-	+
B10.A(5R)	b b b k d	+	-
(B10.A(5R)x B10.A(4R)F$_1$)		+	-

to measure anti-DNP plaques). However, some monoclonal antibodies have been identified, which can distinguish between the two haptens. It is generally accepted that T cells in delayed hypersensitivity clearly distinguish between TNP and DNP derivatives and this has been cited as evidence that receptors of T and B cells are different. Thomas, Mottram and I have examined this at the clonal level with T cell lines from mice sensitized to picrylchloride. While some lines distinguish clearly between the two haptens, TNP and DNP, others react to both. This situation, with respect to fine specificity at the clonal level, is thus similar for both T and B cells.

There is at least one experimental system that points to a thymus influence on the acquisition of responsiveness. Low responder (LR) stem cells differentiating in a thymus grafted from an F$_1$ from a cross between a high responder (HR) and a LR can produce T cells (of LR genotype) which, when presented with antigen in association with the HR haplotype (e.g. on macrophages) can now respond adequatedly. Acquisition of responsiveness has thus been acquired through some thymus influence.

Session V

Induction and Effector Functions of T Cells

Chairman: H. Wigzell

INDUCTION AND EFFECTOR FUNCTION OF T CELLS

Elizabeth Simpson, Phillip Chandler, *F. Y. Liew,
Gerard Farmer, Walter Fierz and Robert Gregory

Clinical Research Centre
Watford Road, Harrow, Middlesex, HA1 3UJ

*Wellcome Research Laboratories
Beckenham, Kent

INTRODUCTION

Immune response (Ir) genes are involved at both the induction
and effector phase of T cell responses.   To induce differentiation
of precursors of effector cytotoxic T cells (Tc) or delayed-type
hypersensitivity cells (Tdh) extrinsic antigen must be presented
in the context of the appropriate major histocompatibility complex
(MHC) determinants.   In addition for induction of Tc and Tdh
extrinsic antigen must activate T helper cells (Th) because the
generation of most T cell effector functions like specific antibody
production of B cells, is helper cell dependent.   Generally Tdh
and Th require the presentation of antigen in the context of class
II MHC molecules (H-2Ia in mouse, HL-D antigens in man) whilst
most Tc similarly use class I MHC molecules (H-2K/D/L in mouse,
HL-A/B/C in man).

The manner in which T cells recognise extrinsic antigen X plus
self MHC determinants is not fully understood.   Two hypotheses
have been put forward, one that of 'dual recognition' whereby the
T cell receptor sees both X and the self MHC molecule: the other
hypothesis is that of 'altered self' for which it is proposed that
the proximity of X and self MHC on the membrane of the antigen
presenting cell creates novel, neoantigenic determinants.   It is
difficult to design experiments to unequivocally distinguish
between these two hypotheses: knowledge of the structure of the T
cell receptor would also certainly help.   However, the pivotal
role of self MHC determinants in presenting extrinsic antigen to

T cells is undisputed.   Both class I and class II MHC molecules
can be regarded as the MHC linked Ir gene products although how they
do so is a matter of discussion.

    The 'association model' (1) proposes that MHC molecules control
immune responses by forming complexes with the extrinsic antigen
in question (leading to responsiveness) whilst other alleles do
not (leading to unresponsiveness).   This is an attractive hypothesis, consistent with much published data concerning H-2 Ir gene
control of helper T cell responses (2) and cytotoxic T cell
responses (3) but it has recently been challenged on the grounds
that some T cells can recognise extrinsic antigen when presented
on allogeneic, H-2 different macrophages which fail to elicit
responses in syngeneic or H-2 matched cultures (4).   It is unclear
at the moment whether the recognition of antigen X in the context
of a non-self H-2 molecule in this situation alters the position.
The association of MHC molecules with the antigen could still define
the antigenic determinant which is presented to the T-cell and the
syngeneic restricted repertoire of the non-responder strain is
likely to be different from the allogeneic restricted repertoire of
the allogeneically responding strain.   But then it is of course
semantic whether one states that the antigen complex does not match
the repertoire or the repertoire does not match the antigen complex
leading to non-responsiveness.   That allogeneic class I molecules
per se are recognised by T cell clones selected to react with self
class I molecules plus X is a common finding (eg 5) and indicates
a structural relationship between self + X and allogeneic H-2
molecules.

    The influence of non H-2 Ir genes in controlling antibody res-
ponses has been reported eg Ir-Ea-1 on chromosome 2 (6).   Of very
great interest have been recent reports of the combined influence
of Gm allotypes and HLA haplotype in man on autoimmune responses,
and on the interactive influence of IgH allotypes and H-2 haplotypes in the anti-gliadin antibody response in mouse (7).   On the
assumption that a helper T cell is involved, it might be argued
that the non H-2 Ir gene(s) could be operating at the level of the
T cell receptor, perhaps coding, in part, for its structure.

H-Y Specific T cell Functions are Controlled by H-2 and non H-2 Ir genes

    The male specific antigen, H-Y, elicits strong T cell responses,
graft rejection, delayed-type hypersensitivity (DTH), host versus
graft, help and cytotoxic T cells (8).   These responses are under
Ir gene control and mice of the H-2^b haplotype give them readily
regardless of non H-2 background genes (9,10).   Some mice of other
H-2 haplotypes can be induced to give H-Y specific responses by
more rigorous immunisation procedures, but the influence of non H-2

genes in determining responsiveness in non H-2^b strains is also apparent.   Thus, some but not all H-2^k strains can make an H-Y specific cytotoxic T cell response after footpad immunisation, and this is also true of H-2^d and H-2^s strains (10).   The pattern of responsiveness amongst mouse strains indicates a combined influence of H-2 haplotype and non H-2 Ir gene(s).

H-2 Ir genes for H-Y responsiveness in both H-2^b and non H-2^b strains are of two types (1) K/D genes, (2) I region genes.   K/D genes determine the cytotoxic T cell specificity and generally for any haplotype either a K or a D end product acts as the H-Y associative antigen.   I region genes determine graft rejection, DTH and help, but it appears that in H-2^b mice, IA^b gene products control help, whilst an IB^b gene controls both graft rejection and DTH, which are very strongly correlated.   In CBA (H-2^k) mice, help is controlled by both IA and IE products (11).

We have recently been investigating the mapping and identity of the non H-2 Ir genes for the H-Y specific cytotoxic T cell response following immunisation in non H-2^b mice.   One candidate was the IgH locus, and for this purpose the IgH congenic strains C57BL/KS(H-2^d, IgH^b) and C57BL/Ks.A20 (H-2^{d}IgH^a) were used.   We already knew that B10.D2 (H-2^d, IgH^b) was a responder strain, whilst BALB/c (H-2^d IgH^a) was not (10): using the congenics, although all 7 of the C57BL/KS made responses, 3 of 8 C57BL/Ks.A20 also responded indicating that the IgH genes were not of sole importance in determining responsiveness in H-2^d mice (12).   This conclusion was reinforced by results using another congenic pair, BALB/c and BALB/c.B20 (H-2^d,IgH^b), neither of which responded (12).   Another approach to mapping the non H-2 Ir genes has been to examine responsiveness in a set of recombinant inbred mouse strains.   For this purpose we used the H-2^d strains of the BXD RI strains derived from the parental strains, B6 and DBA/2.   From the strain distribution pattern (SDP) of ability to respond to H-Y, it is clear that in this genetic combination, the IgH locus exerts no demonstrable effect, but a gene mapping at or close to B2m on chromosome 2 exerts a strong effect (13).   This is a very interesting location, firstly because of the contribution B2m molecules make to class I MHC antigens and secondly because this chromosomal region is a complex including a number of genes coding for cell surface molecules (H-3, Pgp-1; Ly m11) (14).

Finally, it is perhaps of interest to examine the results of experiments designed to overcome *in vivo* non responsiveness to H-Y. The starting point was the finding that CBA (H-2^k) mice previously considered to be non responders to H-Y since females failed to generate cytotoxic T cells after intraperitoneal immunisation by syngeneic male cells and did not reject primary syngeneic male skin grafts, could be induced to make excellent H-Y specific cytotoxic T cell responses after immunisation in the footpad (fp) with syngeneic male spleen cells (15).   We therefore fp immunised the

TABLE 1.   Induction of anti H-Y graft rejection responses
            in mice immunised via the footpad

Strain	Day of graft following		Graft survival time footpad immunisation		
	7	14	21	28	35
C57BL/10	11(x7)	<10(x5) 12,12	<10,10 12,12,15 15,24	<10(x3) 11(x3) 19	<11,12(x3) 15,17 20
CBA	14,14 28 >100(x4)	17(x3) >100(x4)	16(x4) 20,78,	13,13 >100(x4)	13,13,36 >100(x3)
B10.BR	11,11 >100(x4)	<10,11,13(x3),14,16,33,38 40,41,58,61,63,64, >100(x5)***			<11,23 >100(x2)
BALB/c	>100(x5)	>100(x7)	>100(x7)	16 >100(x6)	12,15,78 82,82 >100

*** Mice pooled in these groups

following mouse strains: C57BL/10, CBA, B10.BR and BALB/c and
subsequently grafted groups of each strain, 7, 14, 21, 28 or 35
days after immunisation with syngeneic male skin, and then measured
graft survival.   The results are shown in Table 1.   It is clear
that all C57BL/10 mice give rapid second set graft rejection
responses at all times after immunisation.   In contrast, very few
BALB/c mice make the response at any time after immunisation,
whereas both the $H-2^k$ strains CBA and B10.BR give a response, although it is somewhat irregular amongst animals in a group, and is
quite strongly influenced by the time after immunisation that the
mice were grafted.   It is also a matter of interest that there
was very little correlation between the graft rejection response
and the ability to generate an H-Y specific T cell response after
in vitro stimulation in MLC in the non $H-2^b$ mice.   Almost all CBA
mice generated cytotoxic responses, regardless of whether they had
rejected grafts or not, and in contrast, amongst B10.BR mice which
rejected their grafts, there were many who failed to generate an
H-Y specific cytotoxic response (Table 2)

     In another series of experiments, we examined the effect of
footpad immunisation on the subsequent ability to generate DTH
responses to H-Y.   Previous experiments had shown that subcutaneous
immunisation 6 days before elicitation of DTH allowed C57BL/10 but
not CBA mice to respond (17).   However, following the time course
protocol used in the skin grafting experiment (Table 1), and then
testing for DTH at weekly intervals after priming, we obtained the

TABLE 2.   Relationship between graft survival and ability to generate H-Y specific cytotoxic T cell responses

Strain	Graft* Status	Cytotoxic T cell response (no. +ve/no. tested)
C57BL/10	–	20/20
CBA	+	12/12
	–	13/16
BALB/c	+	8/31
	–	3/3
B10.BR	+	0/13
	–	9/17

* -= graft rejected, + = graft intact.

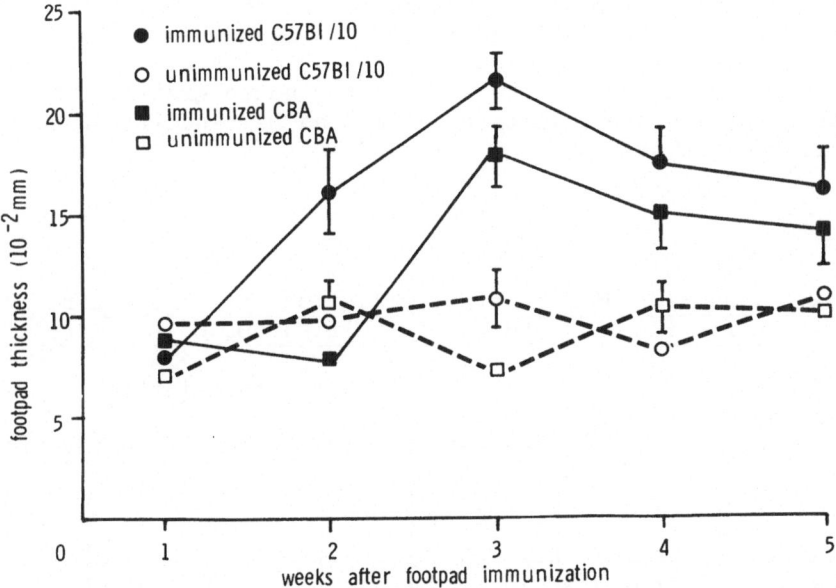

Fig. 1. Immunised female mice received 2×10^7 syngeneic male spleen cells in the front footpads. Mice were challenged at the times indicated with an injection of 1×10^7 syngeneic male lymphocytes into the right hind footpad. Footpad thickness was measured after 24 hours (see ref.17).

results shown in figure 1.   C57BL/10 mice gave DTH responses strongly from d14 after fp priming onwards, whereas for the CBA mice there was a clear peak response at 21 days after priming.   This correlates with the skin graft rejection data shown in Table 1 and suggests that the graft rejection effector cells which are probably Tdh cells are controlled independently of the H-Y specific cytotoxic T cells.   This is consistent with genetic mapping data for H-2^b mice localising the control of help to IA^b and that of DTH and graft rejection to IB^b (8,17).   From the results shown in Table 1 it seems clear that H-2 Ir genes influence the inducibility of the second set graft response after footpad immunisation, but we do not yet have the results from enough strains to determine whether non H-2 genes also have an influence.   The failure of some mice to respond, especially in groups where genetically identical individuals did make a response, suggests either that to some extent responsiveness is determined by random somatic mutation and/or that the delicate balance between responsiveness and non-responsiveness is maintained by a sensitive feedback control mechanism, perhaps involving suppressor cells.   We certainly have evidence for the role of suppressor cells in maintaining tolerance to H-Y in multiparous C57BL/10 females and in C57BL/10 females injected neonatally with small numbers of syngeneic male cells (16).   In addition, we have found that it is possible to break tolerance to H-Y in a proportion of multiparous C57BL/10 females by immunising them in the footpads with syngeneic male cells (Table 3).   Again, there is little correlation between the ability to induce graft rejection in these mice, and the ability to elicit an H-Y specific cytotoxic T cell response (Table 3).

TABLE 3.   Induction of skin graft rejection of H-Y specific cyto-toxic T cell responses in multiparous C57BL/10 females

Anti H-Y cyto-toxic responses tested between d. 24 - 110*	No. footpad immuni-sation	Graft survival time				
		Day of grafting following fp immunisation				
		7	14	21	28	35
Positive		14,14 17			55	15,17 >100
Negative	>100(x12)	>100(x2)	30	<11,29 40	17 >100(x2)	>100(x2)
Not tested	72,80,80 >100(x20)	22 >100	12,12 12	11(x3)		

* Mice which rejected grafts were tested for cytotoxicity within 3 weeks of rejection.   Those which failed to reject were tested at d.110.

SUMMARY

Induction of effector function in T cells, helper, DTH and cytotoxic is dependent on presentation of the antigen in the context of self MHC molecules. In this sense such T cell functions are H-2 restricted, and the restricting elements are the Ir gene products. The MHC restriction of T suppressor cells is less firmly established, particularly at the effector stage since at least some seem to operate via non-specific factors. The use of the minor transplantation antigen, H-Y, which only stimulates responses in some mouse strains, has enabled us to probe the Ir genes controlling several different T cell responses to this antigen. MHC, class I and class II antigens are important in control, but in non H-2^b mice at least, they also appear to interact with non H-2 Ir genes when responses are stimulated by a rigorous immunisation schedule. One non H-2 Ir gene maps to chromosome 2, at or near B2m, the influence of IgH genes, although not totally excluded, is not paramount.

REFERENCES

1. E. Simpson and T. Matsunaga. Physiological function of major histocompatibility complex macromolecules. *Transplantation*, 27: 295 (1979).
2. A.S. Rosenthal. Determinant selection and macrophage function in genetic control of the immune response. *Immunol. Rev.*, 40: 136 (1978).
3. E. Simpson, T. Matsunaga, M. Brenan, C. Brunner, D. Benjamin, C. Hetherington, M. Hurme and P. Chandler. H-Y antigen as a model for tumour antigens: the role of H-2 associative antigens in controlling anti H-Y immune responses. *Trans. Proc.*, 12: 103 (1980).
4. N. Ishii, C.N. Baxevanis, Z.A. Nagy and J. Klein. Responder T cells depleted of alloreactive cells react to antigen presented on allogeneic macrophages from non responder strains. *J. Exp. Med.*, 154: 978 (1981).
5. H. von Boehmer, H. Hengartner, M. Nabholz, W. Lernhardt, M.H. Schreier and W. Haas. Fine specificity of a continuously growing killer cell clone specific for H-Y. *Eur. J. Immunol.*, 9: 592 (1979).
6. D.L. Gasser. Genetic control of the immune response in mice. *J. Immunol.*, 103: 66 (1969).
7. M.F. Kagnoff. Two genetic loci control the murine immune response to A-gliadin, a wheat protein that activates coeliac sprue. *Nature*, 296: 158 (1982).
8. E. Simpson. The role of H-Y as a minor transplantation antigen. *Immunology Today*, 3: 97 (1982).
9. R.D. Gordon, E. Simpson. Immune response gene control of cytotoxic T cell responses to H-Y. *Trans. Proc.*, 9: 885 (1977).

10. W. Fierz, M. Brenan, A. Müllbacher and E. Simpson. Non H-2 and H-2 linked immune response genes control the cytotoxic T cell response to H-Y. *Immunogenetics*, 15: 170 (1982).

11. M. Brenan and A. Müllbacher. Analysis of H-2 determinants recognised during the induction of H-Y immune cytotoxic T cells by monoclonal antibodies *in vitro*. *J. Exp. Med.*, 154: 563 (1981).

12. G. Farmer, W. Fierz and E. Simpson. The influence of IgH-I genes on cytotoxic T cell responsiveness to H-Y in interaction with H-2 genes. In preparation.

13. W. Fierz, G. Farmer, J. Sheena and E. Simpson. Genetic analysis of the non-H-2 linked Ir-genes controlling the cytotoxic T-cell response to H-Y in H-2^d mice. Submitted. 1982.

14. N. Tada, S. Kimura, A. Hatzfeld and U. Hammerling. Ly-m11: the H-3 region of mouse chromosome 2 controls a new surface alloantigen. *J. Immunogenetics*, 11: 441 (1980).

15. A. Müllbacher and M. Brenan. Cytotoxic T-cell response to H-Y in 'non responder' CBA mice. *Nature*, 285: 34 (1980).

16. E. Simpson, D. Benjamin and P. Chandler. Non-responsiveness to H-Y: tolerance in H-1^b mice. *Trans. Proc.*, 13: 1880 (1981).

17. F.Y. Liew and E. Simpson. Delayed-type hypersensitivity responses to H-Y: characterisation and mapping of Ir genes. *Immunogenetics*, 11: 155 (1980).

DISCUSSION

Doherty: Are (CBA/H x B10.BR)F$_1$ mice capable of generating a CTL response?

Simpson: I have tested (CBA/H x AKR)F$_1$, half respond, half do not.

Doherty: Does that not mean that you cannot make a preclusion argument for deletion of T cell specificites as a result of molecular mimicry unless it is the case that the non-H-2 gene is allelically excluded, or differentially expressed in individual mice?

Simpson: The fact that F$_1$ hybrids between responder x non-responder, such as (CBA x AKR)F$_1$ can make H-Y specific cytotoxic T cell responses does tend to argue against molecular mimicry as a cause of non-responsiveness. However, the result is not straightforward, since only about 50% of such F$_1$ mice respond, one could still argue that dominant cross reactive clone(s) do not develop in such mice and that in some animals noncross-reactive clones do.

Simpson: On the question as to the proportion of H-Y specific clones which also are specific for cross-reactive antigens, we find that approximately 10% of CBA and B10 female mice make anti-H-Y bulk culture responses which can reactively kill allogeneic female target cells to some extent. To enumerate these it would be necessary to clone these effector cells.

Simpson: The Harald von Boehmer clone which showed specificity for D^b+H-Y and D^d is evidence that molecular mimicry occurs and involves H-2 class 1 molecules.

Sachs: When one sees the same background behaving quite differently in the presence of different non-responder H-2 types, one should consider the possibility of genetic drift in the background, which can of course happen between congenic strains maintained as inbred lines. In this regard, have you examined a variety of sublines of any of your responder and non-responder strains? If numerous genes are involved and subject to drift, I would expect frequent subline differences in responses.

Simpson: This has not been investigated and should be.

Mäkelä: You must have considered the possibility that the Ir gene in chromosome 2 is a structural gene for a T cell receptor. What is your present feeling about this possibility?

Simpson: When we found evidence for the existence of non H-2 Ir genes, we speculated that one might be the gene for the T cell receptor. It is an attractive hypothesis but we still need to find out how the chromosome 2 mapping gene operates.

Uhr: Could you define what you mean by the term molecular mimicry. Is it an explanation for a set of data or is there direct evidence for this concept?

Simpson: The best evidence for molecular mimicry being responsible for non-responsiveness comes from experiments with $(B10 \times CBA)F_1$ and $(B10 \times B10.S)F_1$ hybrid females immunized with syngeneic F_1 male cells. These mice make only $H-2^k$ or $H-2^s$ restricted responses respectively, and not $H-2^b$ restricted H-Y specific cytotoxic cell responses. This result can be attributed to the cross reactivity of D^b+H-Y with H-2s and H-2k class 1 molecules. Such cross reactivity can be shown in bulk cultures of H-Y specific cytotoxic cells from B10 and CBA mice.

Molecular mimicry can also be invoked to explain the failure of CBA females tolerized at birth with $(B10 \times CBA)F_1$ female cells to subsequently make an H-Y cytotoxic response to CBA male cells.

Coutinho: Now that you have raised the point of non-MHC-linked Ir genes, I would like to underline one aspect of helper cell repertoire which is not often considered. In essence, the current conviction that T cells are preoccupied mostly (or exclusively) with MHC may well not be justified for helper T cells. Fitch's laboratory has published strong evidence that the frequency of "factor-producing" helper cell precursors specific for either MHC or the whole non-MHC backgrounds is about 5 times higher for non-MHC antigens. We have similar indications for T cells that help in antibody responses. Certainly, these cells could still be MHC-restricted. However, not only Mls-reactive cells (where controversy exists as to their MHC-restriction) but other types of "background" loci certainly different from Mls-locus, stimulate MHC-unrestricted responses involving high enough numbers of cells in unprimed populations to be easily detected, often at levels similar (or higher than anti-MHC MLC. In any case, those results stand in clear contrast with the frequencies of CTL precursors determined across the same genetic differences.

E. Möller: As to the discussion on molecular mimicry, Teresa Ramos and I have found that bulk cultures with reactivity specific for FITC-modified $H-2D^d$ will crossreact with unmodified $H-2D^d$. This cross reactivity is analogous to von Boehmers H-4 specific D^b restricted cytotoxic clone that reacts with unmodified D^d carrying cells. This cross-reactivity is not universal, since TNP-modified D^b does not seem to cross-react with D^d. Furthermore, there is no serological relationship between D^b and D^d, nor is there HVG cross-reactivity between unmodified D^b and D^d.

Therefore, these experiments are compatible with an "altered self" concept.

Coutinho: Just to add the counter-part to what I said: The same type of involvements for CTL precursors namely, frequencies of anti-MHC or anti-non MHC specificities, the very large majority of all precursors are anti-MHC, in contrast with the helper cell determination.

Svejgaard: The involvement of MHC determinants in the cooperation between various cells belonging to the immune system has also been demonstrated for the HLA system by in vitro studies of MHC restriction. Thus, the proliferative response of T lymphocytes to various antigens requires the presence of monocytes sharing HLA-D/DR antigens with the T lymphocytes (Bergholz & Thorsby, Scand. J. Immunol. 6:779, 1977; Hansen et al., Eur. J. Immunol. 7:520, 1978), whereas cytotoxic T cells only kill haptenized or virus-infected target cells sharing HLA-ABC antigens with the T cells (Goulmy et al., Nature 266:544, 1977; Dickmeiss et al., Nature 270:526, 1977; McMichael et al., Nature 270:524, 1977). More recently, evidence has been presented that even hybrid (combinatorial) D/DR antigens may also be restricting elements in the monocyte-T-lymphocyte cooperation (Hansen et al., J. Immunol. 128:2497, 1982), and the preferential restriction phenomenon known from mice studies has also been demonstrated for cytotoxic T lymphocytes (McMichael et al., J. Exp. Med. 148:1458, 1978; Dickmeiss et al., Scand. J. Immunol. 14:293, 1981).

Because of the ethical problems inherent in immunizing humans with synthetic antigens, direct proof of the existence of immune response (Ir) or suppressor (Is) genes in man has not been obtained, but evidence has recently been provided for the operation of HLA linked Ir (or Is) gene functions on the basis of population and family studies (Sasazuki et al., Nature 272:359, 1978; Sasazuki et al., J. Exp. Med. 152:297, 1980). In any case, on the basis of the above in vitro experiments and on the pronounced homology known to exist between the MHC's of various vertebrates, it would be a great surprise (indeed an exciting one) if the HLA system turned out not to control Ir (and immune suppressor (Is)) functions just like the H-2 system does.

Accordingly, at the present time, it seems as if the major biological function of the HLA-ABC and D/DR antigens is to ensure adequate cooperations between various antigen presenting cells on the one hand and various subsets of T lymphocytes on the other. At the present time, one of the most fascinating problems is why the polymorphic alloantigenic determinants themselves are involved in this cooperation: or else the MHC restriction could not have been demonstrated by the methods used. It is possible that our ideas about the importance of polymorphic HLA antigens are to some extent biased and overestimated just because MHC restriction has been the key tool to understanding these cellular cooperations. It might appear that non-polymorphic HLA factors may be involved in the response to some foreign antigens.

In this context, it is of interest to note that MHC restriction in some cases has been difficult to demonstrate when primary immunization has been made in vitro (Shaw et al., Transplant. Proc. 10:937, 1978), whereas the same hapten gives strict MHC restriction after in vivo immunization (Dickmeiss et al., Nature 270:526, 1977). This phenomenon of increasing specificity for subtypic alloantigens seems to have a parallel when cytotoxic T lymphocytes are generated before and after in vivo immunization to HLA antigens (Malissen et al., Scand. J. Immunol. 14:213, 1981) after immunization, clones are obtained which show precisely the same HLA-A,B, or C specificity as that detected by alloantibodies; in contrast, cell-mediated lympholysis (CML) with cells from non-immunized individuals shows a broad specificity. Thus, it seems as if the HLA alloantigens are selected for during the development of an immune response both against foreign and against alloantigens themselves; what appear to be strong alloantigens in · MHC immunization also seem to be good restricting self-elements within the individual who possesses them.

Another crucial question is whether the pronounced polymorphism of the HLA system is neutral or due to selection mechanisms operating via the various types of cellular cooperations. Advantage of the heterozygotes (who have twice the number of polymorphic MHC determinants to play on as compared to homozygotes) was proposed already by Zinkernagel and Doherty (Nature 248:701, 1974), and such an effect might even be augmented by the existance of hybrid antigens in heterozygotes. In man, however, Hardy-Weinberg analyses of quite large numbers of individuals have not supported the existance of an advantage of heterozygotes. Indeed, there is evidence that some heterozygotes may be at a disadvantage: for example, DR3/4 hetero-zygotes run a higher risk of developing insulin-dependent diabetes that do DR3/3 and DR4/4 homozygotes (Svejgaard et al., Histocomp. Testing 1980:638). However, this disease is so rare that its weight in terms of natural selection is probably small, and it should be empha-zised that Hardy-Weinberg data are not available on sufficiently large numbers of individuals living under strong selective pressures. The many associations between a variety of "autoimmune" diseases and various HLA-DR antigens may reflect untoward "side effects" of Ir determinants in populations under relaxed selective environments, whereas the same determinants may have a protective role in more hostile environments characterized by severe infections.

For the sake of completeness, it should be noted that the

biological function of the HLA system may not be restricted to various immune responses (even if the HLA controlled complement factors are considered part of the immune system). For example, the gene for

Congenital adrenal hyperplasia due to 21-hydroxylase deficiency is located within HLA (close to the HLA-B locus). Moreover, there must be a gene within or closely linked to HLA controlling iron absorption from the gut since idiopathic haemochromatosis has been shown to be both HLA associated at the population level and closely linked to HLA in family studies, Finally, most recently it has been found that human insulin binds to a determinant associated with, or identical to, the monomorphic part of HLA-ABC antigens but not DR antigens (Olsson et al., submitted for publication). It is not known whether this phenomenon reflects another biological function of these antigens, but it is tempting to speculate that it is an example of interaction between MHC antigens and other cell surface molecules, e.g. minor histocompatibility antigens.

Forman: Jo-Ann Keene in my laboratory has used the H-Y antigen to determine what role helper determinats play in the activation of cytotoxic T-cell (CTL) precursors. She has shown that some congenic strains of mice are non responders to the Qa-1 alloantigen. However, this is not due to a lack of anti-Qa-1 CTL precursors in these mice, since the cells can be activated if the animals are primed in vivo with the Qa alloantigen toghether with H-Y. Further, the helper antigen (H-Y) and the CTL antigen (Qa-1) must be presented on the same cell for effective in vivo priming.

Since this response is boosted in vitro by culturing the primed spleen cells with antigen and testing for CTL activity after 5 days, we would determine whether the helper antigen was needed at both the in vivo and for in vitro phase of the response. Our results show that the helper antigen is only needed for in vivo priming and is not needed for in vitro restimulation. Therefore, unprimed CTL precursors have different activation requirements than memory CTL precursors activated in vitro. In addition to H-Y, some but not all minor H-antigens also act as helper determinants. In contrast, H-2 antigens do not act as helpers.

We have proposed a model for CTL precursor activation as follows:
CTL precursors are activated by recognizing antigen and receiving an activating signal from a T helper cell (Th1). Although the signal may be nonspecific, the fact that both helper and CTL antigens need to be on the same antigen presenting cell suggests that the signal can only be transmitted at close range. Once the CTL precursor is activated, it then can receive proliferative signals from a different helper cell (Th2), and expand in numbers. These cells generate memory cells that

are operationally defined as CTL precursor for a signal from Th1. Finally, interaction of the in vivo CTL precursor with antigen but without the helper signal from Th1 may lead to inactivation. Evidence in support of this is our finding that CTL precursor from a portion of animals immunized with Qa-1 also followed by a subsequent re-immunzation with Qa-1 plus H-Y fail to become primed.

Melchers: Can this experiment be performed on H-2K background?

Forman: Our preliminary data indicates the A.Tla^b animals that are non responders to Qa-1^a presented on A spleen cells will respond if H-Y is added as a helper antigen. That is, A.Tla^b female mice can be successfully primed with A male cells.

Coutinho: There is quite compelling evidence that (at least alloreactive) CTL do not require "help" to become reactive to helper "factors". This applies even to prethymic bone marrow cells. I would, therefore, delete the Th1 cell from your model and explain the data in alternative ways which are at least as likely as the possibility that all alloreactive CTL are already "primed".

Forman: We would argue that in vitro CTL activity is dependent on prior in vivo activation. If pre-T cells were available we could further test this model. In addition, CTL precursors found in nude mice may be different than truly naive CTL precursors, since older nude mice have a relatively high number of functional T cells.

Cohn: I previously argued that the germline cannot encode a random repertoire under an "altered-self" model or for that matter any model. We have proposed that the germline encodes, in large measure, anti-allele-specific determinants on R elements. I gave you my arguments for that earlier when discussing polymorphism.

I recall that Jerne argued that the repertoire is derived from the germline encoded anti-self repertoire and from this concluded that the germline encodes anti-MHC. The conclusion is close to being correct, but the argument is wrong. The assumption that the available repertoire is somatically derived from germline encoded anti-self does not predict what the self component would be (why MHC?) and does not account for polymorphism or allele-specific recognition even if one postulates (or guesses) that the self-recognition is for MHC encoded R elements.

However, as we have proposed, if the available repertoire is derived somatically from the totality of the germline encoded anti-allele-specific determinants on R$_F$ (**not** the anti-self R) then not only is polymorphism and allele-specific recognition accounted for, but a rather puzzling finding is explained. There are many examples where a T cell line which restrictively recognizes a given antigen-X shows alloreactivity for one or another R_F. The reason is that the somatic mutation in the germline encoded anti-R_F which results in anti-X activity may no obliterate the anti-R_F specificity. This finding supports the notion that the germline encodes anti-allele specific determinants on R.

I recall that we have seen this phenomenon at the level of the B cell. In discussing Hood's data, I pointed out that the somatic mutants in the anti-PC encoding germline V-genes results in anti-X specificities which are unknown. However, since the experimentor selected hybridomas with anti-PC specificity, we have examples where these new somatically derived specificities retain a memory of their anti-PC origin. For the B cell we know the germline encoded specificity (anti-PC), but not the somatically derived anti-X. In the case of the T cell, we know the anti-X specificity and surmise that the germline encoded anti-R (allele-specific) by the significant proportion of crossreactions.

Svejgaard: It has been said that the specificity of the T lymphocyte receptor for antigen is less strict than that of immunoglobulins. However, under certain conditions, T lymphocytes may show precisely the same strict specificity as antibodies. Thus, Malissen et al. (Scand. J. Immunol. 14:213, 1981) when cloning cytotoxic T cells from a repeatedly HLA immunized individual obtained clones which showed precisely the same allospecificity as the detected antibodies. Accordingly, it is possible that repeated immunizations are necessary for T lymphocytes to develop the same high degree of specificity as immunoglobulins. In any case, the work cited indicate that the T- and B-lymphocyte receptors may be related.

Ohno: Since the subject of H-Y antigen was brought up, I will try to give answers to two questions: 1) What is the function of the Y-chromosome? and 2) What part of the Y-chromosome is transcribed and translated?

The only function of the Y is to organize testes instead of ovaries. Thus, its presence in extragonadal somatic cells is largely irrelevant. Witness the fact that in two genera of australian marsupials, extragonadal somatic cells of the male eliminate the Y to become XO, the Y being retained only in the testis. Since, the task so limited requires only one or few genes, most of the Y-chromosome is dispensable; a microscopically invisible segment on its short arm sufficing for testicular organization; e.g. XX males of man are apparently caused by a meiotic crossing-over of such a Y-segment to an X-chromosome.

Based on a premise that nature is always content to play

variations of the same theme, we have used the snake W-chromosome DNA as probes to identity the male-specific messenger RNA of the mouse and man. The cloned, 2,500-base-pair-long snake W-chromosome DNA sequences by J.T. Epplen of my laboratory contained two potential coding segments. When separately used as Northern hybridization probes on polysomal, poly A$^+$ RNAs obtained from male and female mice, the first probe containing a short coding sequence (80 or so amino acid residues) singled out one only 1,000-base-long messenger RNA from males and females alike. Thus, this gene which was W-linked in the snake has become either X-linked or autosomally inherited in mammals. The other probe, on the other hand, picked up the male-specific messenger RNA roughly 1,600-base-long. This is thought to specify the testis-organizing protein; H-Y antigen.

Hood: Metazoans display cell-surface recognition systems that exhibit the ability to distinguish between self and nonself. One self-nonself recognition system, the major histocompatibility complex of vertebrates, was initially defined by the rejection of foreign skin grafts in mice. This system is now being analyzed at the molecular level. One of the family of genes encoded by this region, denoted class I genes, encode polymorphic cell-surface molecules that fall into two distinct categories. First, the classical transplantation antigens are present on all the cells of the organism and play an important role in mediating T-cell immunosurveillance of virally-infected or neoplastically-transformed cells. A second category includes the hematopoietic differentiation antigens such as Qa and TL, which are closely related structurally to the transplantation antigens, but are only expressed on a subset of bone marrow-derived cells.

The transplantation antigens appear to represent one of the most polymorphic systems studied in eukaryotes. The structure of these molecules is relatively simple. Transplantation antigens or transmembrane proteins composed of two chains-the 45,0000-dalton transmembrane polypeptide encoded by the class I genes of the major histocompatibility complex and a noncovalently associated 12,000-dalton polypeptide, beta$_2$-microglobulin. The class I molecules are divided into three external domains each about 90 residues, a transmembrane region of 40 residues, and the short cytoplasmic domain of about 30 residues. An analysis of the structure of genomic clones encoding class I molecules shows that there is a striking correlation between coding regions or exons and these domains. Separate exons encode the signal peptide, each of the three external domains, and the transmembrane region and three exons encode the small cytoplasmic domain.

We have studied the linkage arrangement and complexity of the class I genes in the mouse by cloning 40-kilobas (kb) fragments of eukaryotic DNA into cosmid vectors. Overlapping cosmid clones isolated from a BALB/c sperm DNA library defined 13 distinct gene clusters with a total of 36 class I genes encompassing 837 kb of DNA. Thus, the class I gene family and the BALB/c mouse is a moderately complex multigene family. We have used single-copy fragments from each of these 13 gene clusters to carry out restriction enzyme site polymorphism mapping to precisely locate each of these gene cluster to a particular region of the major histocompatibility complex. Three of these gene clusters map to the classical H-2 complex which includes the K, D, L, and R transplantation antigen genes. The remainder of these clusters appear to map to the adjacent Tla region which encodes the Qa and Tla genes. Thus, only 5 of 36 class I genes appear to map to the classic H-2 region.

Gene transfer experiments have identified virtually all of the serologically-defined class I genes of the BALB/c mouse. These experiments were carried out by cotransformation of mouse L cells ($H-2^k$ haplotype) lacking the enzyme thymidine kinase with herpes viral thymidine kinas gene and a class I gene. These gene transfer experiments resulted in the expression of cell-surface class I molecules that reacted with monoclonal antibodies to the various serologically-defined class I polypeptides. In this manner we have identified the K^d, L^d, D^d, Qa-2,3, and several TL antigens. These gene assignments also permit us to map the gene clusters in which these class I sequences are contained to precise regions of the major histocompatibility complex and the mapping carried out by restriction enzyme site polymorphism and gene transfer experiments coincide perfectly. We have also established a very sensitive radioimmunoassay for beta$_2$-microglobulin on the surface of cells so that we can detect novel or serologically undefined class I gene products as they are expressed in mouse L cells by the gene transfer experiments. Using this type of analysis we have identified at least ten additional class I genes that appear to synthesize novel gene products. In one particular case, we have used mouse L cells transformed with the novel gene to immunize parental C3H mice and raise alloantisera directed against the novel gene product. These alloantisera precipitate a 45,000-dalton class I polypeptide, These types of immunization procedures will be carried out on each of the other nine novel gene products to determine when in differentiation they are expressed, on what tissue type they are expressed, and ultimately what the function of these novel gene products might be.

The physiological role of transplantation antigens may be to serve as restricting elements in virus-mediated T-cell killing of infected self cells. Virus infection of mice generated killer T cells whose receptors must interact with the foreign viral antigen and a class I molecule a restricting element for the cytotoxic effector function to be activated. Thus, the T-cell receptor recognizes the viral antigen in the context of the class I molecule. To study the interaction between the T-cell receptor and a particular class I restricting element, we have used the mouse L-cell transformant which expresses L^d molecules, K^d molecules, and D^d molecules. If mice are infected with lymphocytic choriomeningitis virus (LCM virus), killer T cells are generated that can see on the target mouse L cells L^d molecules as restricting elements but not K^d or D^d molecules. Thus, the LCM virus infection, under the conditions that we have employed, is absolutely specific for the L^d class I molecule as a restricting element. We are now in the process of shuffling the exons between the L^d (functional) and the D^d (nonfunctional) genes to determine precisely which parts of the L^d molecule interact with the T-cell receptor of lymphocytes in the LCM virus immune response.

A careful analysis of the exons in the class I genes demonstrate that the fourth exon which encodes the third external domain shows striking homology relationships to the constant regions of immunglobulins. This raises the provocative possibility that the class I genes and antibody genes descended in one time from a common ancestral multigene family - perhaps one that carried some type of informational role at the cell surface of early metazoa.

Uhr: Are the H-2 genes incorporated into the L cell chromosomes?

Hood: The class I genes are incorporated directly into the L cell chromosomes, presumably at random sites throughout the genome.

Uhr: Is there an increase in B_2microglobulin synthesis in all instances in which a class I gene is integrated into the transfected cell? I would guess that this coordinate regulation might involve several steps that might not always occur. Hence, your estimation of the number of class I genes could be a minimum figure.

Hood: Our estimates of functional class I genes with the anti-$beta_2$ microglobulin assay clearly may yield false negatives for any one of a variety of reasons. Thus, our estimates of 16-20 functional class I genes represent a minimal estimate.

Doherty: As a recall H-2K^d was associated with an LCMV-specific CTL response, when analyzed by recombinant-inbred mapping techniques. Also, H-2$^{kxd}F_1$ mice responded to H-2K^d+LCMV. Is there any obvious difference in the way that K^d and L^d are expressed on the surface of the transfected L cell?

Hood: In our hands, the BALB/c killer T cells raized to LCM virus can clearly only kill mouse L cells transformed with the L^d gene. They are incapable of killing L cells transformed with either the D^d or K^d genes.

Jones: We have biochemical evidence for a second H-2K^d-encoded class I antigen on spleen cells. It may be present at approximately 1/3 the amount of the classical H-2K antigen. It may be that the H-2K^d gene that Hood's lab transfected doesn't function as target for LCMV recognition is not the appropriate one, thereby providing an explanation for the discrepancy mentioned by Peter Doherty.

Miller: Together with D. Kemp, J. Adams, P. Mottram and W. Thomas at the Walter and Eliza Hall Institute we have used the Northern hybridization approach to determine whether V_H gene expression can be detected in T cells. We used a wide range of T cell populations in order to maximize the chance of detecting V_H-bearing mRNAs. They included thymus cells, concanavalin-A stimulated thymus cells, T lymphomas, purified lymph node T cells, antigen-specific cultured T cell lines and T cell hybridomas. RNA was prepared from 10^8-10^9 cells and poly A$^+$ RNA selected by chromatography on oligo-dT-cellulose. After size-fractionation by gel electrophoresis, the RNA molecules were transferred to diazotized paper filters. The filters were then hybridized with ^{32}P-labelled DNA probes derived from cloned V_H genes; low stringency hybridization conditions were used to maximize cross-hybridization. Any RNA molecule which hybridized to the DNA probe was detected by autoradiography.

Fig. 1A is an autoradiogram of a typical experiment in which a number of T cell RNA preparations have been screened for mRNA complementary to the M11 V_H gene. The tracks with the intense bands were loaded with known amounts of restriction fragments of cloned V_H genes. Since we know the mass of poly A$^+$ RNA loaded and the content of poly A$^+$ RNA per cell we can calculate from the intensity of these control signals that a perfectly homologous sequence would be detected at levels of 0.1-1.0 molecule per cell.

No specific hybridization is evident in any track containing RNA from thymocytes, peripheral T cells or T cell-derived tumour cell lines. Fig. 1B shows that the A8 genomic V_H probe gave weak hybridization with 18S ribosomal RNA and other RNA species present in all of the cells. These irrelevant signals reflect weak homology to repetitive sequences flanking the V_H gene in the probe. Two other faintly hybridizing RNA species are also evident in track h, which contains poly A$^+$ RNA from a transformed line obtained by intrathymic injection of Abelson virus (Cook, W., Proc. Nat. Acad. Sci. 79, 1982). Although many such lines are Thy-1$^+$, this line was entirely Thy-1$^-$ and hence probably is not of the T lineage. To maximize the possibility of detecting V_H-bearing RNA species, two other V_H probes were used. Each of the four probes detects a family of 4-22 V_H genes under stringent hybridization conditions and most or all of these are non-overlapping (Kemp, D.J. et al.,J. Mol. Appl. Gen. 1:245-261, 1982.). In addition, a probe for the Cu gene was used. Results are shown in Table 1, and other T cell lymphomas and hybridomas have also been examined (our unpublished results and Kemp, D.J. et al., Proc. Nat. Acad. Sci. 77:7400-7404, 1980). The general conclusion is clear. In no

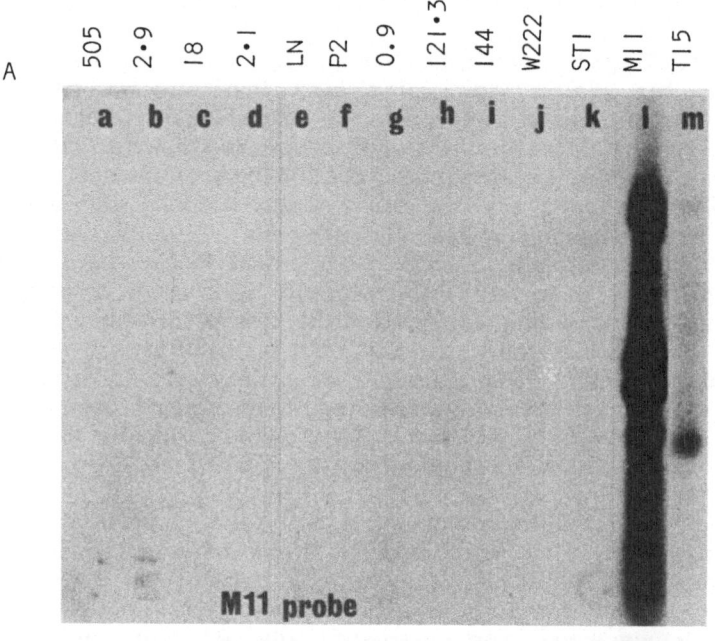

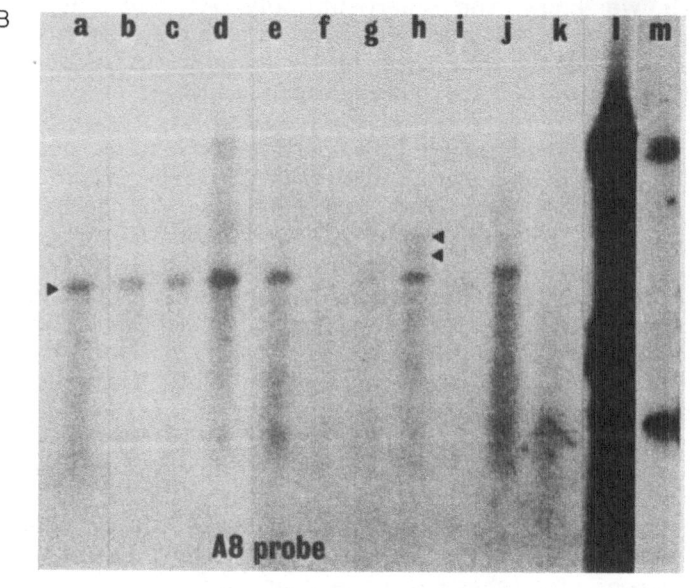

Fig. 1. A search for V_H sequences in T cell mRNA. T cell hybridomas (tracks a-d) were constructed by fusion of EL4 to oxazolone sensitized BALB/c spleen cells (505), EL4 to azobenzenearsonate sensitized A/J spleen cells (2.9 and 2.1) and BW5147 to azobenzenearsonate sensitized A/J spleen cells (18). Lymph node T cells (track e) were purified from in vitro cultures. Antigen-specific T cell lines 09 (oxazolone-specific) and P2 (picrylchloride-specific) (tracks g and f) were obtained as described elsewhere (Thomas, W.R. et al., J. Exp. Med. 156, 1982, in press); both mediated antigen-specific in vivo delayed-type hyper-sensitivity. Abelson virus transformed lines (tracks H and i) were obtained by Cook (Proc. Nat. Acad. Sci. 79, 1982) and briefly described elsewhere (Kemp, D.J. et al., J. Mol. Appl. Gen. 1:245-261, 1982). Poly A^+ RNA was prepared and 5 μg samples were fractionated on 1.5% agarose-methylmercuric hydroxide gels, transferred to diazobezylozymethyl paper and hybridized with nick-translated probes (specific activity 1-2 $\times$ 10^8 cpm per ug) as described (Alwine, J.C. et al., Proc. Nat. Acad. Sci. 74:5350-53, 1977; Kemp, D.J. et al. Proc. Nat. Acad. Sci. 77: 2876-2880, 1980) except that 30% formamide was used instead of 50% in the hybridization. The probes used were (a) V_H-MPC 11; a 0.204 kb Pst fragment corresponding to amino acid residues 4-72 of the V_H region expressed in plasmacytoma MPC 11; the cDNA clone pV(11)^2 described by Zakut, R. et al., Nucleic Acid Res. 8:3591-3600, 1980 was a gift from Dr. David Givol. (b) V_H-A8.2: a 1.1 kp Bgl_2-Pst fragment spanning the complete V_H and D_H regions of a rearranged V_H gene from Abelson lymphoma A8 (Kemp et al., 1981). The clone was sequenced by S. Gerondakis and O. Bernard. As hybridization controls restriction digests of plasmids containing the MPC 11 and TEPC15 V_H regions were loaded (tracks l and m), using 1 ng per kb of DNA - hence the amount of DNA corresponds to 2.0 $\times$ 10^{-4} $\times$ the amount of RNA. The grossly overexposed signals in track l are at least 200 $\times$ greater than the limits of detection. Hence 1 molecule in 10^6 should be detected in the RNA, corresponding to about 0.1 to 1 molecule per cell.

Table 1. mRNA copies per cell complementary to V_H gene probes.

gene probes		HPC 76	A8	TEPC 15	MPC 11	Cu
T cell	P2	-	-	-	-	ND
lines	09	-	-	-	-	ND
T cell	505	-	-	-	-	ND
hybrid-	2.9	-	-	-	-	ND
omas	18	-	-	-	-	ND
T	WEHI 222	-	-	-	-	ca.30
lympho-	ST1	-	-	-	-	-
mas	ST 4	-	-	-	ND	ca.30
B	WEHI 231	2-10	2-10	ND	ND	ca.100
lympho-	WEHI	2-10	ca.100	ND	ND	ca.100
mas						
Abelson	121.3	-	0.1-1.0	-	-	5-10
lymphoma						
thymocytes[a]		-	ND	ND	ND	5-10
Con A thymocytes[b] purified LN		-	-	-	-	ND
T cells[c]		-	ND	ND	ND	5-10
cultured LN T cell (1wk)		-	-	-	-	5-10
unfractionated spleen[a]		5-10[d]	ND	ND	ND	ca.100
T cell depleted spleen[a]		5-10[d]	ND	ND	ND	ca.100
nude spleen cells[a]		5-10[d]	ND	ND	ND	ca.100

- signifies < 1 molecule per cell.

ND = Not done.

[a] Calculated from data in Kemp, D.J. et al. Proc. Nat. Acad. Sci. 77:7400-7404, 1980;
[b] thymocytes cultured for 2h in serum-free medium with 5 ug/ml concanavalin A, then washed and cultured for a further 48 hours;
[c] prepared by treatment of lymph node cells with an anti-B cell hybridoma antigbody, 2A2, plus complement, followed by removal of dead cells;

case could mRNA from a T cell source, either normal or neoplastic, be shown to contain sequences complementary to any V_H probe used.

The four V_H probes we have used each recognize a different spectrum of V_H genes and several observations suggest that, under the low stringency conditions used, they would detect a substantial fraction of the V_H genes expressed in the B linkage.

(1) Spleen B cell mRNA was shown to contain sequences hybridizable with both Cu and V_H probes, while both thymic and lymph node T cell RNA hybridized only to the Cu probe (Table 1). The Cu RNA detected in some T cell is not mRNA, as it encodes no polypeptide and contains no V_H sequence (Alt, F.W. et al., Mol. Cell. Biol. 2:386-400 1982; Kemp, D.J. et al., Proc. Nat. Acad. Sci. 77:7400-7404, 1980; Walker, I.D. and Harris, A.W., Nature 288:290-293, 1980).

(2) The mRNA of B lymphomas WEHI 231 and 279 hybridized with both V_H probes tested, albeit more efficiently with one than the other (Table 1).

(3) Southern hybridization results (Kemp, D.J. et al., J. Mol. Appl. Gen. 1:245-261, 1982) show that the four probes detect a minimum of 52 distinct V_H genes under high stringency conditions out of an estimated 160 V_H genes in the V_H locus.

(4) Under the low stringency conditions used here, an even greater proportion of V_H genes would hybridize - this is clearly true because, for example, cross-hybridization of the M11 probe with TEPC15 DNA was detected (Fig. 1, track m), even though their nucleotide sequences are only 64% homologous in framework regions (Zakut, R. et al., Nucleic Acid Res. 8:3591-3600, 1980) Pairwise comparisons with four other published nucleotide sequences from other V_H gene families shows that they exhibit considerable homology (66 to 87%) with at least one of our probes. Taken together, these observations suggest that our probes can detect a sizeable proportion of the B cell V_H repertoire. It is clear that if even one molecule per cell of mRNA complementary to the V_H probes was present in any of the T cell lymphomas, T cell hybridomas, or antigen-specific T cell lines, its detection by one or more of the V_H probes used would have been anticipated.

---

d detected using 0.5 ug RNA/track whereas all other samples were 5 ug; hence the sensitivity for the T cell RNA should be 10 times greater.

Probes other than those used in Fig. 1 were: V_H-HPC76; a 0.5 kb BamHl fragment extending from amino acid residue 16 through the entire v gene expressed in plasmacytoma HPC76 (Bernard, O. and Gough, N. Proc.Nat.Acad.Sci. 77:3630-3634, 1980) and V_H-TEPC 15: a 1.5 kb BamHl-Eco Rl fragment from embryonic clone M31 (Kemp et al., 1982) which spans the single functional TEPC15 gene (S. Crews, personal communication).

Perhaps the lymphomas and hybridomas simply lacked antigen-specific receptors. This is certainly not the case with the T cell lines (McKimm-Breschkin, J. et al. J. Exp. Med. 155:1204-1209, 1982; Thomas, W.R. et al. J. Exp. Med. 156, 1982, in press) The possibility that these lines are comprised of many T cell clones, each specific for the antigen but using a different V_H gene, cannot yet be ruled out. Individual clones are now being expanded to test this possibility.

There is now mounting evidence that T cell receptor polypeptides are not coded by C_H, D_H or J_H region gene segments. In some cloned cytotoxic effector and helper cell lines, and in T cell hybridomas, these gene segments are not rearranged (Cayre, Y. et al., Proc. Nat. Acad. Sci. 78:3814-3818, 1981; Cory, S. et al., Proc. Nat. Acad. Sci. 77:4843-4947, 1980; Kronenberg, M. et al., J. Exp. Med. 152:1745-1761, 1980; Kurosawa, Y. et al., Nature 290:565-570, 1981) Zuniga, M.C. et al., Proc. Nat. Acad. Sci. 793:3015-3019, 1982). In other "abortive" D_H or J_H rearrangements that cold not encode any functional polypeptide have been reported (Forster, A. et al., Nature 286:879-899, 1980; Kurosawa, Y. et al., Nature 290:565-570, 1981) Whereas these results do not rule out the possibility that the V_H genes code for T cell receptor molecules, they do deprive these genes of all known molecular elements required to assemble a functional antibody.

A notable feature of the results is that we have readily identified V_H-bearing RNA sequences in several B cell preparations studied, but not in any T cells. The results certainly rule out the possibility that peripheral T cells express V_H-coded RNA molecules at any level comparable to that found in B cells. They seriously question whether V_H genes are expressed in T cells.

Baltimore: Is the positive lymphosarcoma a B cell tumor?

Miller: Abelson virus was injected intrathymically in mice by Dr Wendy Cook. Most thymic lymphomas which resulted were Thy-1[+], but the line shown in track h of the autoradiograph was entirely Thy-1[-] and hence probably <u>not</u> of the T cell lineage.

Weigert: How adequate are the V_H probes that you used to detect any V_H gene products?

Miller: Southern hybridization results (Kemp et al. 1982) show that the 4 probes detect a minimum of 52 distinct V_H genes under high stringency conditions out of an estimated 160 V_H genes in the V_H locus. Under low stringency conditions used here an even greater proportion of V_H genes would hybridize. This is seen by the detection of cross-hybridization of the M11 probe with TEPC15 DNA, even though their nucleotide sequences are only 64% homologous in framework regions.

Hood: Under low criteria of hybridization we can use any V_H probe to see virtually any B cell V_H gene. Thus, I believe it is possible to use these conditions to search for B cell V_H gene products in various kinds of T cells.

Baltimore: I agree with Lee Hood.

Honjo: We have done molecular genetic studies on T cell receptor molecules produced by a KLH-specific suppressor T cell hybridoma (34S-70) in collaboration with Dr. M. Taniguchi of Chiba University. Taniguchi and his associates (Taniguchi, M. et al., Nature 283, 227, 1981; Taniguchi, M. et al., J. Exp. Med. 153, 1672, 1981) have shown that the suppressor molecule is composed of two polypeptide chains, one carrying the I-J determinant and the other bearing the antigen binding activity. The latter chain was also shown to react with a monoclonal antibody against the putative constant region of the T cell receptor (Cts) which was originally described by Spurll and Owen (Nature 293, 742, 1981).

The poly(A) containing RNA was isolated from the suppressor T cell hybridoma and fractionated by sucrose density gradient centrifugataion. An aliquot of each fraction was injected into Xenopus oocyte (Taniguchi, M. et al. Nature 298, 172, 1982) The translation products were tested for their ability to inhibit the cytotoxic activity of the monoclonal antibodiés, anti-I-J (F4) and anti-Cts^b (7C5) with the suppressor T cell hybridoma as a target cell.

As shown in Fig. 2, 11S mRNA seems to direct synthesis of a molecule that is capable of inhibiting the cytotoxicity of the monoclonal anti-I-J-^{b} to the suppressor T cell. The translation products of 13S and 18.5S mRNAs seem to react with monoclonal anti-Cts. The molecular weights of the translation products of the 11S, 13S and 18.5S mRNA are 26, 32 and $45-62 \times 10^3$ dalton, respectively. The results suggest that the I-J molecule is encoded by 11S mRNA and has a molecular weight of 26×10^3 dalton. It is unexpected that the Cts-bearing molecules are encoded by two distinct MRNAs. Inasmuch as 13S and 18.5S mRNAs direct synthesis of the Cts-bearing molecules with different sizes, 18.5S mRNA is not the aggregate of 13S mRNA. The small and large Cts-bearing molecules might represent the secreted and the membrane-bound forms, respectively, of the antigen-binding molecules of suppressor T cells like two forms of immunoglobulin heavy chains.

Taniguchi and his coworkers (Nature 283, 227, 1981; J. Exp. Med. 153, 1672, 1981) have shown that the mixture of the dissociated I-J encoded products and the KLH-binding molecules, either of which did not have any suppressor activity by itself, reconstitute the KLH-specific suppressor activity. Similarly, the in vitro translation products of 13S and 18.5S mRNAs exerted the suppressor activity only when the translation products of 11S mRNA were present as shown in Table 2.

Table 2. Antigen-specific suppressor activity of the in vitro translation products[1]

Addition		anti-DNP IgG PFC to	
		DNP-KLH	DNP-EA
Exp I	None	1470	
	11S mRNA translates	1800	
	13S mRNA translates	1450	
	18.5S mRNA translates	1620	
	11S + 13S mRNA translates	210	
	11S + 18.5S mRNA translates	630	
Exp II	None	1730	770
	11S + 13S mRNA translates	90	820

1) Experimental conditions were described elsewhere (Taniguchi, M. et al. Nature 298, 172, 1982)

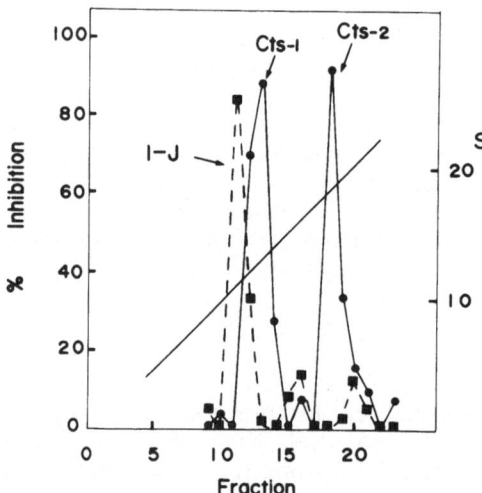

Fig. 2. Fractionation of I-J and Cts-encoding mRNAs by sucrose density gradient centrifugation. Experimented conditions were described elsewhere (Taniguchi et al., Nature 298, 172, 1982).

The suppressor activity of the in vitro translation products was specific to KLH. The translation products of 13S mRNA bind to a KLH-column and the eluate has the suppressor activity in combination with 11S mRNA translation products.

We have made cDNA library from the 13S mRNA to clone the Cts-encoding nucleotide sequence. Pools of 50 clones were grown and screened by the inhibition of the cytotoxicity of the monoclonal anti-Cts as described above. We have obtained five candidates out of 5×10^4 clones. One of the candidates pCt-5 seems hopeful in the following criteria. 1) mRNA purified by hybridization to pCt-5 DNA directs synthesis of molecules that have the suppressor activity when mixed with either 11S mRNA products or I-J-encoded molecules purified from the suppressor T cell. 2) The suppressor activity described above is positive in the DNP-KLH system but negative in the BALB/c system. 3) The translation products of pCt-5-hybridized mRNA have the same molecular weight and the same pI value with those of 13S mRNA. All the functional assays described above were carried out at Taniguchi's laboratory in Chiba.

However, we do not have direct evidence that the pCt-5 insert encodes the Cts molecule. It is still possible that a species of mRNAs cross-hybridizing with pCt-5 has a sequence encoding the Cts protein. In any case, we cannot convince ourselves until we obtain chemical basis for the antigen specificity of the T cell receptor molecule. We wish to obtain cDNA clones from two suppressor T cell lines with different specificities. Structural comparison of these clones will reveal the variable and constant regions of the receptor molecule and eventually elucidate the recognition mechanism of self and not-self by the T cell.

Leder: Which portions of the genomic clones were used to assess rearrangement?

Honjo: The genomic clone has a portion of the cDNA sequence and long introns which contain highly reiterated sequences. As we cannot use most of the fragments as probe, the analysis of DNA rearrangement is limited at this stage.

Baltimore: Does it hybridize to RNA from other cell types?

Honjo: Our clone hybrides 11S-13S mRNA in B cells as well as T cells.

Cohn: If we now agree (or at least are nervous) that the Igh-locus does not encode the MHC restricted T-cell receptor how would we explain the finding of V_H-encoded idiotypes on restricted T-cells?

Hans Wigzell's answer is that the Igh-locus was derived by duplication of the IgT-locus and remains linked but distinct from it. The two evolutionarily related loci could share the encoding of crossreactive idiotypes. This assumption is reasonable, but I do not see how it explains the findings of a one to one relationship between the idiotype of the anti-X on a T-cell and on a B-cell.

If one looks at the idiotypes on given antibodies made by allelic Igh-loci, they have drifted such that the idiotypes are not cross-reactive, e.g. anti-PC or anti-arsanilate in BALB/c and A/J; anti-alpha(1,3) dextran in BALB/c and C57BL/6; etc. Why then should the idiotypes present on a given antibody, e.g. anti-PC, be the same when it is encoded by the IgT- and Igh-loci? What would keep a one to one relationship between combining specificity and idiotype in the IgT- vs. Igh-loci and ignore this relationship between alleles of the Igh-loci? I do not see how your argument explains the presence of Ig idiotypes on T-cells. Clearly, we should search for another explanation of which there are few.

One explanation is artefact. Maybe the anti-Id sera are not specific; or the procedures for assay are suspect; or the experimentor is a Kamikaze bent on fulfilling a categorical imperative. Another explanation applies only to the the physiological evidence, which as yet does not permit a distinction between T-cells anti-Id and Id+ T-cells anti-X. Have you ever wondered why it is so easy to clone antigen-specific T-cells restricted to MHC, yet no one has yet cloned an antigen-specific T-cell, which either is restricted to an idiotype (or isotype) or expresses the idiotype corresponding to that on the B-cell of the same specificity?

Given the many publications that bits and pieces of Ig are expressed on T-cells as part of its restricted receptor and given that these studies have either gone nowhere or are known to be arte-factual, I find that the workers in this area of immunology are in need of much "autocritique" and "self-abnegation".

Session VI

T Cell Regulation

Chairman: B. Benacerraf

T-CELL GROWTH FACTOR, A LYMPHOCYTOTROPHIC HORMONE

Kendall A. Smith

The Department of Medicine
Dartmouth Medical School
Hanover, New Hampshire

INTRODUCTION

Despite an intensive effort over the past twenty years, our
understanding of the process by which the immune response is
regulated remains rudimentary. In part, our difficulties in this
area have related to the morphological homogeneity but functional
heterogeneity of the cells responsible for the immune reaction.
The dissection of the mechanisms that underlie the regulatory
control of the immune response has been facilitated, however, by
the development of cell culture systems that can be made to generate measurable immune reactions, and thus mimic immune responses
as they are thought to occur in vivo. As a result, it has become
apparent that the differentiation of lymphocytes to become functionally competent immunocytes, is dependent upon a complex inter-
cellular communication system that involves not only different
classes and subclasses of lymphocytes, but macrophages as well.
Consequently, considerable attention has focused on the roles
played by each cell type, and the mechanisms operative.

While the isolation of the cells principally involved in the
immune response has permitted considerable progress in our understanding of immune regulation, it has also led to the view that
the immune system exists in isolation, completely internally
regulated. Sir Peter Medawar, almost 10 years ago(1), succinctly
stated the prevailing viewpoint: "We have been operating under the
hypothesis that the immunological process is controlled from
within, essentially by inputs and by outputs, driven by antigen,
and resulting in a number of immunocyte products that control the
progress of the immune reaction by positive or negative feedback
actions." Medawar then went on to say, however, that an internally

regulated immune system seemed conceptually simplistic and "that perhaps the control of the immune process is imposed on it from without, by means of promoting or inhibiting lymphocytotrophic hormones."

In the past few years, owing to the pioneering discovery by Morgan, Ruscetti and Gallo(2) that T-lymphocytes can be grown for extended periods in vitro, we have progressed to the point where the first lymphocytotrophic hormone has been identified and characterized. T-cell growth factor (for review see 3-5), a small polypeptide that has been found responsible for the initiation and maintenance of T-cell proliferation, shares many of the characteristics of a hormone, and may well be the prototype for other, as yet undiscovered, lymphocytotrophic hormones that control and regulate T-cell and B-cell immune responses.

Most of the accumulated evidence indicates that TCGF is a hormone that originates from, and is controlled by the immune system, thus providing further support for the hypothesis that the immune system is isolated and internally regulated. However, that lymphocytes may produce and regulate themselves by molecules that resemble hormones is itself a new concept, and neccessitates a re-evaluation of the relative importance of antibodies and antigen receptors as the primary potential regulators of lymphocyte growth and differentiation. Moreover, the concept that lymphocytotrophic hormones are operative within the immune system provides the rationale for the hypothesis that perhaps lymphocyte hormones are in turn regulated from without, by the hormones of the neuroendocrine system. If so, then for the first time the immune system could be thought of as an integral part of the functioning host, exquisitely internally controlled to be sure, but communicating with, and under the influence of, other physiological control mechanisms.

This review will concentrate on two points; first, the evidence that TCGF has characteristics common to hormones, and secondly, the experimental evidence that suggests TCGF may be influenced by other hormones of the neuoendocrine system. Prior to such a discussion, it is useful to review the accepted definitions of hormones. The term hormone was first used by Bayliss and Starling in 1902 and is derived from a Greek root meaning "to excite" or "to arouse." Hormones have come to be regarded as substances produced by specific glands, secreted directly into the blood, and transported to specific organs and tissues where they exert their effects. Hormones function at low concentrations, generally less than 10^{-8} M, are produced at a variable rate, exert a regulatory function in response to environmental or other variations, and are under feedback regulatory control. A corollary to these characteristics is the requirement that hormones react with receptor molecules, for it has become recognized that receptors

impart the target cell specificity of the hormone effect and by
virtue of their high affinity for the specific ligand, allow the
effect to be mediated at very low concentrations. In turn, to
define a site capable of binding a given hormone as a receptor,
the following minimum criteria should be met. The affinity of the
binding site for hormone must be appropriate for concentrations of
hormone that are biologically or physiologically relevant. The
binding site should be detectable on those cells or tissues that
are hormone responsive and absent from unresponsive cells or
tissues. The hormone binding site should show specificity for
active hormones and their antagonists.

A Single Polypeptide is Responsible for TCGF Activity

One criteria necessary to define a moiety as a hormone resides
in the demonstration that the biological activity can be ascribed
to a single molecule. Early biochemical analysis of human TCGF
revealed that the activity migrated in a uniform fashion upon
molecular gel filtration (Mr = 20,000), however, it appeared
heterogeneous with respect to charge such that the biological
activities appeared to reside in several distinct moieties when
examined by isoelectric focusing(6,7). Although this charge
heterogeneity could result from post-translation modification or
degradation of a single polypeptide, such heterogeneity also
suggested the possibility that several polypeptides might be
responsible for T-cell mitosis.

The activity profile of human TCGF derived from tonsilar
cells after isoelectric focusing is shown in Figure 1. Approximately equal quantities of 3 distinct species are produced by
tonsilar cells with isoelectric points evenly spaced 0.3 pH units
apart(8). Figure 2 depicts that this charge heterogeneity can be
explained by variable sialylation. Isolation of each of the more
acidic moieties (pI 7.9 and pI 7.6) followed by treatment with
neuraminidase results in a shift in the biological activity profile to the more basic isoelectric point (pI = 8.2). Treatment of
this species with neuraminidase results in no further shift in pI.
As well, production of TCGF in the presence of 2-deoxy D-glucose,
an inhibitor of N-linked glycosylation, results in the appearance
of primarily a species with an isoelectric point identical to that
obtained after digestion with neuraminidase (Figure 3).

Human TCGF activity also appears heterogeneous with respect
to molecular size when analyzed by sodium dodecyl sulfate polyacrylamide gel eletrophoresis (SDS-PAGE), but again, this heterogeneity can be ascribed to variable glycosylation and sialylation(8).
As shown in Figure 4A, tonsilar-derived TCGF activity isolated by
molecular gel (Sephadex G-100) chromatography followed by SDS-PAGE
analysis separates into two major species. Treatment with neuraminidase prior to SDS-PAGE analysis results in the loss of the

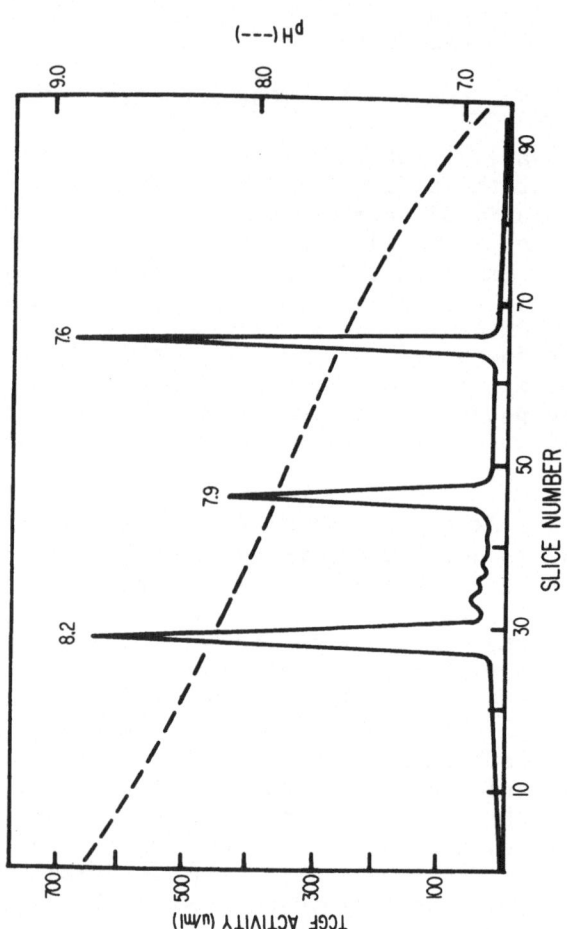

Fig. 1   Isoelectric focusing gels (pH 6.5-9) of Sephadex G-100 pool of tonsil-derived TCGF (4000 units loaded). The TCGF sample was equilibrated with ampholines (0.5% Pharmolyte) and focused for 10 hrs at 1000 V on 0.6 x 10 cm polyacrylamide tube gels (7% acrylamide, 6.25% Pharmolyte) after which the gels were cut into 2 mm slices and eluted with 1 ml 10 mM Tris, pH 7.5, 0.15 M NaCl, 1 mg/ml polyethylene glycol 6,000. From Robb and Smith (8).

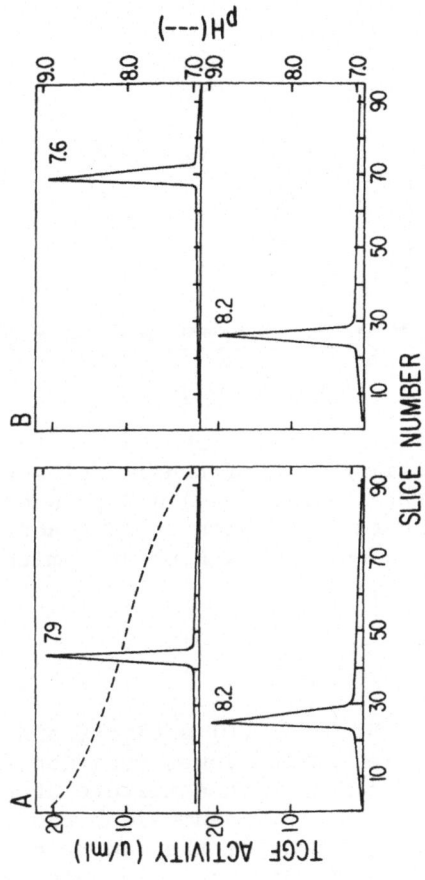

Fig. 2   Isoelectric focusing gels (pH 6.5-9) of tonsil-derived TCGF activity isolated from an IEF gel
as in Figure 1 that focused at pI 7.9 (A) and pI 7.6 (B). Upper panels represent material
not treated with neuraminidase whereas lower panels represent material treated with neuraminidase. From Robb and Smith (8).

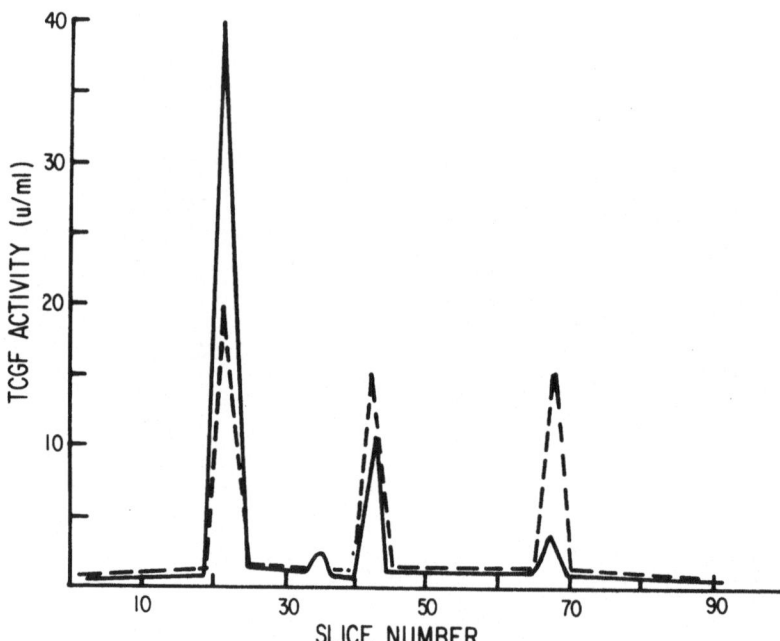

Fig. 3   Isoelectric focusing gels (pH 6.5-9) of TCGF prepared by
            PHA and PMA stimulation of tonsil cells from a single in-
            dividual in the absence (---) and presence (——) of 7 mM
            2-deoxy-D-glucose (120 units of TCGF activity from each
            preparation loaded). From Robb and Smith (8).

higher molecular weight (Mr = 16,500) activity and the appearance
of a closely spaced doublet at the lower position (Mr 15,500 to
14,500) (Figure 4B). Treatment with a mixture of neuraminidase
and exo- and endoglycosidases (D. pneumoniae) converts all biological activity to a single peak at the low Mr position (Figure
4C). Although differences in amino acid sequence or small differences in size may have remained undetected by this methodology,
the combined results from IEF and PAGE analysis demonstrate that
the heterogeneity of human TCGF is primarily due to variable
glycosylation and sialylation. The electrophoretic behavior of
the deglycosylated TCGF (i.e. migration at the lower molecular
size) is consistent both with the loss of carbohydrate and binding
of a larger number SDS molecules thus contributing to a greater
net negative charge. Of interest is the observation that reduction of TCGF results in a loss of biological activity and migra-

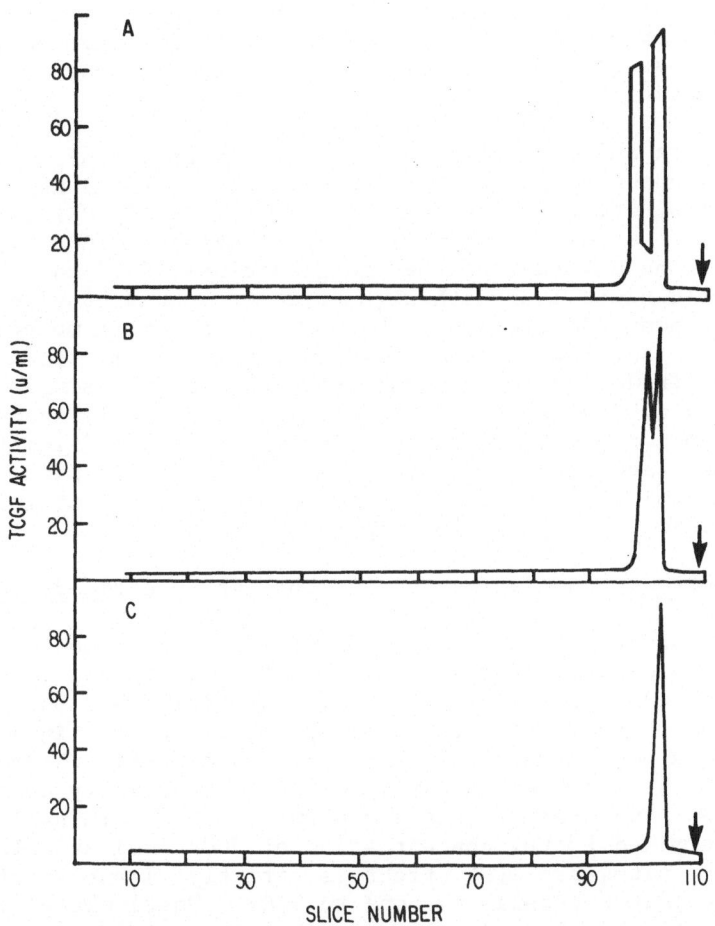

Fig. 4   Sodium dodecyl sulfate-polyacrylamide gel electrophoresis
          (SDS-PAGE) of; (A) Sephadex G-100 pool of tonsil-derived
          TCGF, (B) after incubation with neuraminidase, (C) after
          incubation with neuraminidase and a mixture of glycosidases
          (D. pneumoniae). Lyophilized TCGF samples were dissolved
          in sample buffer (2% SDS, no 2-mercaptoethanol) and heated
          at 60°C for 15 min followed by electrophoresis on 0.6 x
          12 cm tube gels (12% acrylamide, 0.1% SDS). The gels were
          cut into 1 mm slices and eluted with 0.25 ml RPMI 1640, 10%
          fetal calf serum, 10 mg/ml bovine serum albumin followed by
          serial titration for TCGF biological activity(24). From
          Robb and Smith (8).

tion to a larger molecular size (i.e. from 14,500 to 15,500 Mr) on
SDS-PAGE analysis. Thus, the cumulative data indicate that TCGF
acitivity can be ascribed to an entity that is uniform with respect
to size and charge and is most consistent with a single polypeptide
chain that possesses an internal disulfide bond necessary for
biological activity.

These data and conclusions have recently been confirmed by an
alternative approach. Using human TCGF derived from JURKAT T-
leukemia cells, which is identical to nonsialylated TCGF derived
from normal cells, several monoclonal antibodies to TCGF were
derived(9). One antibody of the IgG_{2a} subclass (designated DMS-3)
binds JURKAT-derived TCGF with high efficiency when coupled to
Sepharose. Upon acid elution of bound TCGF, a single molecular
entity can be isolated that contains biological activity, migrates
at 15,500 Mr (reducing conditions), and appears as a single spot
when analyzed by 2-dimensional PAGE (Figure 5). Preliminary data
obtained from amino acid sequence analysis of immunoaffinity-
purified TCGF have revealed a single amino terminal residue (N-
terminus = alanine).[1] As a result of these data TCGF activity can
now be ascribed to a single polypeptide.

TCGF Interacts with Activated T-cells Through Specific Receptors

Another prerequisite for the definition of a hormone is
target cell specifity. Early studies on the biological activity
of TCGF revealed exquisite target cell specificity and suggested
that TCGF interacted with cells by means of receptors, in a fashion
similar to the more classically recognized polypeptide hormones.
For example, the mitogenic activity of TCGF is strictly concentration-dependent such that the rate and extent of T-cell proliferation is determined by the concentration of TCGF available(10).
Moreover, the mitogenic TCGF effect is strictly tissue specific in
that only activated T-cells respond to TCGF. Unstimulated lymphocytes, activated B-cells or cells of other lineages do not proliferate in response to purified TCGF(10,11). In addition, TCGF is
consumed by proliferating T-cells. This observation led to attempts
to absorb TCGF activity from conditioned media and it was readily
found that activated T-cells absorb TCGF activity in a time-, tem-
perature-, and cell concentration-dependent fashion(11-13). As
well, the fact that glutaraldhyde-fixed cells(10) or cells treated
with metabolic inhibitors(13) also absorbed TCGF activity pointed
towards the presence of TCGF-specific membrane binding sites.

To provide a direct demonstration of TCGF-specific receptors,
biosynthetically radiolabeled TCGF was prepared and purified
either by conventional biochemical separative procedures (molecular

---

1 Smith, K. A. and W. North. Unpublished Observation.

Fig. 5   2-dimensional PAGE of immunoaffinity-purified human TCGF.
            TCGF was isolated from the supernatant (4 L) of PHA- and
            PMA-stimulated high producer subclone (6.8) JURKAT T-leu-
            kemia cells by passage through a 1 ml column of Sepharose-
            bound DMS-3 IgG$_{2a}$ anti-TCGF monoclonal antibody (8 mg anti-
            body/ml Sepharose) followed by elution with 5 ml 0.2 N
            acetic acid. Material was subjected to nonequilibrium pH
            (7-9)-gradient electrophoresis in the first dimension
            followed by SDS-PAGE (12% acrylamide). The gel was stained
            by the silver method (Biorad Laboratories, Richmond, CA).
            From Smith et al. (9).

gel filtration and isoelectric focusing)(14) or by immunoaffinity
chromatography with the aid of the IgG$_{2a}$ anti-TCGF monoclonal
antibody(9). With either procedure all radioactivity and biological activity present in purified material resided in a 15,500 Mr
peptide (reducing conditions) when analyzed by SDS-PAGE (Figure
6). Thus far it has not been possible to express the specific
activity directly, owing to the small amounts of protein in

Fig. 6   Fluorograph of biosynthetically radiolabeled immuno-
          affinity-purified human TCGF.   TCGF was radiolabeled by
          stimulating JURKAT subclone 6.8 cells in the presence of
          0.5 mCi/ml [^{3}H]-leucine (110 Ci/mM, New England Nuclear
          Boston, MA) and 0.5 mCi/ml [^{3}H]-lysine (110 Ci/mM).
          Radiolabeled TCGF was isolated from the supernatant by use
          of the immunoaffinity column as described in Figure 5.
          Radiolabeled material (8000 DPM, 2 μl) was dissolved in
          sample buffer (2% SDS, 5% 2-mercaptoethanol), electro-
          phoresed on a 12% acrylamide slab gel and visualized by
          fluorography using EN^{3}HANCE (New England Nuclear).   From
          Smith et al. (9).

biosynthetically radiolabeled material. An estimate of the specific
activity, however, has been possible by measuring the biological
activity and protein content of larger amounts of unlabeled TCGF.
Protein content has been measured by amino acid analysis and
protein dye binding assays on several preparations purified
biochemically or by the monoclonal antibody affinity column. The
results from both procedures have consistently yielded a value of

TCGF activity in the range of 7-8 ng/unit. By measuring the biological activity of several biosynthetically radiolabeled preparations (radiolabeled either with [^{35}S]-methionine or [^{3}H]-leucine and [^{3}H]-lysine), TCGF with specific activities of 7-8 x 10^{6} DPM/ug protein have consistently resulted.

Binding experiments performed with either whole cells(14) or isolated, purified plasma membranes(15) from TCGF-responsive cells yield similar results, and indicate that such cells express high affinity membrane binding sites that satisfy the criteria usually required of a true hormone receptor. The binding is tissue specific for those cells where a mitogenic effect of TCGF can be demonstrated; only activated T-cells express detectable binding sites. As well, radiolabeled TCGF binding is hormone specific in that a variety of other polypeptide hormones and growth factors fail to compete for binding. When the rates of radiolabled TCGF association and dissociation are performed, either with whole cells or with isolated plasma membranes, the results indicate that the binding is of high affinity. Equilibrium binding studies over a wide range of radiolabeled TCGF concentrations confirm these data and reveal that the binding sites detected are of a single class with remarkably high affinity (Kd = 5-20 pM). Moreover, radiolabeled TCGF binding is saturable such that less than 4% of the radiolabeled material bound is nonspecifically associated with the cells. Finally, binding of radiolabeled TCGF occurs at concentrations that closely correlate with the concentrations found to mediate cytolytic T-cell proliferation. All of these data support the conclusion that TCGF interacts with activated T-cells by means of specific membrane receptors that share the characteristics of biologically relevant polypeptide hormone receptors(14,15).

The time course of association and dissociation of radio-labeled TCGF to whole cells and to isolated, purified plasma membranes is shown in Figure 7. When performed with near satura-ting TCGF concentrations (= 120 pM), binding occurs rapidly at 37°C with maximum levels attained within 15 minutes. (t 1/2=4 min) At 4°C the kinetics of association are slower, although by 60 minutes the same maximum level of binding is observed (Figure 7A,B). Utilizing whole cells, dissociation rates were determined after binding for 60 minutes at 4°C to prevent internalization of the hormone-receptor-complex, followed by the addition of a 100-fold excess of unlabeled TCGF to promote exchange when the temperature was raised to 37°C (Figure 7C). From this experimental approach, the half-time for dissociation from whole cells is 45 minutes. However, this value can only be considered approximate, since as detected by TCA precipitation, degradation of radiolabeled TCGF occurs progressively during the conduct of the experiment (Figure 7C). In contrast, as shown in Figure 7D the half-time is 25 minutes for dissociation of radiolabeled TCGF from isolated plasma membranes, where internalization of the hormone-receptor

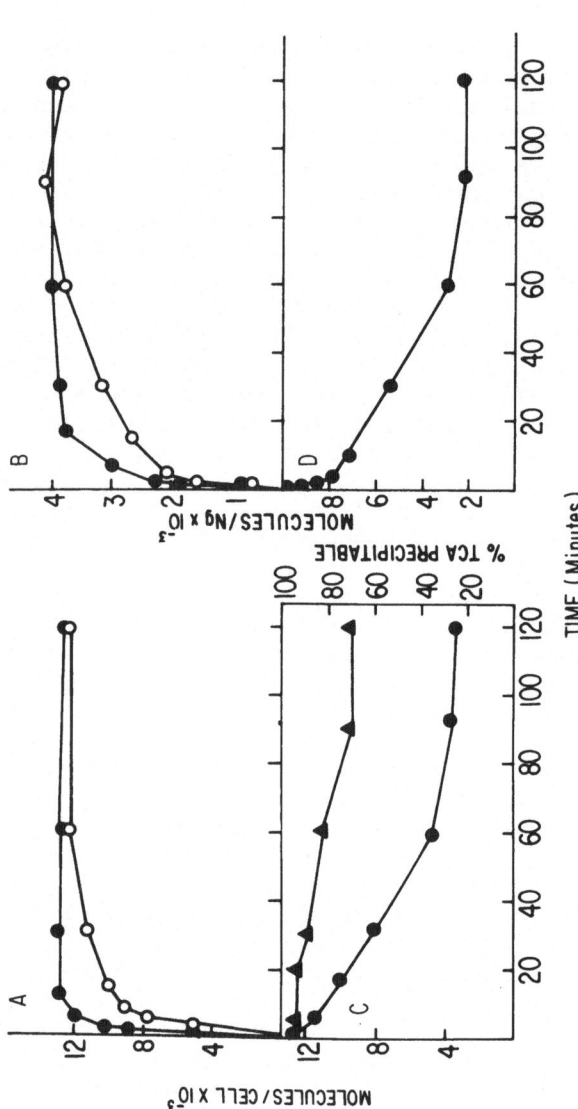

Fig. 7   Time course of association and dissociation of radiolabeled TCGF from whole cells and
isolated plasma membranes.   (A) Association kinetics of radiolabeled TCGF to murine CTLL
clone 15H cells at 37°C (0) and 4°C (0).   (B) Association kinetics of radiolabeled TCGF
to plasma membranes isolated from HUT-102 B2 cells at 37°C (0) and 4°C (0).   (C) Dissociation of radiolabeled TCGF from CTLL-Cl 15H cells at 37°C in the presence of 25 nM
unlabeled TCGF.   (D) Dissociation of radiolabeled TCGF from HUT-102 B2 plasma membranes
at 37°C.   From Robb et al. Smith (15).

complex is not a consideration. Thus, association of radiolabeled
TCGF with TCGF-responsive T-cells is reversible and is characterized
by rapid binding and slow dissociation.

Calculations employing the rate constants of association and
dissociation of radiolabeled TCGF from isolated plasma membranes
results in a value for the dissociation equilibrium constant of 6
pM (human TCGG-responsive HUT-102 B2 cells)(15). In accord with
this, a similar value is obtained when either cells (Figure 8A) or
isolated plasma membranes (Figure 8B) are exposed to increasing
concentrations of radiolabeled TCGF and the data analyzed by the
method of Scatchard (Figure 8C,8D). The close correlations of the
dissociation equilibrium constants obtained from binding to whole
cells (Kd = 5 pM) and to isolated plasma membranes (Kd = 2.7 pM)
together with the resulting linear plots by the method of Scatchard
validates the interpretation that TCGF receptors are identical in
that they all have an equal affinity for TCGF. Moreover, the data
indicate that each receptor functions thermodynamically independently, such that occupation of one site has no effect on binding
to any other site. As well, as shown in Figure 8A for binding to
whole cells, when nonsaturable binding was estimated by including
an excess (25 nM) of unlabeled TCGF, the level of binding that
remained is linearly dependent upon the concentration of free
radiolabeled TCGF and generally constitutes only 4% of the total
bound fraction in the absence of unlabeled TCGF.

The tissue specificity of radiolabeled TCGF binding is shown
in Table I. Consistent with the observations by ourselves(3) and
others (4,16,17), whereby only lectin/antigen-activated T-cells
are responsive to the mitogenic effects of TCGF, radiolabeled TCGF
binds only to TCGF-responsive T-cells(14). Our experience with
the cellular specificity of TCGF binding is of interest, since it
illustrates that even a very small number of contaminating, activated T-cells might cloud the interpretation of which (or how
many) lymphokines are acting on B-cells. In our initial experiments on the TCGF receptor, we found that lipopolysaccharide
(LPS) - activated murine splenocytes expressed a low number
(approximately 1000) of detectable binding sites. Since it had
been shown clearly that LPS activation does not result in T-cell
proliferation this was certainly an unexpected result. Moreover,
in previous experiments we had found that LPS-activated B-cell
blasts did not absorb TCGF activity(11). We felt, therefore, that
the most plausible explanation was that a small number of T-cells
had become activated, perhaps as a result of components in the
serum during the generation of the B-cell blasts. This conclusion
was reinforced by recent experiments performed in collaboration
with Dr. Max Schreier: LPS activation in the presence of fetal
calf serum led to the generation of a significant fraction of TCGF
responsive T-cells, whereas in serum-free conditions, contamina-

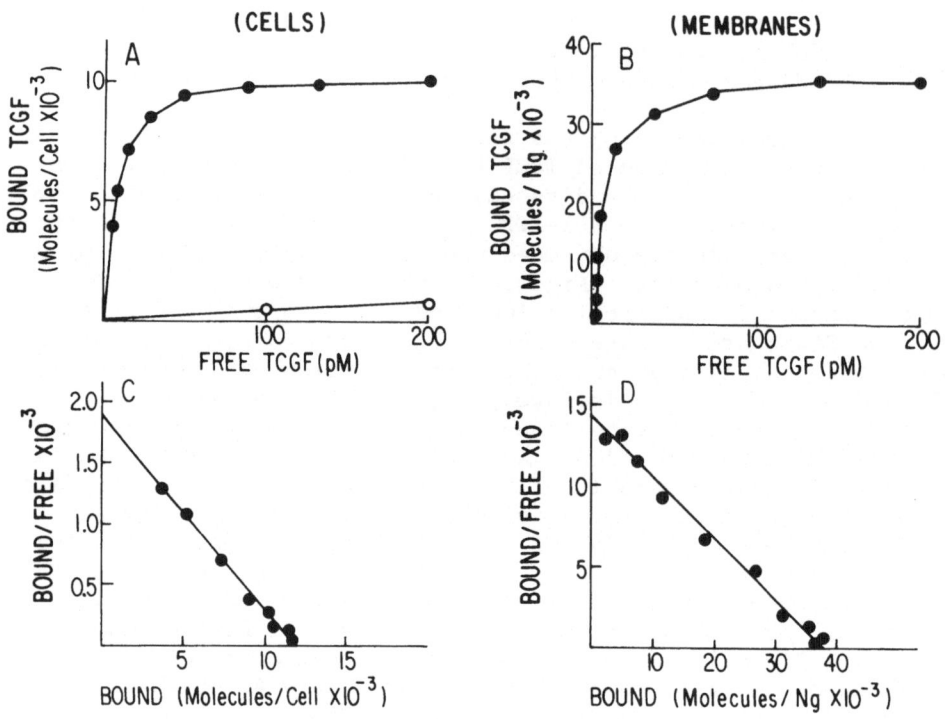

Fig. 8   Binding of radiolabeled TCGF to whole cells and isolated
          plasma membranes. (A) Binding to human PHA blasts in the
          absence (0) and presence (0) of unlabeled TCGF. (B)
          Binding to plasma membranes isolated from HUT-102 B2 cells.
          (C) Scatchard plot of the data in A after correction for
          nonsaturable binding. (D) Scatchard plot of the data in
          B after correction for nonsaturable binding. From Robb
          et al. (14) and Cummings and Smith (15).

ting activated T-cells were considerably less noticeable.[2] To
examine the phenotype of cells binding TCGF, splenocytes were
exposed to monoclonal anti-thy-1 antibody and complement before
and after LPS activation and isolation of the blast cells. Our
results are consistent with the conclusion that LPS-activated B-
cells do not express detectable TCGF receptors. Moreover, LPS-
activated B-cell blasts derived from splenocytes of athymic nu/nu
mice do not express detectable TCGF receptors. These results are
thus consistent with the observations and conclusions that TCGF
binds to, selects for, and promotes only T-cell growth.

---

2   Smith K.A. and M. H. Schreier. Unpublished Observations.

Table I. TCGF Binding is T-Cell Specific*

CELL TYPE	STIMULANT	TCGF BINDING	
MURINE		SITES/CELL	$Kd \times 10^{-12}M$
Splenocyte	–	<60	–
Splenocyte	Con-A	10,000	20
Splenocyte	LPS	<60	–
Splenocyte	LPS	<60	–
HUMAN			
PBL	–	200	7
PBL	PHA	10,000	5
HUMAN CELL LINES			
T-ALL (10)	–	<60	–
B-CELL(4)	–	<60	–
Myeloid	–	<60	–
HUT-102	–	13,000	6
MLA-144		8,000	8

*From Reference 14.

Noteworthy was the finding that although murine and human activated T-cells expressed similar numbers of TCGF binding sites (5,000 to 15,000), murine cells bound human TCGF with a 3-4 fold lower affinity than did activated human cells (Kd = 20 pM and 5-8 pM respectively) (Table I). The greater affinity of the human TCGF receptor for radiolabeled human TCGF may account for the low levels of detectable binding sites on unstimulated human peripheral blood lymphocytes (< 200 sites/cell) in contrast to the absence of detectable binding sites on unstimulated murine lymphocytes. As well, since the TCGF binding assay yields an average level of binding in the whole cell population, the value of 200 binding sites/cell for unstimulated human lymphocytes could represent a low level of receptor sites on most or all of the cells, or a high

level of sites on a small fraction (< 2%) of activated cells
within the population.

The hormone specificity of radiolabeled TCGF binding is shown
in Table II. Of the various growth factors and polypeptide hormones tested, only TCGF competed for binding of the radiolabeled
moiety. Moreover, recent experiments using TCGF isolated by
immunoaffinity column chromatography reveal a concentration-
dependent competition of radiolabeled TCGF that is identical to
competition using biochemically purified unlabeled TCGF(9). This
finding further substantiates the impression that the substance
responsible for the competition, as well as the binding, is TCGF,
and not a contaminant in the biochemically purified TCGF preparations.

A comparison of the binding and biological response curves
upon exposure of a murine cytolytic T-cell clone is shown in
Figure 9. The concentration of radiolabeled TCGF that yields one
half maximal binding (20 pM) closely correlates with the concentration of TCGF that yields one half of the maximum biological
response (16 pM). As well, the maximum biological response occurs
at a concentration (= 120 pM) where greater than 90% of the
receptors are fully saturated. The close correlation between the
biological response curve and binding curve is at variance with
the experience derived from similar experiments performed with
polypeptide hormones where it is known that the biological response

Table II.   TCGF Binding is TCGF-Specific

COMPETITOR	CONCENTRATION	% COMPETITION*
TCGF	2 μM	99
EGF	2 μM	0
NGF(2.5s)	0.5 μM	0
MSA	1 μM	0
FGF	1 μM	3
LAF	60 μ/ml	0
IFN-α	40,000 μ/ml	3
IFN-γ	40,000 μ/ml	0
CSA	–	2
EP	5 μ/ml	0
Insulin	10 μ/ml	0

*Competition of a near saturating concentration of TCGF (120pM)
 From Reference 14.

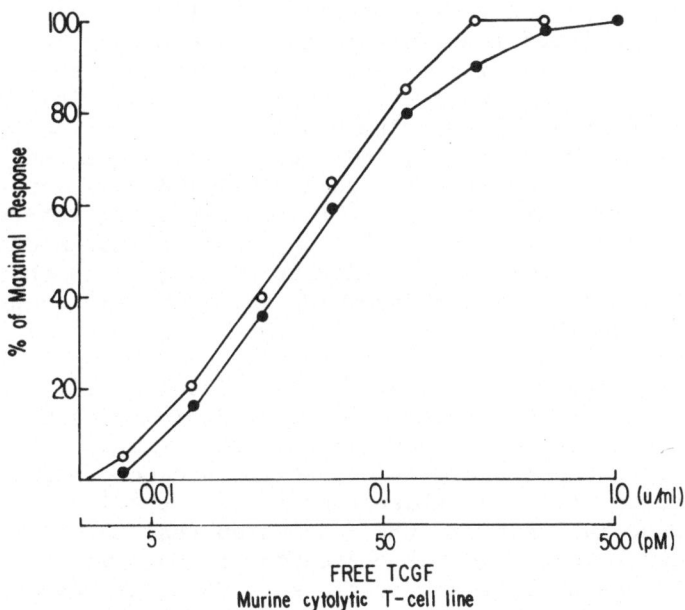

Fig. 9   A comparison of radiolabeled TCGF binding (0) and biologi-
          cal response (0). Murine CTLL Cl 15H cells were exposed
          to increasing concentrations of radiolabeled TCGF for 20
          min and to equivalent concentrations of unlabeled TCGF for
          20 hr prior to a 4 hr pulse of [3H]-thymidine. From Robb
          et al. (14).

is dependent upon the generation of a secondary mediator such as
cyclic AMP(18). In this case biological responses become maximal
at hormone concentrations well below those required for a comparable
degree of receptor saturation. Without invoking concepts of
negative cooperativity, the difference between the hormone-concen-
trations required for half-maximal receptor saturation and those
required for half-maximal biological response can be explained by
the concentration of the secondary mediator formed as a result of
membrane receptor occupancy, and the rate constant for the secondary
mediator reaction, both of which ultimately determine the biological
response(18). The implication, therefore, is that in the case of
TCGF, the physiologically limiting variables that determine the
biolgoical response can be reduced to the hormone concentration,
receptor concentration, and receptor affinity. As well, the close

correlation of the equilibrium dissociation constants determined
by equilibrium binding to either whole cells or isolated plasma
membranes (Figure 8) and those determined by kinetic binding
experiments to isolated membranes (Figure 7), indicate that the
interaction of TCGF with its receptor obeys the same physiochemical
principles that govern ligand-polymer interactions. This fact,
together with the finding that the binding and biological response
curves are virtually identical, indicate that TCGF-driven T-cell
proliferation is the result of an initial ligand-cell interaction
that is no more complex than a simple ligand-polymer interaction.
Consequently, future studies of the mechanism of TCGF-mediated T-
cell proliferation should be far simpler than would be the case
for a more complicated system involving bioenergentic cooperativity
between several soluble factors.

In summary, the high affinity of radiolabeled TCGF binding to
activated T-cells, the restriction of the binding to TCGF responsive T-cells, the lack of competition by other growth factors and
hormones, and the close correlation between the concentrations of
TCGF that bind to cells and those that mediate the T-cell proliferative response, all support the conclusion that the binding site
detected by our studies is on the receptor through which the
biological effects of TCGF are initiated. Moreover, the data also
add to the impression that TCGF, in a fashion similar to polypeptide hormones, interacts with its target tissue via true receptor
molecules, which impart not only the specifity of the reaction,
but also by virtue of the very high affinity of TCGF binding,
enable the mitogenic effects of the T-cell growth hormone to occur
at very low concentrations.

Possible Mechanisms of the Regulation of TCGF Action

The concept that T-cell clonal expansion after antigen activation is mediated by a T-cell specific growth hormone immediately
implies several areas of potential regulatory influences that
could modulate the magnitude of the clonal expansion, and consequently, the magnitude of the resultant immune response. One such
influence would be the concentration of TCGF available to the
activated T-cells, and as well, the duration that adequate concentrations are present. From earlier studies we had observed that the
TCGF concentration decreased as the cell concentration increased(19).
A representative experiment demonstrating this phenomenon is shown
in Figure 10. Cell-mediated degradation of the hormone after it
has bound to the receptor is one possible explanation for this
phenomenon. Pinocytotic internalization of the hormone receptor
complex followed by lysosomal fushion and hydrolysis by acidic
proteases has been shown to occur with a variety of polypeptide
hormones, including insulin, growth hormone, and epidermal growth
factor(20-22). We have explored this possibility and have found

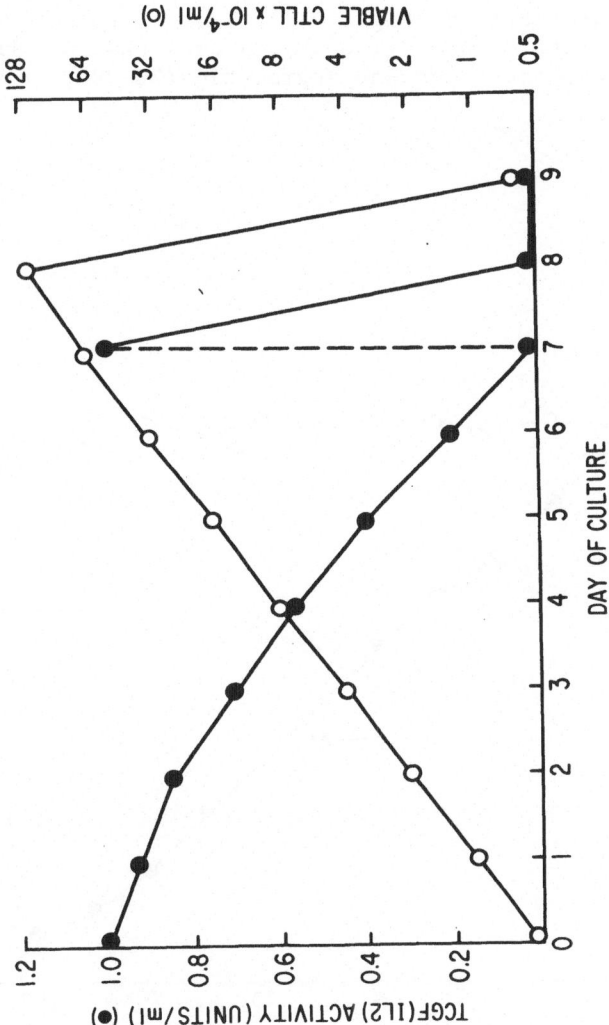

Fig. 10   T-cell growth factor (TCGF) activity present in cultures of cytolytic T-lymphocyte lines (CTLL-Cl 15H) as a function of cell concentration. From Smith and Ruscetti (5).

that cell associated TCGF is converted to a TCA-soluble form at
37°C with a half-time of 60-70 min (Figure 11).   The degradation
to a TCA-soluble form requires receptor binding, since if binding
is prevented by performing the experiment in the presence of a
100-fold excess of unlabeled TCGF, no degradation of radiolabeled
TCGF occurs.   As well, if the experiment is performed at 4°C, a
temperature that prevents internalization, no degradation to a
TCA-soluble form is observed (Figure 11).   Moreover, ammonium
chloride (10 mM) or chloroquin (100 uM), agents that are known to
inhibit lysosome-dependent hormone degradation(20-22), prevents

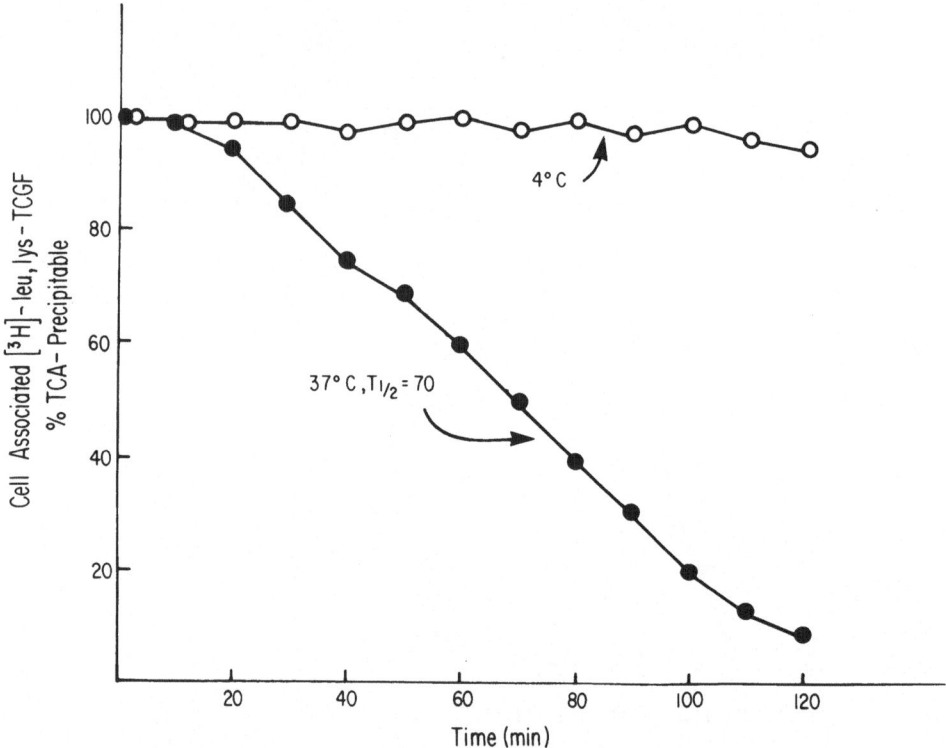

Fig. 11   Degradation of cell associated radiolabeled TCGF.   TCGF was
          bound to cells for 60 min at 4°C followed by washing and
          incubation at 37°C (0) and 4°C (0).   At the time intervals
          indicated aliquots of the whole cell suspension were re-
          moved and adjusted to 10% TCA to determine the level of
          precipitable radiolabeled TCGF.

the conversion of radiolabeled TCGF to a TCA-soluble form at 37°C. Thus, TCGF degradation requires receptor binding, is temperature dependent, and most probably involves internalization and lysosomal association. The implication of these observations is that the maintenance of adequate TCGF concentrations necessary to support continued T-cell clonal expansion, must result from sustained TCGF production in the face of continuous TCGF degradation by responding T-cells.

Another possible physiologically relevant mechanism of regulation of TCGF action relates to the signals required for continued TCGF receptor expression, and as well, TCGF receptor turnover rates. Our preliminary data indicate that once maximum TCGF receptor levels appear on lectin-activated T-cells, the number of receptor sites/cell progressively decreases over time despite the maintenance of adequate concentrations of TCGF. A representative experiment performed with phytohemagglutinin-(PHA)-activated human peripheral blood lymphocytes is shown in Figure 12, and depicts the decline in receptor levels once the peak number is attained after 3 days of culture. Although the mechanism underlying the decline in receptor levels remains obscure, these data correlate with the decline in growth rate of PHA-activated human lymphocytes that we and others have observed despite the continued addition of TCGF(5). At least one possible mechanism that would explain this phenomenon relates to receptor down regulation upon continued hormone exposure as has been observed with other polypeptide hormones(20). It is also possible that reactivation is necessary for receptor reappearance after each successive mitotic event. Consistent with this possibility is the empiric observation that periodic addition of adherent cells together with lectin/antigen often restores the growth rate of T-cell blasts that have slowed in their proliferative rate(5).

Another mechanism that may have particular physiological significance relates to the effects of other polypeptide hormones on TCGF receptors. Using absorption to quantify TCGF receptors rather than the radiolabeled TCGF assay described here, Kumagai et al.(23) found that insulin added to PHA-activated cells on the third day of culture maintained the TCGF absorptive capacity of the T-cell blasts. In addition, utilizing serum-free conditions, Strom and coworkers(24) have recently demonstrated synergistic effects of transferrin and insulin on human T-cell proliferation. These studies may be the forerunners of our understanding of the factors present in serum that are necessary for cell growth, and as well, for the first time, we may begin to uncover their mechanisms of action as they relate to TCGF receptor physiology.

Possible Mechanisms of Regulation of TCGF Production

One final axiom that should be satisfied before one can be

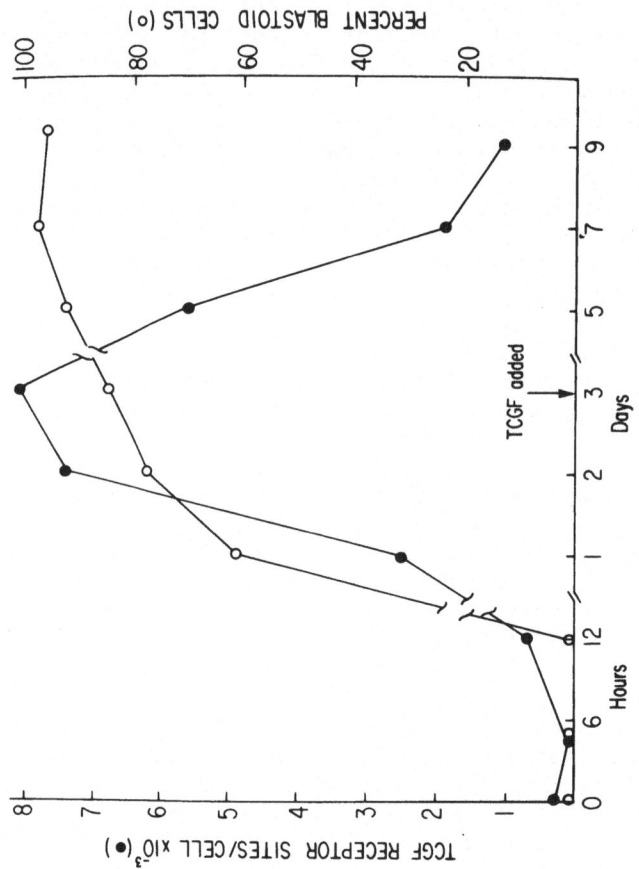

Fig. 12   The kinetics of TCGF receptor appearance. Human peripheral blood lymphocytes were stimulated with PHA (1.5 μg/ml). At the time intervals indicated aliquots of cell suspension
were removed for determination of TCGF receptors and the percentage of blastoid cells
(Wright-Giemsa Stain). After 3 days of culture the cells were diluted to 2 x 10⁵ cells/
ml and JURKAT-derived TCGF (1 μ/ml) was added. Thereafter, the culture was diluted and
TCGF was replenished as the cells attained a concentration of 1 x 10⁶ cells/ml.

sure of the hormonal nature of a biologically active polypeptide
is that of feedback control of hormone production. In our early
experiments(25) where we had noted that TCGF activity reaches
peak concentrations within 24-48 hours after lectin/antigen stimulation followed by a progressive decline, we searched for the
presence of an inhibitor of TCGF activity. Several experimental
approaches failed to demonstrate an inhibitor, and as detailed
in the preceding discussion, the loss of TCGF activity was subsequently found to be due to internalization and degradation.
Consequently, we have yet to discover the presence of a TCGF-
specific or -nonspecific feedback inhibitor that might function to
regulate the TCGF-driven clonal expansion of T-cells in vitro.
However, these experiments were designed to uncover an inhibitor
of TCGF action. Consequently, we have not directly approached the
possibility that inhibitors of TCGF production are released upon
activation of the cultured cells.

An unexplored explanation for the apparent cessation of TCGF
production after lectin/antigen activation would be end-product
inhibition such that occurs in enzymatic reactions. It has been
shown that T-cells responsible for TCGF production also express
TCGF receptors and will proliferate continuously in response to
TCGF supplied exogenously(26). However, if cloned TCGF producer
cells are stimulated to produce TCGF by lectin/antigen stimulation,
TCGF production appears to be finite such that the cells will not
continuously produce TCGF and proliferate in response to their own
growth promoting product(5,26). In addition, cloned TCGF-producer
cells do not continuously produce TCGF if cultured in the presence
of TCGF but in the absence of activating signals. It is possible,
therefore, that TCGF binding to TCGF receptors on TCGF producer
cells functions to shut down continued TCGF production. Exploration
of this possibility will, of course, depend upon the development
of methods to quantify the synthetic rates of TCGF as they occur
intracellularly.

An alternate, or equally plausible level of regulation of
TCGF production that would lead to an immunocyte internal regulatory
control would be through the activation and TCGF-dependent clonal
expansion of suppressor cells that function to down-regulate TCGF
production. There has been at least one report(27) that suggests
such a mechanism, however again, a definitive approach to the
demonstration of this mechanism will necessarily rest with the
study of cloned cells that express suppressive activity and the
methods to measure the rate of TCGF transcription, translation and
secretion.

Possible Neuroendocrine Regulation of TCGF Production

Although TCGF definitely appears to be an example of a lymphocytotrophic hormone that is an antigen-driven immunocyte product,

thus providing an example of how the immune system may be internally
regulated, since we have yet to discern an internally regulated
feedback inhibition of TCGF production, it is possible that
immunocyte-derived polypeptide hormones are primarily regulated by
physiological control systems that are external to the immune
system. In this regard, it may be that we have been hampered by
our in vitro systems for the study of the immune response, having
isolated the cells primarily involved in immune reactions, and
quite excluded any impingement by other systems that could be
operative in vivo: by definition we would not be in a position to
discern any external factors that are operative to modulate the
system.

While considering the possible involvement of other systems
that might function to regulate the clonal expansion of T-cells
through control of TCGF production, the neuroendocrine system
appears to be the most likely candidate. Moreover, among the
neuroendocrine hormones that may be operative, we already have a
great deal of evidence indicative of glucocorticoid hormones
playing a subtle, yet important role in lymphocyte physiology.
For example, glucocorticoid excess results in lymphoid hypoplasia
and immunosuppression(28,29), whereas glucocorticoid deficiency
results in lymphoid hypertrophy and immunopotentiation(29-33). It
is noteworthy that among the hematopoietic cells, the suppressive
effects of glucocorticoids are selective for lymphocytes. The
administration of pharmacologic doses of glucocorticoids for
prolonged periods does not result in anemia, granlocytopenia or
thrombocytopenia. As well, detailed studies of granulocyte and
monocyte turnover rates in the presence of glucocorticoids have
confirmed that there is no suppressive effect of glucocorticoids
of the proliferative capacity of these cells in vivo(34,35).

For glucocorticoids to be operative as feedback regulators of
antigen-driven TCGF production, of necessity, a mechanism must
exist whereby lymphocytotrophic hormones that are released as a
result of antigenic stimulation lead to enhanced corticosteroid
secretion. In this regard, a possible link between the immune
system and the hypothalamic-pituitary-adrenocortical axis has
recently been suggested by the findings of Sorkin and his coworkers,
Adriana Del Ray and Hugo Besedovsky(36). These investigators
found that administration of lymphokine-containing conditioned
medium to rats evoked a 3-4 fold increase in blood corticosterone
levels within 30 minutes to 2 hours. Although the mechanism of
this effect remains to be elucidated, as well as the identification
of the active moiety(s) in the conditioned medium, it is of interest
that changes in glucocorticoids levels of the same magnitude are
reached at the peak of the immune response after injection of
antigens(37).

In contrast to the embryonic information relevant to the possible stimulation of corticosteroid secretion by lymphocytotrophic hormones, we have made considerable progress in our understanding of the mechanism of inhibitory action of glucocorticoids on T-cell proliferation. Early studies on the in vivo immunosuppressive effects of glucocorticoids suggested that some early event in the generation of a competent immune response was suppressed, in that a primary immune response was suppressed to a far greater extent than a secondary immune response(38,39). Moreover, it was noted that if the administration of glucocorticoids was delayed for even a few days after antigenic challenge, the immunosuppressive effects were markedly diminished. These pioneering studies were correctly interpreted as consistent with the hypothesis that glucocorticoids act by delaying the accumulation of a sufficient number of antigen-responsive cells, rather than by preventing the function of already activated immunocytes(38,39).

Lacking in vitro systems to further study the mechanisms of interaction of glucocorticoids and immune reactions, these early observations remained unexplored. It is noteworthy, however, that the very first experiments reported by Nowell, once he had demonstrated the mitogenic effect of PHA, concerned the effect of glucocorticoids on this phenomenon(40,41). His series of experiments, which in retrospect represent classic observations, revealed the same phenomenon that had already been observed in vivo. If present at the initiation of the culture, glucocorticoids markedly suppressed PHA-stimulated lymphocyte proliferation. However, when the addition of glucocorticoids was delayed, even a few hours, their inhibitory effects became progressively less noticeable.

It took almost twenty years to provide an explanation for the critical timing of the glucocorticoid suppressive effects on T-cell proliferation. The resolution of this issue, of necessity, required a further reduction of the immune system, so that homogeneous cloned lymphocyte populations could be studied. Once it was understood that T-cell mitosis was actually triggered by a polypeptide hormone rather than by the interaction of antigen or lectin with the lymphocyte surface, the experimental possibilities could be reduced to two; i.e. glucocorticoids could act either by preventing the production of the hormone, or by preventing the action of the hormone. Since it is possible to separately assay these two parameters of the T-cell proliferative response, the results of the very first experiments were decisive(42,43). Glucocorticoids at receptor-saturating concentrations, completely inhibit the production of TCGF, yet the same concentrations have only a minimal effect on TCGF-dependent proliferation of cloned T-cell populations, provided TCGF is supplied exogenously. A representative experiment that depicts the glucocorticoid concentration-dependent inhibition of TCGF production and resultant suppression of proliferation of Concanavalin-A-stimulated rat splenocytes is shown in

Figure 13.   Recent studies utilizing a cloned population of neoplastic T-cells (MLA-144) that spontaneously produce TCGF confirmed
these observations (Figure 14)(44).   That the inhibitory effect of
glucocorticoids on proliferation of either lectin activated normal
T-cells or cloned neoplastic TCGF-producer T-cells was primarily
mediated by an inhibition of TCGF production, was conclusively
demonstrated by the fact that exogenous TCGF supplementation
completely reversed the glucocorticoid effect.   Figure 15 depicts
the effect of exogenous TCGF supplementation on the inhibitory
effect of glucocorticoid on PHA-stimulated human peripheral blood
lymphocytes.   Identical results were obtained upon TCGF supplementation of the MLA-144 cell line that had been pre-treated with
glucocorticoids to inhibit proliferation (Figure 16).   These
results readily explain the loss of the glucocorticoid effect upon
delayed addition of the hormone: since the primary action of

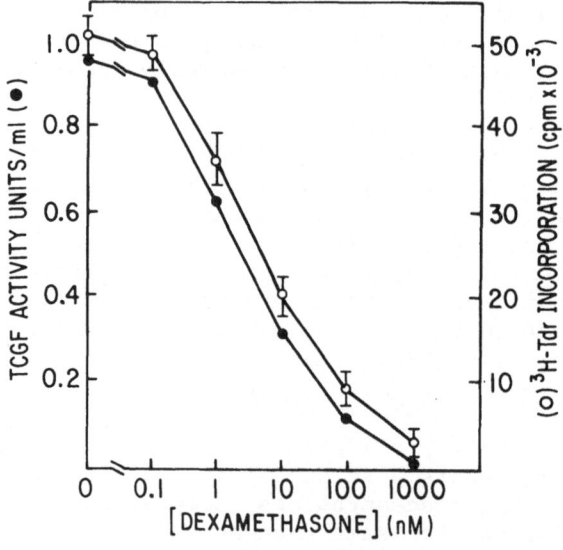

Fig. 13   The effect of dexamethasone on Concanavalin-A-stimulated
           rat splenocyte TCGF production (O) and [^{3}H]-thymidine
           incorporation (O).   Redrawn from Gillis et al. (42).

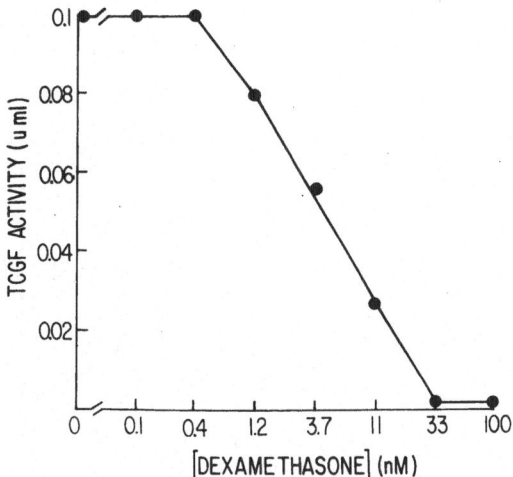

Fig. 14   The effect of dexamethasone on MLA-144 (45) TCGF produc-
           tion. MLA-144 clone 15T cells (5 x 10^5 cells/ml) were
           cultured for 24 hours prior to removal of supernatant
           aliquots for TCGF assay. Redrawn from Smith (44).

glucocorticoids is at the level of TCGF production, there is a
progressive diminution of suppression as adequate quantities of
TCGF are produced. As well, because the glucocorticoid inhibition
of proliferation can be prevented by supplementation with exogenous
TCGF, the data indicate that glucocorticoids do not suppress the
acquisition or functional expression of TCGF receptors.

The selective nature of the suppression of T-cell function
(i.e. the prevention of TCGF production without an effect on TCGF
receptor appearance or the capacity of the cell to respond to
TCGF) indicates that glucocorticoids do not inhibit lymphocyte
metabolism in a general sense. This realization, which is contrary
to the prevailing dogma of the effects of glucocorticoids on
lymphocytes, may have considerable physiological significance.

Future Directions in the Exploration of Lymphocyte Physiology

It is apparent from the foregoing discussion that although we
have established that TCGF shares most of the characteristics of a
hormone, we have yet to unravel the physiological feed back control
mechanisms that must be operative to control TCGF production and

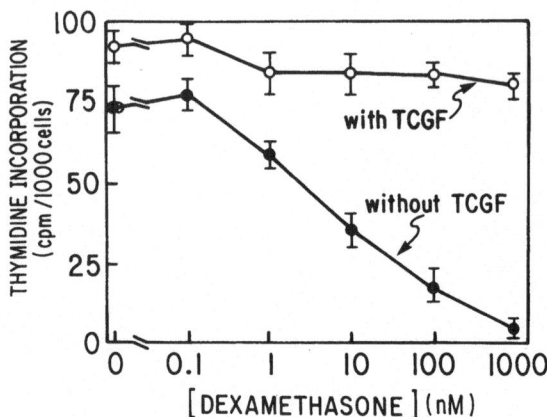

Fig. 15   The effect of TCGF supplementation on dexamethasone-
           induced inhibition of proliferation of PHA-stimulated
           peripheral blood lymphocytes. Cells were cultured in the
           absence (0) and presence (0) of 1 µ/ml TCGF and dexametha-
           sone at the concentrations indicated for 3 days prior to a
           4 hr pulse of [^{3}H]-thymidine. Redrawn from Gillis et al.
           (42).

action, and thus check the continuous clonal expansion of T-cells
after an antigenic challenge. It seems likely that there are
several levels of control, some that relate to internal regulatory
systems operating to diminish both TCGF production and TCGF receptor
expression. In addition, as indicated by our studies on the
profound and specific suppressive effects of glucocorticoids on
TCGF production, it appears likely that the functional expression
of lymphocytotropic hormones, exemplified by TCGF, is also subjected
to broader regulatory controls of the neuroendocrine system.

To approach the mechanisms of TCGF production, and thus begin
to unravel the regulatory influences, our attention must turn to
the control of TCGF gene expression and the molecular mechanisms
of polypeptide transcription, translation and secretion. In this

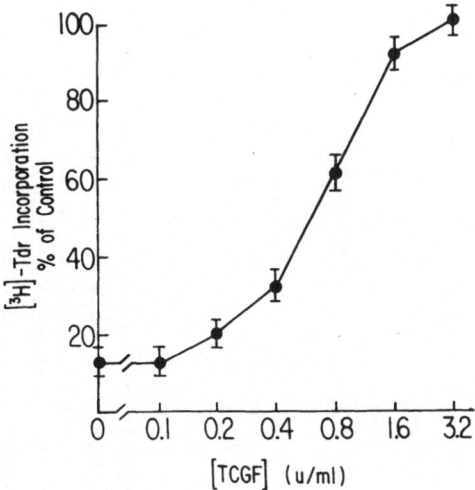

Fig. 16   The effect of TCGF on MLA-144 clone 15T proliferation.
Cells were cultured for 18 hr. with 100 nM dexamethasone,
then continued in culture for 44 hours with dexamethasone
and the concentrations of TCGF indicated. Data are expressed as a percent of control [^{3}H]-thymidine incorporation
without TCGF or dexamethasone.

regard, our studies of the molecular biology of TCGF will clearly
be aided by the availability of cloned T-cell populations capable
of producing and responding to TCGF, in much the same way that the
study of monoclonal plasmacytomas allowed the molecular approaches
that have contributed so much to our understanding of immunoglobulin
expression. We have just begun to study the kinetics of the
appearance of intra- and extracellular TCGF in preparation to
begin an analysis of the mechanism of TCGF production. Figure 17
depicts a representative time course of the appearance of intracellular and extracellular TCGF as identified by immunoprecipitates
using anti-TCGF monoclonal antibody. A high TCGF producer JURKAT
subclone was stimulated with PHA and phorbol myristic acetate for
4 hours prior to the introduction of radiolabeled methionine.
Within 5 minutes, 2 polypeptides (Mr = 17,500 and 15,000) are

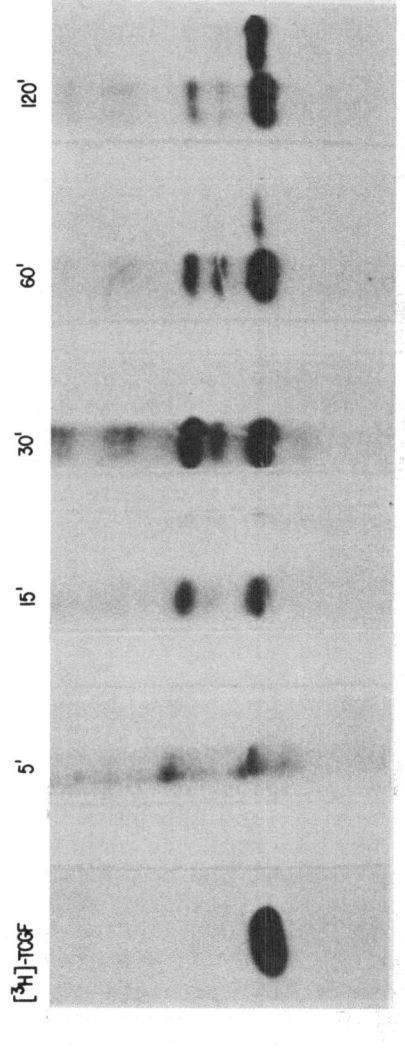

Fig. 17 Kinetic analysis (SDS-PAGE) of radiolabeled immunoprecipitable products derived from JURKAT cytosol (C) and supernatants (S). JURKAT subclone 6.8 cells were stimulated with PHA and PMA for 4 hrs prior to the addition of [^{35}S]-methionine (1010 Ci/mM, Amersham, UK). Aliquots of cell suspension were removed at the time intervals indicated and immunoprecipitates of cytosol and supernatant were formed using monoclonal anti-TCGF antibody (DMS-3) and Staphylococcal A. SDS-PAGE (12% acrylamide) was performed after dissolving precipitates in the presence of 2% SDS and 5% 2-mercaptoethanol. Biosynthetically radiolabeled ([^{3}H]-leucine, [^{3}H]-lysine) TCGF was included as a marker.

precipitable from the cytosol. Both peptides increase in the
cytosol over time, and by 30 minutes the 15,000 (Mr) species is
first barely discernable in the supernatant; after 1 hr. it is
readily appreciated.

 A comparison of in vivo and in vitro translated TCGF is shown
in Figure 18. Whereas there are at least two discernable in vivo
translated peptides, immunoprecipitation of in vitro translated,
poly-A-selected mRNA derived from JURKAT cells, results predominantly
in the peptide migrating at 17,500 (Mr). Identical results have
been obtained from immunoprecipitates of in vitro translated MLA-
144 mRNA. We are hopeful, therefore, that continued effort in
this direction will provide the framework with which to begin a
dissection of the molecular events surrounding the transcription,
translation, glycosylation and secretion of TCGF. It is also
hoped that the insight these studies will provide, together with

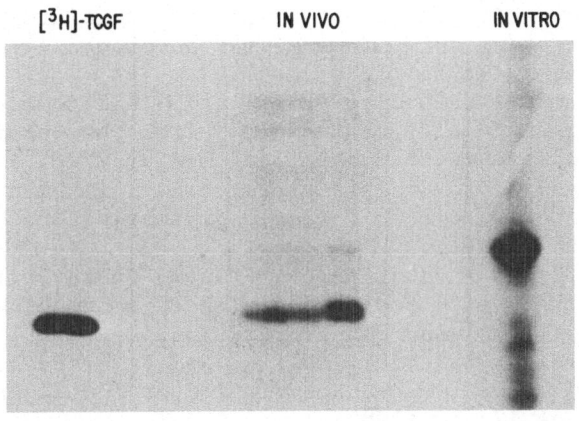

Fig. 18 Comparison of radiolabeled products of JURKAT cells after
in vivo and in vitro translation. In vivo translation was
performed for 1 hr as described in Figure 17. In vitro
translation of JURKAT mRNA was performed by means of re-
ticulocyte lysates. RNA was extracted from PHA- and PMA-
stimulated (4 hr) JURKAT cells by the guanidine HCL method
(46) followed by poly-A selection of mRNA by oligo-dT-
cellulose chromatography (47). SDS-PAGE of immunoprecipitates was performed as described in Figure 17.

an exploration of TCGF physiology and pathophysiology, will ultimately allow meaningful diagnostic approaches and therapeutic inter-
vention in disease states where disorders of T-cell function
predominate.

REFERENCES

1.   P. B. Medawar, in: "Immunopotentiation," Associated Scientific
     Publishers, Amsterdam p.343 (1973).
2.   D. A. Morgan, F. W. Ruscetti, and R. Gallo, Selective in vitro
     growth of T-lymphocytes from normal human bone marrows,
     Science (Wash. D.C.) 193:1007 (1976).
3.   E-L. Larsson, A. Coutinho and C. Martinez-A, A suggested mecha-
     nism for T lymphocyte activation: Implications on the
     acquisition of functional reactivities, Immunol. Rev. 51:61
     (1980).
4.   F. W. Ruscetti, and R. C. Gallo, Human T-lymphocyte growth
     factor: regulation of growth and function of T lymphocytes,
     Blood 57:379 (1981).
5.   K. A. Smith, and F. W. Ruscetti, T-cell growth factor and the
     culture of cloned functional T-cells, Adv. Immunol 31:137
     (1981).
6.   S. Gillis, K. A. Smith, and J. D. Watson, Biochemical and bio-
     logical characterization of lymphocyte regulatory molecules.
     II. Purification of a class of rat and human lymphokines,
     J. Immunol, 124:1954 (1980).
7.   J. W. Mier, and R. C. Gallo, Purification and some characteris-
     tics of human T-cell growth factor from phytohemagglutinin-
     stimulated lymphocyte-conditioned media, 77:6134 (1980).
8.   R. J. Robb, and K. A. Smith, Heterogeneity of human T-cell
     growth factor(s) due to variable glycosylation, Mol. Immu-
     nol. 18:1087 (1981).
9.   K. A. Smith, M. F. Favata, and R. Franza, Characteristics of
     human T-cell growth factor isolated by a monoclonal anti-
     body affinity column. In preparation.
10. K. A. Smith, P. E. Baker, S. Gillis, and F. W. Ruscetti, Func-
     tional and molecular characteristics of T-cell growth factor,
     Mol. Immunol 17:579 (1980).
11. K. A. Smith, S. Gillis, P. E. Baker, D. McKenzie, and F. W.
     Ruscetti, T-cell growth factor mediated T-cell proliferation,
     Ann. N. Y. Acad Sci. 332-423 (1979).
12. A. Coutinho, E. L. Larsson, K-O Gronvik, and J. Anderson,
     Studies on T-lymphocyte activation. II. The target cells
     for concanavalin-A-induced growth factors, Eur. J. Immunol
     9:587 (1979)
13. G. D. Bonnard, D. Yasaka, and D. Jacobson, Ligand- activated
     T-cell growth factor-induced proliferation: Absorption of
     T-cell growth factor by activated T-cells, J. Immunol,
     123:2704 (1979).

14. R. J. Robb, A. Munck, and K. A. Smith, T-cell growth factor receptors: quantitation, specificity, and biological relevance, J. Exp. Med. 154:1455 (1981).

15. D. E. Cummings and K. A. Smith, Characteristics of radiolabeled T-cell growth factor binding to isolated plasma membranes. In preparation.

16. F. W. Ruscetti, D. A. Morgan, and R. C. Gallo, Functional and morphologic characterization of human T-cells continuously grown in vitro, J. Immunol, 119:131 (1977).

17. E. L. Larsson, and A. Coutinho, On the role of mitogenic lectins in T-cell triggering, Nature (Lond.), 280:239 (1979).

18. S. Strickland, and J. N. Loeb, Obligatory separation of hormone binding and biological response curves in systems dependent upon secondary mediators of hormone action, Proc. Nat. Acad. Sci. USA, 79:1366 (1981).

19. K. A. Smith, Continuous cytotoxic T-cell lines, in: "Contemporary topics in immunobiology," N. L. Warner, ed., Plenum Publishing Corporation, New York (1980).

20. M. Krupp, and M. D. Lane, On the mechanism of ligand-induced down-regulation of insulin receptor levels in the liver cell, J. Biol. Chem. 256:1689 (1981).

21. P. J. Gorden, L. Carpentier, P. Freychet, and L. Orci, Internalization of polypeptide hormones. Mechanism, intracellular location, and significance. Diabetolgia 18:263 (1980).

22. A. C. King, and P. Cuatrecasas, Peptide hormone-induced receptor mobility, aggregation, and internalization, New Eng. J. Med. 305:77 (1981).

23. J. Kumagai, H. Akiyama, S. Iwashita, H. Iida, and I. Yahara, In vitro regeneration of resting lymphocytes from stimulated lymphocytes and its inhibition by insulin, J. Immunol. 126:1249 (1981).

24. T. B. Strom, and J. D. Bangs, Human serum-free mixed lymphocyte response: the stereospecific effect of insulin and its potentiation by transferin, 128:1555, J. Immunol.(1982).

25. S. Gillis, M. Ferm, W. Ou, and K. A. Smith, T-cell growth factor: parameters of production and a quantitative microassay for activity, J. Immunol, 120:2027 (1978).

26. M. H. Schreier, N. N. Iscove, R. Tees, L. Aarden, and H. von Boehmer, Clones of killer and helper T-cells: growth requirements, specificity and retention of function in long-term culture, Immunol. Rev. 51:315, (1980).

27. H. Northoff, C. Carter, and J. J. Oppenheim, Inhibition of concanavalin A-induced human lymphocyte mitogenic factor (interleukin-2) production by suppressor T lymphocytes, J. Immunol. 125:1823, (1980).

28. T. F. Dougherty, and A. White, Influence of hormones on lymphoid tissue structure and function. The role of the pituitary adrenotrophic hormone in the regulation of the lymphocytes and other cellular elements of the blood, Endocrinology, 35:1 (1944).

29. M. Ishidate, Jr., and D. Metcalf, The pattern of lymphophoiesis in the mouse thymus after cortisone administration or adrenalectomy, Austral. J. Exp. Biol, 41:637 (1963).

30. J. B. Murphy, and Ernest Sturm, The lymphoid tissue and antibody formation, Proc. Soc. Exp. Biol. 66:303, (1947).

31. R. J. Graff, M. A. Lappe, and G. D. Snell, The influence of the gonads and adrenal glands on the immune response to skin grafts, Transplantation, 7:105, (1969).

32. J. E. Castro, D. N. H. Hamilton, Adrenalectomy and orchidectomy as immunopotentiating procedures, Transplantation, 13:614 (1972).

33. C. B. Streng, and P. Nathan, The immune response in steroid deficient mice, Immunology, 24:559 (1973).

34. C. R. Bishop, J. W. Athens, D. R. Boggs, H. R. Warner, G. E. Cartwright, and M. M. Wintrobe, XIII. a non-steady-state kinetic evaluation of the mechanism of cortisone-induced granulocytosis, J. Clin. Invest. 47:249 (1968).

35. J. Thompson, and R. Van Furth, The effect of glucocorticosteroids on the proliferation and kinetics of promonocytes and monocytes of the bone marrow, J. Exp. Med. 137:10 (1973).

36. H. O. Besedovsky, A. Del Rey, and E. Sorkin, Lymphokine-containing supernatants from con A-stimulated cells increase corticosterone blood levels, J. Immunol. 126:385 (1981).

37. H. O. Besedovsky, E. Sorkin, M. Keller, and J. Muller, Changes in blood hormone levels during the immune response Proc. Exp. Biol. Med., 150:466 (1975).

38. R. E. Billingham, P. L. Krohn, Effect of cortisone on survival of skin homografts in rabbits, Brit. Med. Journal, 1:4716, 1951.

39. P. B. Medawar, and E. M. Sparrow, The effects of adrenocortical hormones, adrenocorticotrophic hormone and pregnancy on skin transplantation immunity in mice, J. Endocrinol. 14:240 (1956).

40. P. C. Nowell, Phytohemagglutinin: An initiator of mitosis in cultures of normal human leukocytes, Cancer Research 20:462 (1960).

41. P. C. Nowell, Inhibition of human leukocyte mitosis by prednisone in vitro, Cancer Research, 21:1518 (1961).

42. S. Gillis, G. R. Crabtree, and K. A. Smith, Glucocorticoid-induced inhibition of T-cell growth factor production. I. The effect on mitogen-induced lymphocyte proliferation J. Immunol. 123:1624 (1979)

43. S. Gillis, G. R. Crabtree, and K. A. Smith, Glucocorticoid-induced inhibition of T-cell growth factor production. II. The effect on the in vitro generation of cytolytic T-cells. J. Immunol.123:1632 (1979).

44. K. A. Smith, T-cell growth factor and glucocorticoids: opposing regulatory hormones in neoplastic T-cell growth, Immunobiol. 161:157 (1982).

45. H. Rabin, R. F. W. Ruscetti, R. H. Neubauer, R. L. Brown, and T. G. Kawakami, Spontaneous release of a factor with T-cell growth factor activity from a continuous line of primate tumor T-cells, J. Immunol. 127:1852, (1981).

46. R. G. Deeley, J. I. Gordon, A. T. H. Burns, K. P. Mullinix, M. Binkstein and R. F. Goldberger, Primary activation of the vitellogenin gene in the rooster, J. Biol. Chem. 252:8310 (1977).

47. H. Aviv and P. Leder, Purification of biologically active globin messenger RNA by chromatography on oligo-thymidylic acid-cellulose, Proc. Nat. Acad. Sci. USA. 69:1408 (1972).

ACKNOWLEDGEMENTS

This work was supported in part by National Cancer Institute grants CA-17643, CA-17323, CA-23108, CA-26273, and grant CH-167 from The American Cancer Society. The author is indebted to Drs. Robert Gallo, Allan Munck, Frank Ruscetti and Maurice Landy for their interest and suggestions throughout. The technical assistance of Ms. Margaret Favata is gratefully acknowledged.

DISCUSSION

Benacerraf: I would like to ask a question of nomenclature. Is the molecule you call TCGF the same molecule sometimes referred to as IL-2, at least as far as its effects on T cells are concerned?

Smith: That is a very good question. There are two reasons that I continue to refer to the factor as TCGF rather than IL-2. First, the characteristics of IL-2 of human origin have not yet been defined. At the time of the 2nd International Lymphokine Workship no data were available on the biochemical characteristics of IL-2. Consequently, the nomenclature was restricted to IL-2 of murine origin. Secondly, because biochemical heterogeneity of murine IL-2 was discovered subsequent to the meeting, IL-2 came to be referred to as a class of molecules (rather than a single molecule) with diverse activities for B-cells as well as T cells. As you have seen from the data that I presented, human TCGF activity can be ascribed to a moiety that is uniform with respect to size (Mr = 15,500) and charge (pI = 8.2). Moreover, human TCGF clearly has no activity for B cells and does not bind to B cells. I am forced, therefore, to continue to refer to the human-derived T cell activity as TCGF rather than IL-2. If one restricts the definition to T cells, then human TCGF could be termed IL-2.

G. Möller: What is known about the serum concentration of TCGF?

Smith: We have not yet tried to measure TCGF from normal serum samples, although we have developed a competitive binding assay to precisely do that experiment. I am somewhat pessimistic, however, in being able to detect serum levels except in situations of chronic antigenic stimulation, especially since TCGF appears to be internalized and degraded after it binds.

Benacerraf: How do T cells without receptors to TCGF grow?

Smith: I really do not know. We have yet to find normal T cells that are unresponsive to TCGF. However, it remains possible that subsets of T-cells exist that respond to some other growth factor. For example it is still an open question whether TCGF-producer T cells also respond to TCGF.

Forman: How do you explain your finding that the amount of proliferation varies linearly with the amount of T-cell growth factor added. Since you are using a short term thymidine pulse you might expect a more all or none effect. Is this due to the heterogeneity in the number of receptors expressed per cell?

Smith: We really need to do more experiments before we can answer that question. Based on binding of radiolabelled TCGF to whole cells, and more importantly, on binding to isolated membranes, we can say that the biological response, measured by the rate of proliferation, is determined by the proportion of occupied receptors at equilibrium. However, these data do not tell us whether the response depends upon the proportion of occupied receptors or the rate at which they are occupied. As well, the biological response may ultimately depend upon the rate at which the TCGF-receptor complexes are degraded intracellularly.

Doherty: I seem to recall that the Mainz group published a paper saying that IL-2 is effectively neutralized by mouse serum. One might, on teleological ground, wish to believe that that is the case. Otherwise there would be a tendency for polyclonal activation if high concentrations were present in serum. It could be more appropriate for high concentration of IL-2 to occur only in a local site of antigen stimulation. Is ther any evidence for presence of such neutralizing substances in human serum?

Smith: We have no data that would suggest the presence of either a TCGF-serum binding protein or an inhibitor, but we have not yet directly searched for such phenomena.

Vitetta: Does mouse IL-2 bind to human cells?

Smith: Human TCGF will bind to, and have activity on mouse cells, however, mouse TCGF will not bind to, or have activity on human cells.

Ohno: Since there is an internalization of TCGF+receptor complexes, how can you measure the dissociation constant of TCGF on live cells?

Smith: You are absolutely right. That is the reason we isolated plasma membranes to perform the kinetic and equilibrium binding assays. The importance of the binding data is the almost exact correlation found for the equilibrium dissociation constants and numbers of binding sites per cell, determined using either whole cells or membranes, because it means that the biological response depends upon the variables of (H), (R) and Ka from the equilibrium binding equation.

Benacerraf: Does the cell that produces TCGF also possess membrane receptors for the TCGF it produces? I.e. can it regulate itself as well as other T cells in this manner?

Smith: At this time it is unclear whether all T cells may have the capacity to produce TCGF but do so only under the appropriate circumstances. Several groups have now found that 10-15% of cytolytic T cell clones can produce TCGF.

G. Möller: Dr Ronald Palacios has a T cell line secreting TCGF (IL-2), but lacking TCGF receptors.

Nabholz: Andy Glasebrook and other people have isolated CTL-clones which produce TCGF, and also require it for growth.

Sachs: Dr Bluestone in my laboratory has recently developed a series of cytotoxic T cell clones, many of which are TCGF in-dependent. Perhaps of relevance is the fact that immunization across a K-only difference (in fact across a K^b mutant difference) led to a much larger percentage of such TCGF independent killer cells than did immunization across an entire H-2 difference.

Melchers: How do T cells without the receptor for TCGF grow?

Coutinho: Fritz Melchers' question is very relevant, namely, the mechanism of T helper cell growth. For several years that we have been very doubtful about TCGF being a growth factor for helper cells in general, and quite certain that it is not the growth factor for the cells which produce it. Current opinions were contrary, however, and considered it (IL-2) the universal lymphocyte - even for B cells - growth factor. This has finally been directly proven to be wrong and I expect the same to happen soon for helper cells (we have actually suggested before that TCGF should be called TKCGF). Fritz Melchers' point goes further: whatever the growth factor for the helpers is, it will still be a factor produced and used by the same cell (and this would perhaps result in uncontrolled growth). There are in fact tumors like this. This is only a problem, however, if the rules of induction which apply to cytotoxic cells (maintenance of growth receptor expression after initial induction, even in the absence of antigen recognition) would also apply for helpers. This is probably not the case.

G. Möller: Dr. Palacios cell line required a growth factor initially that was neither IL-1 or IL-2. With time the line last its dependence of this factor, possibly because the factor was synthesized by the cells themselves.

Benacerraf: In the last few years our laboratory has been engaged in the analysis of T cells concerned with specific suppression of cellular immunity (Germain, R.N. and Benacerraf, B., Scand. J. Immunol. 13, 1, 1981), i.e., delayed type hypersensitivity (DTH) and cytolytic T cell (CTL) responses. We have selected for these studies immunological systems characterized by the presence of predominent cross-reactive idiotypes on specific antibody, such as the azobenzenearsonate (ABA) system in mice with the Igh^e linked CRI (Nisonoff, A. et al., Immunol. Rev. 34, 89, 1977) or the 4-hydroxy-3-nitrophenyl acetyl (NP) system in mice with the Igh NP^b idiotype (Imanishi, T. and Mäkelä, O., J. Exp. Med. 140, 1498, 1974).

The studies of ABA specific suppression were carried out by a group headed by Mark Greene and involving Man-Sun Sy, Al Nisonoff, and Ronald Germain, while the studies on NP specific suppression were performed by Martin Dorf's laboratory. It is remarkable that except for some details unique to each system, essentially identical results were obtained independently by both laboratories and identical conclusions were reached.

The salient findings are that:

1) The specific suppression phenomena involve the interactions of three sets of T cells Ts$_1$, Ts$_2$, Ts$_3$ with defined properties and characteristic surface markers.

2) These T cell subsets each produce specific factors which can be shown to mediate their precise regulatory function.

3) Their specificity is either for the antigen or for the immuno-globulin idiotypes which determine certain aspects of their interactions.

4) Certain of the suppressor T cells in these circuits bear determinants coded for by the I-J subregion of the murine H-2 complex, which also appear to restrict the interactions at certain critical steps in the pathway, in a way similar to the restrictions imposed by I-A and I-E subregions on helper T cell interactions.

Properties of Ts$_1$, Ts$_2$, and Ts$_3$ and their respective factors:

The intravenous injection of haptenated syngeneic spleen cells in both ABA and NP systems stimulates cyclophosphamide-sensitive pre-Ts cells to develop into antigen-binding Ts$_1$ cells (Table I). These Ts$_1$ cells in the ABA system have been shown to express the Ly 1$^+$,2$^-$ phenotype. Ts$_1$ cells are idiotype-positive in both systems and function as afferent and not efferent suppressors (Weinberger, J.Z. et al., J. Exp. Med. 150, 761, 1979; Green, M.I. and Benacerraf, B., Immunol. Rev. 50, 163, 1980; Sy, M-S. et al., J. Exp. Med. 151, 1183, 1980; Dietz, M.H. et al., J. Immunol. 125, 2374, 1980). ABA and NP specific Ts$_1$ cells have been successfully hybridized with the lymphoma BW5147 and stable hybridoma lines have been produced with the characteristic properties of the hapten specific Ts$_1$ factors (Okuda, K. et al., Proc Natl. Acad. Sci. 78, 4557, 1981; Whitaker, R.B. et al., Proc. Natl. Acad. Sci., in press, 1981). Such hybrid lines bear the respective idiotypic determinants and produce in their culture supernatant suppressor factors (TsF$_1$) which are idiotypic, antigen-binding and bear

TABLE I

PROPERTIES OF Ts_1 (SUPPRESSOR INDUCER)

1. Lyt 1^+, I-J$^+$

2. Antigen binding and idiotypic
   (CRI for ABA: NP^b for NP)

3. Induced by tolerizing regimes
   (e.g. haptenated syngeneic spleen cells i.v.)

4. Precursor is cyclophosphamide sensitive

5. Not H-2 nor V_H restricted

6. Afferent suppressor

7. Produces a soluble factor TsF_1 which mediates its activity

TABLE II

PROPERTIES OF Ts_2

1. Lyt 2^+, I-J$^+$

2. Anti-idiotypic (anti-CRI for ABA, anti-NPb for NP)

3. Induced by TsF_1 or by idiotype + antibody coupled spleen cells

4. Precursor cyclophosphamide insensitive

5. Shows functional H-2 (I-J) and V_H (Igh-1) restrictions

6. Efferent suppressor

7. Produces a soluble factor TsF_2

8. Requires interaction with Ts_3 for suppression of cell mediated responses

TsF$_1$ products in both ABA or NP systems function by stimulating non-immune cyclophosphamide (CY) resistant T cells to become Ts2 cells which in these two systems are anti-idiotypic rather than antigen specific (Sy M.-S. et al., J. Exp. Med. 151, 1183, 1980; Weinberger, J.Z. et al., J. Exp. Med. 152, 161, 1980). This has been demonstrated with TsF$_1$s obtained from either immune spleen cell populations or from Ts1 hybridoma cell lines (Takaoki, M. et al., J. Immunol. 128, 49, 1981). In the latter case it could be verified that in these two system hybridoma derived ABA or NP TsF$_1$ factors stimulate Ts2 cells in the absence of antigen.

Ts2 cells differ radically from Ts1 cells in their properties and function. In the ABA and NP system, Ts2 cells are anti-idiotypic and can be shown to bind to idiotype coated plates: they bear Ly 2$^+$ determinants and as shown in the NP system, I-J coded specificities and they function as efferent suppressors, i.e. they are able to suppress DTH reactions and plaque forming cell responses in an already immune animal (Table II). Another very important difference between Ts1 and Ts2 concerns the genetic restrictions which govern their interactions with their targets. Ts2 are restricted by both V$_H$ genes and by the I-J subregion of the MHC in expressing their suppressive activity (Dietz, M.H. et al., J. Exp. Med. 153, 1450, 1981; Minami, M. et al., J. Exp. Med. 154, 1390, 1981).

T cell hybridomas with the properties of Ts2 have been produced in the NP system (Minami, M. et al., J. Exp. Med. 154, 1390, 1981). Such T$_s$ hybridomas have all the properties of the Ts2 parent. Ts2 factors function by producing a soluble factor, TsF$_2$, which in these two systems are anti-idiotypic and also bear I-J subregion coded determinants. TsF$_2$ suppress in the efferent mode and are I-J and V$_H$ restricted in their ability to mediate suppression.

The efferent property of Ts2 led us to consider that these cells might be the final effectors. However this proved not to be the case. Earlier work by Sy et al. (J. Exp. Med. 149, 1197, 1979) in the DNP system had revealed the need for an additional cell, which they called the auxilliary cell, in the final effector pathway. Such a cell, which for internal consistency we termed Ts3, was soon identified in both ABA and NP systems (Sy. M.-S. et al., J. Exp. Med. 153, 1415, 1981; Sunday, M.E. et al., J. Exp. Med. 153, 811. 1981).

The discovery of Ts3 was stimulated by the observation that the injection of Ts2 or TsF$_2$ did not result in suppression of an immune animal if the recipient mouse had been treated with low doses of cyclophosphamide shortly after immunization. It was apparent therefore that a highly CY sensitive cell is the target of TsF$_2$ in the suppressor circuit. Moreover, this Ts3 subset is always induced as part of the conventional immunization which stimulates DTH sensitivity, i.e., immunization with adjuvant or percutaneous sensitization. Antigen activated T_s cells are inactive until appropriately triggered by Ts_2 or TsF_2.

Ts_3 cells in both ABA and NP systems are antigen specific, and MHC (I-J) restricted. They express the Ly 2^+ phenotype and bear, as verified in the NP system, I-J- coded determinants. Ts_3 cells produce an antigen specific TsF_3 which mediates efferent suppression in these systems (Table III). The suppressive activity of Ts_3 and TsF_3 in the NP system can be demonstrated in cyclophosphamide treated recipients and, as in the case of TsF_2, it is restricted by both V_H and MHC (I-J) genes.

Ts_3 hybridomas have been obtained by Dorf in the NP system (Okuda, K. et al., J. Exp. Med. 154, 1838, 1981). In some systems the specific activation of Ts_3 cells results in suppression which is to some extent non-specific. Thus in the ABA specific Ts_3 results in suppression of mice differing at the Igh-1 locus (Sy. M-S. et al. J. Exp. Med. 153, 1415, 1981), and even in suppression of a DTH reaction of a different specificity.

MHC restriction in suppressor T cell interactions in the ABA and NP systems:

Previous studies had indicated the existence of MHC (I-J) restriction in the interaction of T_s and TsF_2 with their Ts_3 targets for these cells to be triggered and suppression to be observed. More recently, we have investigated whether there are MHC restriction in the induction of Ts_3 cells (Takaoki, M. et al. Submitted for publications, 1982; Minami, M. et al. Submitted for publication, 1982). Two sort of experiments were carried out.

To generate Ts_3 cells, (A.BY x A/J)F_1 mice were immunized with ABA coupled A/J cells or ABA coupled A.BY cells. Suppression of DTH and CTL responses in the mice was then attempted with either A/J-TsF_2 or A.BY-TsF_2. As shown in Table IV, suppression was selectively limited by the type of ligand coupled cells used for priming Ts_3 cells. Effective suppression was only observed when ABA-coupled cells, used to sentsitize and to induce Ts_3, and TsF_2 had the same genetic origin - whereas when (A.BY x A/J)F_1 mice were immunized with ABA coupled to (A.BY x A/J)F_1 cells, ABA-specific DTH and CTL responses were equally suppressed by either A.BY-TsF_2 and A/J-TsF_2.

A similar experiment was carried out by Dorf and associates in the NP system, with identical results. Ts_3 cells were generated in (B6 x A)F_1 mice by priming with NP-coupled C57BL/6 or B10.BR spleen cells. After 5 days, the (B6 x A)F_1 lymph node Ts_3 cells were

TABLE III

PROPERTIES OF Ts_3 (EFFECTOR SUPPRESSOR)

1. Lyt 2^+, $I-J^+$

2. Antigen specific and idiotypic
   (CRI in ABA and NPb in NP)

3. Precursor cyclophosphamide sensitive

4. Induced in lymph nodes during conventional immunogenic priming regimen

5. H-2 (I-J) restricted at induction and at interaction with TsF_2

6. Activated by anti-idiotypic TsF_2

7. Suppresses in idiotype and antigen non-specific manner once specifically triggered.

TABLE IV

I-J RESTRICTION IN SELECTIVE SUPPRESSION BY TsF_2 in (A.BY x A/J)F_1 HYBRID MICE

Exp. I

TsF_2 induced in	Priming stimulus for Ts_3	Suppression of DTH
A.BY	ABA-A.BY	yes
	ABA-A/J	no
A/J	ABA-A.BY	no
	ABA-A/J	yes

Exp. II

B10.A (3R)	ABA-A.BY	yes
	ABA-A/J	no
B10.A (5R)	ABA-A.BY	no
	ABA-A/J	yes

transferred to either C57BL/6 or B10.BR cyclophosphamide treated recipients along with $H-2^b$ TsF_2 or $H-2^k$ TsF_2. Suppression of DTH was only observed when the antigenic stimulus for Ts3 induction and the TsF_2 were of the same parental type.

In another series of experiments we evaluated the role of I-J coded determinants in the MHC restriction of Ts3 and TsF_2 cells. (57BL6 x A/J)F_1 mice were primed for Ts3 induction with ABA coupled B10.A (3R) or ABA coupled B10.A (5R) mice. The hapten coupled cells used for Ts3 induction and the TsF_2 used to trigger these cells were required to share I-J for suppression to be observed. Similar experiments with identical results were carried out by Dorf et al. in the NP system.

The results of these experiments illustrate that I-J determinants may in selected systems act as restriction specificities for the induction of effector suppressor T cells (T_s3) and for the interaction of these cells with the appropriate TsF_2 factor required to trigger their suppressive activity.

Miller: 1. Are the adherent cells required for the activation of Ts3 cells $I-J^+$?

2. Can you detect the idiotype on your Ts_1 and Ts3 hybridomas and if so by what method and can you estimate the approximate number of molecules per cell surface?

Benacerraf: Many of the NP specific Ts hybridomas produced by Martin Dorf expressed idiotype on their surface. However, this was not quantitated. The idiotype was detected by susceptibility to lysis in the presence of complement. The expression of surface idiotype decreased with time that the lines were maintained.

The F_{12} Ts_1 ABA specific hybridoma never expressed the idiotype on its surface although it produced idiotype possitive suppressor factor.

Wigzell: Do yo know whether the restriction (I-J and Igh) between Ts_2 and Ts3 is opportune, that is capable of adaptive differentiation?

Benacerraf: We have not carried out the experiment you refer to and therefore we do not know whether the I-J restriction of Ts_2-Ts3 interaction is susceptible to adaptive differentiation.

Honjo: Are there any differences in chemical natures of TsF_1 and TsF_2?

Benacerraf: I regret that at the present time we do not have definite information on the chemical structure of the suppressor factors produced by the T cell hybridomas generated in our laboratory.

Cohn: I cannot help having doubts about the existence of a normally functional suppressor circuit of the type you (and many others) have described.

There seems to be no way to rationalize a pathway of alternating self-Id reactions in order to suppress DTH to a foreign pathogen. I do not see what might be the role in a normal response to antigen of a single and major T cell suppressor pathway that goes **obligatorily** and indirectly via an anti-Id interaction. I am suspicious of a proposed pathway that involves an exquisitely specific cascade of stable factors, i.e. TsF_1 (anti-X,Id^+, not MHC restricted), and TsF_2(anti-Id, MHC-restricted) but has an effector output to the protective arm of the immune system that is a nonspecific, stable factor clearly capable by experiment (i.v. injection) of long range suppression. This takes out of the hands of the immune system the concordance between antibody response to be suppressed and the antigen contacted and requires further guesses, e.g. the role of topology or architecture, as to how control of specificity must be effected. Yet even this is contradictory for it is experimentally obvious that no control whatever is operating. It is necessary to invoke functional lack of concordance or non-specificity of the output of the circuit in order to explain your finding that the **totality** of the DTH response anti-Ars is suppressed when the Id Ars you are manipulating is neither the major nor the high affinity Id class expressed on anti-Ars. I wonder to what extent this suppressor pathway will turn out to be a laboratory construct of no physiological significance in the regulation of the normally specific immune response.

Benacerraf: It is not surprising to me that the last step in the suppressor pathway that we have studied proves to be immunologically non-specific. This is similar to the release of histamin or heparin from mast cells triggered by an IgE-antigen interaction at the mast cell surface. Our observations imply the similar release of a non-specific mediator or mediators by an unspecified cell at the term of the suppressor T cell circuit.

Miller: Wayne Thomas and I have indeed demonstrated the existence of a non-specific effector suppressor T cell in a system quite different from the one described by Dr. Benacerraf. While the initial activation was antigen specific the final result was mediated by a non-antigen specific T cell - (Thomas et. al., J. Exp. Med., 1980).

Cohn: I will make two points: First, I question the existence of I-J-restricted suppressor factors or, for that matter, I-J-restricted suppressor T-cells.

As an example, in the arsanilate case which you have described, the TsF_1 (anti-Ars) is not MHC restricted but the TsF_2 (anti-Id Ars) is said to be MHC restricted. This conclusion is not required from your data. The reference Id^+ anti-Ars is the low affinity population of anti-Ars. It is revealed after heavy immunization with Ars-KLH at a time when the T^H anti-KLH is so high that the more numerous low affinity Id^+ anti-Ars is induced. Such a situation would be expected to be under an observable IR-1 gene control and in fact the A/J mouse responds with a more than 3 fold higher proportion of Id^+ anti-Ars than the A.BY/Sn congenic. This can be seen in spite of the aggressive immunization of both strains with a "strong" immunogen; that is, even heavy immunization does not obliterate the difference in responsiveness in the Id^+ anti-Ars class between A/J and A.BY. In your case, you are using a "weak" immunogen so that the difference could be enormous, i.e. A.BY might not be induced at all to express the Id^+ anti-Ars. Obviously, in order for TsF_2 anti-Id^+ to function, there must be Id^+ targets in the animal. If the presence or absence of the Id^+ anti-Ars target is determined by H-2 (IR-1) then the suppressive activity of TsF_2 will depend on the H-2 allele, **not** because TsF_2 is MHC restricted in its function but because there is no target for it. Besides it is doubtful that TsF_2 could be restricted to the I-J determinant that it expresses. This above argument makes it equally unlikely that TsF_2 is restricted by the Igh-locus. There are no T-cells or T-cell factors anti-X restricted by the Igh-encoded idiotype.

Second, this suppressor pathway is constructed using an experimental system which is inadequately defined. We know too little about the mechanism of the assay of DTH by footpad swelling; the chemistry of the idiotype and its associated combining specificity is shrouded in contradictions; and the I-J encoded determinant believed to be present on the suppressor T-cell receptor (factor) is essentially uncharacterized.

I recall that in systems analogous to your Ars-spleen cell (SC) model, e.g. DNP/TNP-SC, FITC-SC, SAD-SC, etc. the usual response is a cytotoxic T^K-response. In the case of the DNP-SC system, DTH is class I restricted implying that it is T^K-mediated while in the Ars-SC case DTH seems to be class II restricted implying that it is T^{DH}-mediated. Further, under conditions where the animal mounts a cytotoxic response, the humoral response to the same antigen is suppressed. If the suppression of the humoral response were mediated by T^K-cells, no contribution by factors could be invoked.

In order to interpret your findings, we must know whether the footpad swelling assay of DTH has a humoral component or is entirely T-cell-mediated. Further, we must know the relationship between the mechanism of suppression of the humoral Id^+ anti-Ars response to Ars-KLH and of the cell-mediated DTH response to Ars-spleen cells.

There are too many contradictions between the behaviour of the idiotype (Id Ars) and the combining specificity (anti-Ars) when studied on immunoglobulin and on suppressor factors. It is even worse for the heteroclitic NP-system. When studied on Ig, both the idiotype and the combining activity require specific $V_L V_H$ complementation. The affinity for Ars of the Id Ars$^+$ is already low and must be significantly lower in the case of a factor containing V_H alone. Yet this idiotype and its associated combining specificity when studied on Ig has a totally different behaviour than when studied on TsF$_1$ anti-Ars. No V_{kappa} is required for the idiotype or combining specificity. Only V_H is required and its combining affinity for arsanilate must be high given that TsF$_1$ is monovalent and acts to suppress DTH **in vivo** at what must be homeopathic levels (10^{-9}-10-$^{-10}$M).

Finally, all of this must be tied into the relationship with the I-J bearing subunit; nothing of a consistent or reproducible nature can be said about that.

Third, I question the logic of Benacerraf's approach to analyzing suppression.

If you immunize an animal with an antigen, you get **per force** an antibody carrying an idiotype (TsF$_1$). Since these injections could have no other outcome than observed, how do you arrive at the conclusion that this represents a single, major and normal suppressive pathway which upon injection of antigen passes **obligatorily** via TsF$_1$(anti-X) to TsF$_2$(anti-IdX) to some nonspecific output?

Benacerraf: The expression of id$^+$ by only a fraction of the cells is not a problem. Since the last step of the suppressor circuit is non-specific and idiotype non-restricted, the interaction of the anti-idiotype Ts$_2$ with only a limited number of idiotype bearing Ts$_3$ is capable of suppressing DTH mediated by a large number of idiotype negative effector cells. We have indeed demonstrated this point experimentally by showing that anti-id Ts$_2$ cells, which otherwise would be incapable of suppressing an id-recipient, will suppress it if a limited number of id$^+$Ts$_3$ cells are transferred.

Sprent: Do the two subsets of I-J-restricted T$_s$ cells found in normal F$_1$ mice exist in F$_1$--<parent chimeras?

Benacerraf: We have not carried out experiments involving chimeras as yet, although I would expect that such chimeras would behave similarly to those that you have studied.

Miller: W.R. Thomas, P.C. Mottram and I have grown cell lines from mice sensitized to the contact sensitizing agents oxazolone (OX), picryl chloride (PCl) and azobenzene arsonate (ABA) that have been shown to mediate delayed hypersensitivity (DH) (Thomas, W. R. et al., J. Exp. Med. 156: in press, 1982). A feature of this reactivity was the ability of the cells to respond to hapten presented on mouse cells or foreign proteins. Further evidence for hapten-specificity is given here. It shows that T cells react in vitro with a monovalent hapten-amino acid conjugate.

Cells from a CBA anti-OX T cell line were incubated in RPMI containing 40 ug/ml OX coupled glycine on ice for 1 hour, washed and injected into mice to test their ability to produce local DH reactions to OX. This treatment inhibited transfer of DH by the anti-OX cell line, 018, but not the activity of cells from the anti-ABA line, AA3 (Table 1). The ability of AA3 to mediate ABA-specific DH could, however, be inhibited by pre-incubation with 10 ug/ml ABA-BSA. This demonstration of direct interaction of T cells with a monovalent hapten agrees with experiments of Moorhead, (J. Exp. Med. 154, 1811, 1981) using cells taken directly from immune mice. It has also provided a model for testing antisera for the presence of anti-antigen receptor specificities.

We injected CBA mice intraperitoneally repeatedly with the 018 anti-OX cell line and serum from these mice was incubated with the cell line for 15 minutes at 37°C at a 1/20 dilution. OX-conjugated glycine (40 ug/ml) was then added and the incubation continued at 4°C for a further hour. Cells were washed and tested for their ability to mediate DH. The anti-cell line antiserum, but not normal CBA ascites fluid, abrogated the ability of the OX-glycine to inhibit transfer of DH indicating the presence of anti-receptor activity in the antiserum (Table II). Previous work had shown that anti-idiotypic sera prepared against immune anti-DNFB cells prevented DH transfer if incubated with cells in the absence of complement (Moorhead, J.W., J. Exp. Med. 155, 820, 1982). This is, however, a suppressor phenomenon dependent on the presence of Ia-bearing T cells which have not been detectable in our T cell lines. The mechanisms of both the effect of monovalent hapten and its reversal by antisera have not been investigated. The system does, however, have the potential for demonstrating anti-idiotypic or anti-receptor activity even in the presence of other antibody specifities.

Evidence for anti-idiotypic activity in antisera prepared against cell lines has been shown by a different design of experiment. Antiserum from CBA mice, given repeated injections of the CBA T6T anti-OX cell line, 010, was injected in the footpads and 4 dorsal subcutaneous sites of normal CBA mice, a total of 0.2 ml of 1/20 dilution of antiserum being given. Challenge with OX, 3,5 and 7 days later, showed the induction of anti-OX DH peaking on day 5 (Fig. I). Challenge with PC1 did not elicit DH showing the specificity of the induction. To date immunization of mice with 2 of 6 cell lines has produced antisera capable of inducing DH to an antigen with the same

Table 1.   Effect of soluble hapten and of anti-T cell idiotype on
                DTH T cell lines

Line	Antigen specificity	In vitro treatment	Ear increment* 10^{-2}mm $\pm$ SE	
O18	oxazolone	medium	5.9	0.8
O18	oxazolone	medium + ox-glycine (40g/ml)	0.5	0.5
·O18	oxazolone	CBA anti-O18 + ox-glycine	7.0	0.1
AA3	ABA	TNP.BSA	6.5	0.9
AA3	ABA	ABA.BSA	2.6	0.4
AA3	ABA	ox-glycine	6.1	1.1

*For naive mice challenged with OX = 1.0 $\pm$ 0.5
 For naive mice challenged with ABA = 2.0 $\pm$ 0.6

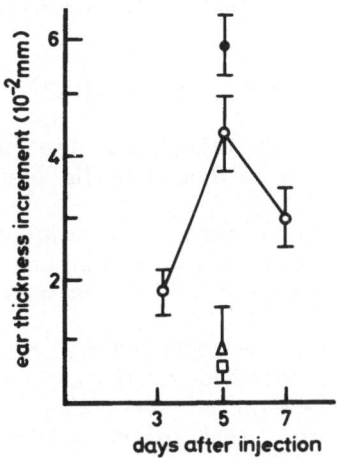

Fig 1. Anti-idiotypic activity in antiserum prepared against T cell
lines. Injection of antiserum against an anti-OX cell line (O10) induces
primary (O) or secondary (●) delayed hypersensitivity responses to OX
but not to PCl (△). □ , response of naive mice to OX.

specificity as the cell line. However, several sera from mice injected with 4 other cell lines have not induced activity.

Anti-idiotypic antibody against antibody variable regions can readily be defined because the antibody is available for detailed serological analysis. This type of analysis is not possible for T cells where the nature of the antigen-receptor molecule is unknown. Antiserum from mice injected with hapten-specific T cells does appear to contain anti-idiotypic activity by at least two criteria: (I) by its ability to induce antigen-specific DH, and (2) by its ability to interfere with an interaction between hapten and T cells in vitro. Similar results have been reported by Infante, A.J. et al. (J. Exp. Med. 155, 1100, 1982) who showed that similarly prepared antiserum could induce T cell clones to proliferate and produce IL-2. It is thought that this approach, combined with hybridoma techniques, may develop suitable probes for examining antigen-receptors on T cells.

Vitetta: Do the antisera precipitate anything?

Miller: It has not been done yet.

Vitetta: Do the antisera precipitate cell surface antigens?

Miller: It is too early for us to give an answer to this important question.

Jones: Do the antibodies made to the T_{DTH} cell lines bind (detectably) to the cells and if so, is the binding hapten-inhibitable?

Miller: We have not yet produced any evidence for this but the work is at an early stage.

Cohn: Do the lines show helper activity?

Miller: One of our ABA DTH cell line has been able to help primed B cells in vitro in an antigen specific manner.

Cohn: I would like to venture an oversimplification which might sharpen the issues. Let us assume as a minimum that
1) there are only two types of MHC restricted effector T cells, namely $T^I(T^{K/S})$ and $T^{II}(T^{H}/DH)$.
2) T^I cells are RI restricted; T^{II} cells are RII restricted.
3) T^{II} cells are required for the activation of all antigen-sensitive cells, T or B, to the T^*- and B^*-state (the associative recognition model) where they become responsive to interleukins for further proliferation and differentiation.
4) T^I cells mediate suppression of a humoral response by killing activated T^* and B^* cells which bind antigen. Antigen-sensitive T and

B cells are resistant to T^I activity. Only T^* and B^* cells are sensitive.

T^{II} cells interacting with accessory cells induce the production of interleukins, responsible for the proliferation and differentiation of activated T^* and B^* cells. This activity can override the killing activity (suppression) by T^I cells. Induction or suppression depends upon the balance between these two activities acting at the level of the activated T^* or B^* cells.

The physiological role of suppression (T^I-activity) is to regulate the class of the response, CMI or humoral, **not** the self-nonself discrimination (i.e. tolerance).

In this view, the T^I and T^{II} cells mediate their function via cell-cell interactions involving restrictive recognition of antigen and communicate a signal to the target either via a direct membrane contact or via a transmitter that only acts over synaptic distances. In the case of T^{II} cells, the known interleukins play no role in this first step of activation of T and B cells.

I question whether the presently described antigen-specific and MHC restricted factors play a normal role in the regulation of the self/nonself discrimination or class of the response by substituting for T^I or T^{II} cell-cell interactions with antigen-sensitive T or B cell targets. It is doubtful that MHC restricted, antigen-specific, T^I and T^{II} cells secrete their receptors as do B cells in order to mediate their function. It is possible that there is another class of T cells which secrete antigen-specific factors that arm target cells, e.g. macrophages, much like immunoglobulin by binding via Fc type receptors. Under certain conditions, these armed cells might suppress, enhance or mediate effector functions of the immune system. However, at the moment we have too many factors and too few functions.

Benacerraf: The systems that we have developed in our laboratory concerning the suppression of ABA and NP DTH revealed an I-J restriction whereas the system studied by Klein showed an MHC restriction until map in I-E. There can indeed be several loci which restrict suppressor T cells of different specificities. Indeed our earlier studies on the GT specific suppressors showed that in that system suppressor cells were restricted by complementing genes in I-A and I-E. Besides this point the systems that Jan Klein and I described have many analogies. Both identyty an Ly_1 T_{s1} induce and a Ts effector cell for instance.

Coutinho: Also from my ignorance of suppressor cells: 1) are these different cell types successive differentiation stages along the same pathway?

How many of these suppressor cells are there in a normal spleen

T cell compartment? 1%, 10%? If they can be cloned, it shold be possible to calculate their frequences and so far, there are not even very rough indications on these numbers.

Benacerraf: We do not have any information on the number of suppressor T cells of the various subclasses.

E. Möller: Teresa Ramos and I have studied genetic control of both cellular and humoral immunity against hapten-modified syngeneic cells. Cell-mediated immunity was measured as CTL response. Humoral immunity is a typical thymus-independent IgM response that peaks already day 4-5 and is completely gone by day 7, and is followed by a long duration of specific suppression.

What I would like to bring up now is an interesting finding that both cell-mediated immunity and humoral immunity responsiveness is genetically controlled, the CTL response by H-2 linked genes, the humoral immunity response by as yet undefined genes.

However, those strains that are high CTL responders are without exception so far low humoral immunity responders. This is probably not due to CTL's affecting antibody forming cell precursors, since responses are dominant in F_1 hybrids between high responder parental strains for the two types of immunity. This leaves us with the possibility that the repertoires in T and B cells respectively are non-overlapping and thus dependent upon each other. How this occurs is as yet not explicable in any scheme of development of immunological repertoires. (Ramos, T. and Möller, E., Immunogenetics, in press, 1982)

Session VII

B Cell Differentiation

Chairman: J. Uhr

STIMULATION OF A B CELL SUBSET BY ANTI-IMMUNOGLOBULIN AND T CELL-DERIVED REGULATORY MOLECULES

William E. Paul, Anthony L. DeFranco, Kenji Nakanishi, Elizabeth S. Raveche, John Farrar, and Maureen Howard

Laboratory of Immunology, NIAID, Laboratory of Experimental Pathology, NIADDKD, and Laboratory of Microbiology and Immunology, NIDR, National Institutes of Health, Bethesda, Maryland 20205

INTRODUCTION

B lymphocytes may be divided into distinct subpopulations which differ from one another in the membrane antigens they express, in the immunogens to which they respond, and in their sensitivity to distinct regulatory mechanisms. The appreciation that such subpopulations exist is based, to a very large extent, on studies of mice which have an immunologic defect determined by the <u>xid</u> gene. This X chromosome gene, when present in the hemizygous or homozygous state, leads to a series of B lymphocyte abnormalities among which are unresponsiveness to soluble polysaccharides and other type 2 antigens,[1] depressed serum IgM and IgG3 concentrations,[2] and failure of B lymphocytes to proliferate upon stimulation with anti-immunoglobulin (Ig) antibodies.[3] Mice with the <u>xid</u> defect lack B lymphocytes which bear the Lyb3,[4] Lyb5,[5] Lyb7,[6] and Ia.W39[7] antigens. These lymphocytes, which are found in all normal strains, will be referred to as Lyb5$^+$ B lymphocytes. The defects of xid-mice can be accounted for by the absence of Lyb5$^+$ B cells.

The properties of the two major B lymphocyte populations now recognized (i.e. Lyb5$^+$ and Lyb5$^-$ B lymphocytes) are summarized in Table 1. These assignments of function have been based on the relative properties of cells from mice with the xid-determined defect ("xid-mice"), which only possess Lyb5$^-$ B cells, and of genetically related normal mice, which possess both Lyb5$^-$ and Lyb5$^+$ B cells. In many instances these assignments have been verified by testing the functions of normal Lyb5$^-$ B cells, prepared by treating

205

Table 1. Properties of Lyb5$^+$ and Lyb5$^-$ B Cells

	B Cell Populations	
	Lyb5$^-$	Lyb5$^+$
Membrane Ig	IgM>IgD	IgD>IgM
Differentiation antigens	Lyb3$^-$, 5$^-$, 7$^-$ Most express antigen recognized by 14G8 (Ref. 8)	Lyb3$^+$, 5$^+$, 7$^+$ Most are 14G8$^-$
Responsiveness to mitogens		
1. Anti-μ	Activation without proliferation	Activation with proliferation
2. LPS	Proliferation	?
Responsiveness to antigens		
1. Type 1 antigens (e.g. TNP-Brucella abortus)	Responsive	?
2. Type 2 antigens (e.g. TNP-Ficoll)	Unresponsive	Responsive
3. Thymus-dependent antigens	Responsive	Responsive
MHC-restricted T cell-B cell interactions	Responsive (Ref. 9)	?

B cells from normal mice with anti-Lyb5 and complement (C).
Although these functional assignments appear to reasonably reflect the properties of the two B lymphocyte subpopulations, one
should be aware of some of the assumptions underlying these conclusions. First, it is assumed that Lyb5$^-$ B cells from xid mice
are similar in their properties to Lyb5$^+$ B cells from normal
donors. Second, the properties of Lyb5$^+$ B cells have been de-
duced from a comparison of normal and xid B cells or of normal B
cells and Lyb5$^-$ normal B cells; no approach to purify and directly
study Lyb5$^+$ B cells has yet been developed.

As indicated above, B lymphocytes from xid-mice fail to
incorporate tritiated thymidine in response to culture with a
variety of anti-Ig reagents, including anti-μ, anti-δ, and anti-
κ. Since these antibodies act upon B cells by binding to their
receptors, the activation caused by them would appear to provide a

polyclonal analog for the activation of B cells by antigen. The
failure of xid B cells to proliferate in response to anti-Ig
implies a fundamental difference between Lyb5$^-$ and Lyb5$^+$ B cells
in the means through which they respond to antigens. Indeed,
this is consistent with the observation that responses to soluble
polysaccharides and other type 2 antigens are limited to Lyb5$^+$ B
cells.

In using responsiveness of B lymphocytes to anti-Ig antibodies
as a model system, it became clear to us that reliance on thymidine
uptake as the sole measure of response was inadequate. In our recent studies, we have divided B cell responses to anti-Ig into three
distinct stages: 1) activation or the transition of the resting
(G$_0$) B cell into G$_1$ phase and the stimulation of its progress
through G$_1$ phase; 2) proliferation, or the stimulation of the activated (G$_1$) B cell to enter S phase and thence to divide; 3)
differentiation, or the stimulation of the proliferating or,
possibly, the G$_1$ B cell to develop into an antibody secreting cell.

We have been interested in a more detailed analysis of the
processes which regulate growth, proliferation and differentiation
of Lyb5$^+$ lymphocytes in response to anti-Ig antibodies. These
events do not appear to involve "MHC-restricted" or "cognate" T
cell-B cell interactions. In this communication, we will review
our recent work on this topic.

RESULTS AND DISCUSSION

Separate Control of Entry into G$_1$ Phase and of S Phase of Resting
B Cells

Resting B cells purified by density gradient centrifugation
were found to remain essentially constant in volume for at least 24
hours when cultured in serum-free Iscove's/F-12 medium.
Culture with specifically purified goat anti-mouse IgM (anti-μ)
antibodies for as brief a time as one hour leads to a distinct
enlargement of these cells. This enlargement is progressive and
quite synchronous for the first 24 hours of culture, provided that
anti-μ is present continuously. We believe that this enlargement
process reflects entry into and transition through G$_1$ phase as it
correlates well with both increased RNA synthesis and acquisition
of the ability to enter S phase upon receipt of the appropriate
additional signal. B cell enlargement is stimulated by stoichio-
metric concentrations of anti-μ in contrast to the very high
concentrations generally used in proliferation studies.

This new approach to the study of B cell activation by anti-
Ig has provided an important new insight into this process. While
previous studies showed that only Lyb5$^+$ B cells proliferated in
response to anti-μ, it is now clear that all B cells, including
those of xid mice, enter G$_1$ phase in response to this stimulus.

This suggests that a second stimulus controls entry of anti-μ activated B cells into S phase.

To measure the entry of anti-μ activated B cells into S phase, we stained intact nuclei with the DNA-binding dye propridium iodide and used flow microfluorometry to identify, on the basis of DNA content, those cells in G_0 and G_1, in S, and in G_2 and M phases of the cell cycle.[12-14] When this approach is used to examine dense B cells incubated with anti-μ, several important points emerge. First, such B cells do not enter S phase in any numbers until ∿30 hours after the addition of anti-μ. The entry into S phase occurs over a period of about 15 hours, indicating considerable asynchrony among the cells. Only a portion of the B cells enter S phase in response to anti-μ. This proportion ranges between 30 and 60 percent of normal B cells, depending upon the strain of mouse and reflecting experiment-to-experiment variation. Essentially no cells from xid-mice enter S phase as a result of stimulation with anti-μ. The concentration of anti-μ required to cause entry into S phase is relatively high. Ten micrograms/ml is very much better than 1 ug/ml, although these concentrations are essentially equivalent in stimulating B cell activation. Finally, anti-μ may be withdrawn approximately 6 hours before cells enter S phase without effecting this process. In contrast, removal of anti-μ during early G_1 leads to immediate cessation of the activation process.[15]

Each of the points alluded to about regulation of entry into S phase in response to anti-μ represents an instance of difference in comparison to control of activation (Table 2). These observations lead us to conclude that activation and proliferation are independently controlled processes.

Table 2. Distinct Control of Entry of B Cells into G_1 and S
          Phases in Response to Anti-μ

	$\underline{G_0 \rightarrow G_1}$	$\underline{G_1 \rightarrow S}$
Percent of adult B cells responding	All including xid B cells	30-60%; xid B cells do not respond
Concentration of anti-μ required	Low	High
Requirement for continuous presence of anti-μ	Yes	No
Is process synchronous	Yes	No
Dependent on T cells or growth factors	No	Yes

Table 3. Anti-µ Prepares Separate Populations of B Cells to
          Enter S Phase to Anti-µ or to LPS

Additions		Number of Cells in S Phase at 48 h
0 h	24 h	
–	–	10%
1 µg/ml anti-µ	–	17%
–	50 µg/ml anti-µ	12%
–	50 µg/ml LPS	13%
1 µg/ml anti-µ	50 µg/ml anti-µ	40%
1 µg/ml anti-µ	50 µg/ml LPS	43%
1 µg/ml anti-µ	50 µg/ml anti-µ + 50 µg/ml LPS	52%

A substantial fraction of B cells enter G_1 but not S in response to anti-µ. At least some of these cells appear to have been made responsive to the signals provided by another stimulant, lipopolysaccharide (LPS). To study this, we took advantage of the fact that a low concentration of anti-µ (1 µg/ml), even if present from the beginning of a 2 day culture caused almost no B cells to enter S phase and that LPS (50 µg/ml) present for the last 24 hours of the culture also failed to stimulate an appreciable fraction of the cells to enter S phase. However, stimulation of normal cells with anti-µ at the beginning of a 48 hour culture and adding LPS at 24 h led to a very substantial fraction of the cells entering S phase. Furthermore, these cells appear to be at least partially distinct from the population that entered S phase in response to a high concentration of anti-µ alone since the number of cells which entered S phase in response to 1 µg/ml of anti-µ at the beginning with 50 µg/ml of LPS and 50 µg/ml of anti-µ added at 24 hours were greater than the number of cells which entered S phase to each combination separately (Table 3).

These data are consistent with the concept that anti-µ, and possibly antigen, stimulates both Lyb5$^+$ and Lyb5$^-$ B cells to enter G_1; high concentrations of anti-µ appear to act directly or indirectly to cause many (? all) Lyb5$^+$ B cells to enter S phase. High concentrations of LPS appear to generate signals which cause many Lyb5$^-$ B cells, in G_1 phase, to enter S phase.

Growth Factor Control of B Cell Proliferation

The previous section has considered B cell activation and proliferation without reference to the possible involvement of other cell types as possible sources of growth factors which might play critical roles in these processes. It was initially believed that B cell proliferation in response to anti-µ was

Table 4. EL-4 Supernatant Contains a B Cell Growth Factor (BCGF)

Additions to culture	Tritiated thymidine uptake $(5 \times 10^4$ B Cells/well)
0	939
Anti-μ (5 μg/ml)	1,462
EL-4 supernatant (1:10)	2,886
Anti-μ + EL-4 supernatant	17,601

largely independent of the need for T cells and, possibly, macrophages.[5,16]   Indeed, when very highly purified B cell populations are cultured at high cell density (2×10^5 cells/ 0.2 ml) with specifically purified anti-μ antibody (50 ug/ml), a very striking stimulation of tritiated thymidine incorporation is observed.[17]   However, if the cell density is reduced to 5×10^4 cells/0.2 ml, almost no stimulation of thymidine uptake occurs. This suggested that another cell, or its products, might be required for B cell activation to anti-μ and that the likelihood of the interaction of the two cells was substantially diminished as a result of reducing their concentrations. We found that the addition of an induced supernatant from the C57BL/6 T cell line EL-4 reconstituted the capacity of anti-μ to stimulate tritiated thymidine uptake by B cells cultured at low density (Table 4).

    The EL-4 supernatant was prepared by stimulating these cells with phorbol myristate acetate (PMA, 10 ng/ml) for two days. This supernatant is known to contain several biologically active factors, including interleukin 2 (IL-2) and colony stimulating factor (CSF).[18]   The factor capable of stimulating B cell proliferation in response to anti-μ can be separated from both IL-2 and CSF and thus appears to be a distinct entity which we have designated B cell growth factor (BCGF).[17,18]   BCGF has an approximate Mr by gel filtration of 18,000, and is clearly resolved from IL-2 by this means. It can also be separated from IL-2 by phenylsepharose chromatography, isoelectric focusing (IEF), and sodium dodecyl sulfate-polyacrylamide gel electrophoresis. It fails to be absorbed by cells which bear IL-2 receptors. BCGF has no apparent action on resting B cells and its effect on anti-μ activated B cells is polyclonal, not MHC-restricted, and, seemingly limited to stimulation of DNA synthesis without the induction of Ig production. Table 5 presents a summary of the properties of BCGF and some sources of this material.

    There is considerable evidence which suggests that BCGF acts in G_1 on B cells which have been stimulated from the G_0 state by anti-μ. We have not yet determined precisely when in G_1 BCGF acts, nor have we yet developed an assay for BCGF receptors. One explanation which would integrate the results we have obtained with high

Table 5. Properties of BCGF

---

    1. T cell derived.
    2. M_r 18,000 (Gel filtration).
    3. Not mitogenic for resting B cells.
    4. Induces polyclonal proliferation by anti-μ activated
       B cells.
    5. Does not induce Ig secreting cells but is involved in
       responses leading to Ig secretion.
    6. Activity is not MHC-restricted.
    7. Sources: EL-4 supernatant
               FS6 14.13 supernatant
               Long term T helper cell line supernatants

      Not found in: B151k12 supernatant
                 C.C3.11.75 supernatant
                 Con A/PHA induced spleen cell supernatant
                 (24 h stimulation)

---

and low cell density conditions is that BCGF generated endogenously
is responsible for the proliferation of B cells, cultured at high
density, in response to high concentrations of anti-μ. However,
this has not been directly demonstrated. Stimulation of B cells
cultured at low density with anti-μ plus BCGF resembles stimulation of B cells cultured at high density with anti-μ alone in
that xid B cells fail to respond under either condition. We cannot exclude from the above studies the possibility that other
lymphokines or monokines may be involved in enhancing, modifying
or regulating anti-Ig induced B cell proliferation. Indeed, we
have evidence that interleukin 1 (IL1)-containing supernatants
significantly enhance BCGF-dependent anti-Ig induced B cell proliferation measured at lower cell densities than in the above
experiments. It is not yet clear however whether IL-1 exerts a
direct or secondary effect on the B cell.

<u>Regulation of IgM Synthesis in Response to Anti-μ</u>

    B cells stimulated with anti-μ and BCGF proliferated but failed
to develop into Ig-secreting cells[19] as monitored by staining cells
for cytoplasmic (c)IgM with a fluoresceinated monoclonal anti-IgM
antibody.[20] Others have shown that antigen and anti-Ig driven
differentiation into antibody secretion requires additional factors,
such as "T cell replacing factor" (TRF) and/or IL-2.[21-24] We found
that the development of specific plaque-forming cells by B cells
stimulated with sheep erythrocytes[17] and the appearance of cIgM[4]
cells in cultures of anti-μ stimulated B cells[19] required the
addition of three distinct T-cell derived factors: BCGF, purified
from induced EL-4 supernatants by either IEF or phenylsepharose

Table 6.   Role of Growth and Differentiation Factors in
            Appearance of cIgM$^+$ Cells in Response to Anti-μ

Cultures contain anti-μ (5 μg/ml) plus:	Cell Yield (day 4)	cIgM$^+$ cells (day 4)
0	+/-	+/-
BCGF	++	+/-
B15-TRF	+/-	+/-
EL-TRF	+/-	+/-
BCGF+B15-TRF	+++	+/-
BCGF+EL-TRF	++	+/-
B15-TRF+EL-TRF	+/-	+/-
BCGF+EL-TRF+B15-TRF	+++	++

chromatography; a supernatant obtained from the T cell hybridoma B151K12[22] (designated B15-TRF); and the pI-4.5 fraction from the IEF of an induced EL-4 supernatant (designated EL-TRF). The addition of any one or two of these factors to cultures of B cells stimulated with anti-μ produced few, if any, cIgM$^+$ cells (Table 6).

Interestingly, while neither B15-TRF nor EL-TRF caused proliferation of anti-μ activated B cells, B15-TRF substantially enhanced cell yields in cultures also containing anti-μ and BCGF. While the relative roles of these three co-factors in B cell development are not fully understood, preliminary results indicate that BCGF and B15-TRF are required early in the culture while EL-TRF appears to be a late-acting differentiation factor. Although EL-TRF preparations contain IL-2, our initial results indicate the active factor is not IL-2, since other preparations rich in IL-2 have very limited EL-TRF activity. EL-TRF may be identical to the recently described differentiation factor BCDF-μ.[25]

CONCLUSIONS

The studies presented here can be primarily regarded as forming a foundation for the fuller understanding of the cellular and molecular biology of the activation of Lyb5$^+$ B cells. They also allow us to propose a model for the action of various factors which regulate the activation, proliferation and differentiation of these cells. We suggest that agents which can cross-link membrane Ig receptors in an appropriate manner, such as anti-Ig antibodies and certain antigens, cause resting B cells to become activated and to enter the G_1 phase of the cell cycle. As a result of this activation, these G_1 B cells become sensitive to certain lymphokines and interaction with these agents induces the cells to enter S phase. The sensitivity of G_1 B cells to such growth factors is most likely determined by the expression of growth factor receptors on the cell membrane. Lyb5$^+$ B cells stimulated to enter G_1 by anti-μ are sensitive to the action of BCGF, a T cell derived factor, and possibly also to a macrophage-derived factor closely resembling IL-1. The differentiation of these cells into antibody-secreting cells requires two additional factors: B15-TRF, which apparently acts as a growth factor, and a differentiation factor in EL-4 supernatant (EL-TRF).

REFERENCES

1. D. E. Mosier, I. M. Zitron, J. J. Mond, A. Ahmed, I. Scher, and W. E. Paul, Surface immunoglobulin D as a functional receptor for a subclass of B lymphocytes. Immunol. Rev. 37:89 (1977).
2. R. M. Perlmutter, M. Nahm, K. E. Stein, J. Slack, I. Zitron, W. E. Paul, and J. M. Davie, Immunoglobulin subclass-specific immunodeficiency in mice with an X-linked B-lymphocyte defect. J. Exp. Med. 149:993 (1979).
3. D. G. Sieckmann, I. Scher, R. Asofsky, D. E. Mosier, and W. E. Paul, Activation of mouse lymphocytes by anti-immunoglobulin. II. A thymus-dependent response by a mature subset of B lymphocytes. J. Exp. Med. 148:1628 (1978).
4. B. Huber, R. K. Gershon, and H. Cantor, Identification of a B cell surface structure involved in antigen-dependent triggering: Absence of this structure on B cells from CBA/N mutant mice. J. Exp. Med. 145:10 (1977).
5. A. Ahmed, I. Scher, S. O. Sharrow, A. H. Smith, W. E. Paul, D. H. Sachs, and K. W. Sell, B-lymphocyte heterogeneity: Development and characterization of an alloantiserum which distinguishes B-lymphocyte differentiation alloantigens. J. Exp. Med. 145:101 (1977).
6. B. Subbarao, A. Ahmed, W. E. Paul, I. Scher, R. Lieberman, and D. E. Mosier, Lyb 7, a B cell alloantigen controlled by genes linked to the IgC$_H$ locus. J. Immunol. 122:2279 (1979).
7. B. T. Huber, Antigenic marker on a functional subpopulation of B cells, controlled by the I-A subregions of the H-2 complex. Proc. Natl. Acad. Sci. USA 76:3460 (1979).
8. J. T. Kung, S. O. Sharrow, A. Ahmed, R. Habbersett, I. Scher, and W. E. Paul, By lymphocyte subpopulation defined by a rat monoclonal antibody 14G8. J. Immunol. 128:in press.
9. Y. Asano, A. Singer, and R. J. Hodes, Role of the major histocompatibility complex in T cell activation of B cell subpopulations. MHC restricted and unrestricted B cell responses are mediated by distinct B cell subpopulations. J. Exp. Med. 154:1100 (1981).
10. N. N. Iscove, and F. Melchers, Complete replacement of serum by albumin, transferrin, and soybean lipid in cultures of lipopolysaccharide-reactive B lymphocyte. J. Exp. Med. 147:923 (1978).
11. D. E. Mosier, Primary in vitro antibody responses by purified murine B lymphocytes in serum-free defined medium. J. Immunol. 127:1490 (1981).

12. A. L. DeFranco, E. S. Raveche, R. Asofsky, and W. E. Paul, Frequency of B lymphocytes responsive to anti-immunoglobulin. J. Exp. Med. 155:1523 (1982).

13. A. Krishan, Rapid flow cytofluorometric analysis of mammalian cell cycle by propidium iodide staining. J. Cell Biol. 66: 188 (1975).

14. A. Gazdar, DNA content analysis by flow cytometry and cytogenetic analysis in Mycosis Fungoides and Sezary Syndrome. J. Clin. Invest. 65:1440 (1980).

15. A. L. DeFranco, E. S. Raveche, and W. E. Paul, manuscript in preparation.

16. D. G. Sieckmann, R. Habbersett, I. Scher, and W. E. Paul, Activation of mouse lymphocytes by anti-immunoglobulin. III. Analysis of responding B lymphocytes by flow cytometry and cell sorting. J. Immunol. 127:205 (1981).

17. M. Howard, J. Farrer, M. Hilfiker, B. Johnson, K. Takatsu, and W. Paul, Identification of a T-cell derived B-cell growth factor distinct from interleukin 2. J. Exp. Med. 155:914 (1982).

18. J. J. Farrar, W. R. Benjamin, M. L. Hilfiker, M. Howard, W. L. Farrar, and J. Fuller-Farrar, The biochemistry, biology, and role of interleukin 2 in the induction of cytotoxic T cell and antibody-forming B cell responses. Immunol. Rev. 63: 129 (1982).

19. K. Nakanishi, M. Howard, A. Muraguchi, J. Farrar, K. Takatsu, T. Hamaoka, and W. E. Paul, Manuscript in preparation.

20. J. T. Kung, S. O. Sharrow, D. G. Sieckmann, R. Lieberman, and W. E. Paul, A mouse IgM allotypic determinant (Igh-6.5) recognized by a monoclonal rat antibody. J. Immunol. 127: 873 (1981).

21. D. Parker, Induction and suppression of polyclonal antibody responses by anti-Ig reagents and antigen-nonspecific helper factors. Immunol. Rev. 52:115 (1980).

22. K. Takatsu and T. Hamaoka, DBA/2Ha mice as a model of an X-linked immunodeficiency which is defective in the expression of TRF-acceptor site(s) on B lymphocytes. Immunol. Rev. 64: 21 (1982).

23. H. J. Leibson, P. Marrack, and J. W. Kappler, B cell helper factors. I. Requirement for both interleukin-2 and another 40KD factor. J. Exp. Med. 154:1681 (1981).

24. S. Swain, G. Dennert, J. Warner, and R. Dutton, Culture supernatants of a stimulated T cell line have helper activity that syngergizes with IL-2 in the response of B cells to antigen. Proc. Natl. Acad. Sci. USA 78:2517 (1981).

25. E. Pure, P. C. Isakson, K. Takatsu, T. Hamaoka, S. L. Swain, D. W. Dutton, G. Dennert, J. W. Uhr, and E. S. Vitetta, Induction of B cell differentiation by T cell factors. I. Stimulation of IgM secretion by products of a T cell hybridoma and a T cell line. J. Immunol. 127:1953 (1981).

DISCUSSION

Cohn: I would like to attempt an interpretation of the Xid mutation.

First, I must congratulate Bill Paul on dropping the TI-1 and TI-2 versus TD designation of antigens. I recommend the designations Type 1, 2 and 3. The distinction between Type 1 substances, like LPS, and Types 2 or 3 is qualitative in that Type 1 substances are Signal (2) substitutes, whereas Types 2 and 3 require T^H sources of Signal (2). The difference between Types 2 (TNP-Ficoll) and 3 (TNP-KLH) is quantitative in that repeating polymers are very efficient utilizers of T^H activity.

The second point is that the **Xid** mutation affects the inherent inducibility of the B and possibly the T cell. The demonstration that the mutation acts at the level of the antigen-sensitive cell and not at the level of a humoral factor or hormone comes from Joe Davies who reported at the Hammer Symposium this year that in heterozygous Xid/+ females, the response to Type 2 antigens is due to only those B cells expressing the wild type X chromosome. **Xid** B cells do not respond in heterozygous females.

Given these two points then the simplest assumption, it seems to me, is that the **Xid** mutation raises the threshold level of Signal (2) required to activate the antigen-sensitive B cells (possibly T cells also) to the B^* state. It probably also raises the threshold level for the triggering of accessory cells by T^H to secrete interleukins. In this case, Type 1 substances (not antigens) like LPS induce, because they are Signal (2) substitutes; Type 3 antigens (TNP-KLH) induce because they are very effective inducers of T^H-activity. Type 2 antigens (TNP-Ficoll) generate levels of T^H-activity too low to induce the **Xid** mutant B cells, but high enough to induce wild type B cells. If the **nude** mutation is combined with **Xid**, as Wortis showed, the animal does not respond even to Type 1 substances (LPS). This implies that this unresponsiveness is due to a raised threshold for response to Signal (2) and an insufficiency of interleukins needed to drive B cell proliferation and differentiation. This latter effect is a consequence of the **nude** mutation which reduces T cell function, the source of many interleukins.

Paul: A critical point is the relation of Lyb-5⁻ to Lyb-5⁺ B cells. It has been suggested that Lyb-5⁺ B cells might be the precursors of Lyb-5⁺ B cells. This is based on the fact that Lyb-5⁻ B cells appear earlier in the life of the mouse than do Lyb-5⁺ B cells and on the related observations that many of the immune defects of Xid-mice resemble the defective immune responses of neonates.

However, the fact that Lyb-5⁻B cells appear before Lyb-5⁺ B cells does not establish a precursor-product, which simply expand at different times in the maturation of the animal.

Baltimore: Please clarify the basis for suggesting the switching pathway characteristic of Lyb-5⁺ cells.

Paul: TNP-Ficoll immunization of nu/nu C57BL/10 mice leads to a pattern of isotype expression within the anti-TNP antibodies in which IgM>IgG3>IgG1>IgG2b>IgG2a. A similar hierarchy in clonal precursors which yield daughter cells expressing these classes of anti-TNP antibody, in response to TNP-Ficoll, exists since this response is uniquely a feature of Lyb-5⁺ B cells. We have concluded that type 2 antigens stimulating Lyb-5⁺ B cells in the absence of "overt" T cell help engage a switching pathway which, among the Igh-gamma genes, leads to a pattern of expression which follows the order of these genes on the chromosom.

Vitetta: In collaboration with Peter C. Isakson, Ellen Prué, Kathryn Brook and Peter H. Krammer I have studied T cell-derived B cell growth and differentiation factors.

Several years ago, (Dutton, R., Transplant. Rev. 23:6, 1975) and Schimpl and Wecker (Transplant. Rev. 23:176, 1975) observed that cell free supernatants obtained from activated T cells could replace T cells in the induction of antibody secretion by B cells. With the development of long-term T cell clones and hybridomas, it has become possible to characterize lymphokines which affect the growth and differentiation of B cells. B cell growth factor (BCGF) has been described in both human (Ford, R. et al., Nature 294:261, 1981) and murine (Howard, M. et al., J. Exp. Med. 155:914, 1982) systems and sustains the growth of purified B cells after their activation by either anti-Ig (Howard, M. et al., J. Exp. Med. 155:914, 1982) or mitogens (Ford, R. et al., Nature 294:261, 1981). In addition, two B cell differentiation factors have been described, termed $BCDF_u$ (Pure, E. et al., J. Immunol. 127:1954, 1981) and $BCDF_{gamma}$ (Isakson, P.C. et al., J. Exp. Med. 155:734, 1982), which induce the polyclonal secretion of IgM and IgG, respectively. In the case of $BCDF_u$, the secretion of IgG is induced in LPS-stimulated B cells that do not bear sIgG (Isakson, P.C. et al., J. Exp. Med. 155:734, 1982). In this report, we describe the effects of these lymphokines on the growth and differentiation of mature and immature B cells and discuss the implications of these results for B cell activation and isotype switching.

Identification and Description of $BCDF_u$

We previously reported that cells from the non-secreting **in vivo** BCL_1 tumor line can be induced to secrete IgM by soluble T cell

127:1954, 1981). More recently, we and others have assayed supernatants from several monoclonal populations of T cells (lines, hybridomas, and tumors) to identify the factors which mediate this effect.
Some of these monoclonal sources of $BCDF_u$ are summarized in Table
I. Three of the most potent producers of $BCDF_u$ are the FS7-6.18
hybridoma (stimulated with Con A) (Harwell, L. et al., J. Exp. Med.
152:734, 1980), the EL-4 thymoma, (stimulated by phorbol myristate
acetate) (Farrar, J. et al., J. Immunol. 125:2555, 1980) and the long-
term alloreactive (AKR anti-C57BL/6) T cell line, designated 7.1
(stimulated with Con A) (Krammer, P.H. et al., In: Isolation, Characterization and Utilization of T lymphocytes. Fathman, G., and Fitch, F.,
Eds., Academic press, New York, pp. 252-262, 1982). When BCL_1 cells
or normal (T-depleted) B cells from adult or neonatal mice are
cultured with supernatants from either 7.1 or EL-4, there is a 10 to
30-fold increase in the number of IgM PFC (Table II) and a 5-fold
increase in the concentration of IgM in the culture medium (Fig. 1).
$BCDF_u$-mediated IgM secretion occurs in the absence of either anti-
immunoglobulin or LPS. Since the cells which can be induced to secrete
IgM are essentially free of T cells, the data suggest that $BCDF_u$ acts
directly on B cells. Furthermore, the 7.1 cells do not produce IL-2,
IFN-gamma, or conventional (Schimpl, A., and Wecker, E., Transplant.
Rev. 23:176, 1975) TRF (Krammer, P.H., et al., In: Isolation, Characterization and Utilization of T lymphocytes. Fathman, G. and Fitch,
F., Eds., Academic press, New York, pp. 252-262, 1982) suggesting that
$BCDF_u$ is distinct from these lymphokines and that they are not
obligatory for the induction of $BCDF_u$-mediated IgM secretion. In
recent experiments, we have demonstrated that the addition of purified
IL-2 to BCL_1 cells neither induces IgM secretion itself nor enhances
the effect of the 7.1 supernatant (Pure, E., Isakson, P., Paetkau, V.,
Vitetta, E.S. and Krammer, P., 1982, Submitted for publication).
Furthermore, using a cloned line of BCL_1 cells maintained **in vitro**,
macrophages, or their products (Brooks, K., Uhr, J., Krammer, P.H.
and Vitetta, E.S., 1982, Manuscript in preparation).

These studies provide evidence that $BCDF_u$ acts directly on B
cells to induce their differentiation. Preliminary studies using gel
filtration columns suggest that $BCDF_u$ has a molecular weight of
30,000-60,000 (Pure, E., Isakson, P., Krammer, P.H. and Vitetta, E.S.,
1982, Submitted for publication), which is larger than that reported for
B cell growth factor (15,00-20,000) (Ford, R. et al., Nature 294:261,
1981).

Identification and Description of BCGF

BCGF has been defined by its capacity to sustain the growth and
proliferation of anti-Ig-stimulated B cells (Ford, R. et al., Nature
294:261, 1981). Since both the EL-4 and 7.1 supernatants contain
BCGF, we have compared the effects of these supernatants on normal

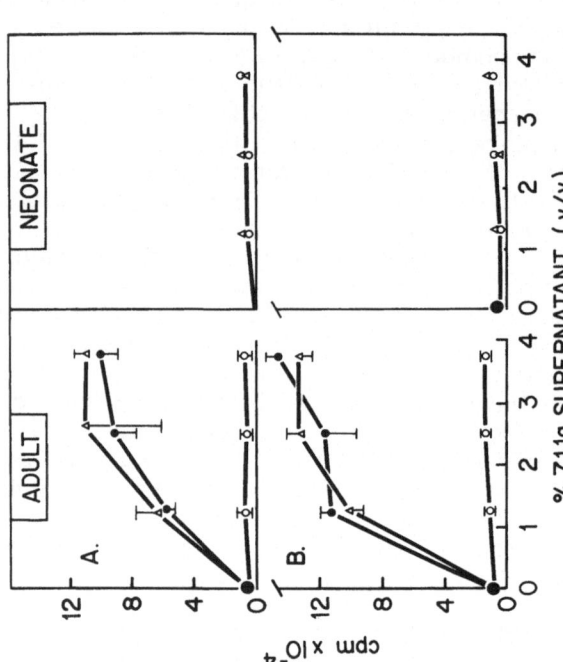

Figure 1. Response of B cells from adult and 13 day old neonatal BALB/c mice to BCGF. Splenic B cells were cultured at (A) 12.5 × 10^5/ml or (B) 5 × 10^5/ml in the presence of Sepharose-coupled ● anti-u, △ anti-delta, or ○ normal Ig. 7.1.1a supernatant was added and 3 days later cells were pulsed for 16 hours with ^{3}H-TdR. Results are expressed as mean cpm ± S.D.

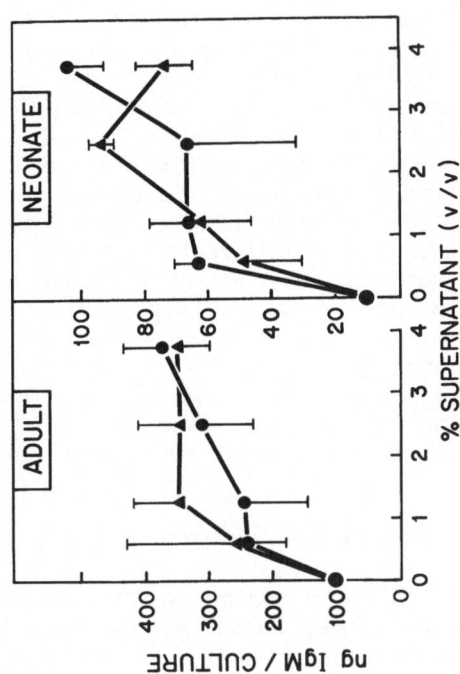

Figure 2. Response of B cells from adult and 13 day old neonatal mice to BCDFμ. Splenic B cells were cultured for 4 days at 5 x 10⁵/ml with ● 7.1.1a or ▲ 7.1.2 supernatant. IgM secretion was determined by a solid phase radioimmunoassay.

B cells from adult and neonatal mice (Pure, E., Isakson, P., Krammer, P.H. and Vitetta, E.S., 1982, Submitted for publication). This comparison was of particular interest since neonatal B cells give a poor proliferative response to some mitogens, such as LPS, but, nevertheless, can be induced to secrete IgM and IgG by the same mitogens (Kearney, J.F. and Lawton, A.R., J. Immunol. 115:677, 1975). From these results, it could be predicted that neonatal cells would respond to BCDF but not to BCGF. To test this possibility directly, neonatal and adult B cells were treated with either anti-u or anti-delta coupled to Sepharose, and cultured in the presence of these BCGF-containing supernatants. Three days later, cells were pulsed with ^{3}H-thymidine and the stimulation index was determined. As seen in Fig. 2, adult B cells respond to BCGF, but neonatal B cells do not despite the fact that they can be induced to differentiate to IgM-secreting cells in the presence of BCDF$_u$. As defined by their molecular weights, BCGF and BCDF$_u$ appear to be different lymphokines (Pure, E., Isakson, P., Krammer, P.H. and Vitetta, E.S., 1982, Submitted for publication). These results suggest that the interaction of anti-Ig with immunoglobulin receptors on neonatal B cells in the presence of BCGF, does not result in clonal expansion despite the fact that the cells can be induced to differentiate into IgM secreting cells. In contrast, adult B cells can both clonally expand and differentiate. These differences are depicted in the model described in Fig. 3. To what extent terminal differentiation in the absence of clonal expansion is physiologically relevant to the immuno-incompetence and ease of tolerance induction in immature B cells (Metcalf, E.S. and Klinman, N.R., J. Exp. Med. 143:1327, 1976) is at present unclear. However, it is conceivable that such a mechanism might prevent the expansion of immature self-reactive B cell clones until the normal suppressor network becomes operational.

Identification and Characterization of BCDF$_{gamma}$

Small IgM$^+$ IgD$^+$ B cells can switch to the production of other classes of immunoglobulin (Nossal, G.V.J. et al., Cell Immunol. 2:41, 1971; Pernis, B., XLI Cold Spring Harbor Symposium on Quantitative Biology. Origins of Lymphocyte Diversity. 41:175, 1976; Wabl, M.R. et al., Science 199:1978, 1978). This switch can be induced by either antigenic (Press, J.L. and Klinman, N.R., J. Exp. Med. 138:300, 1973; Gearhart, P.J. et al., Proc. Natl. Acad. Sci. 72:1707, 1975) or mitogenic stimulation and is relatively T cell dependent (Braley-Mullen, H., J. Immunol. 113:1909, 1974; Torrigiani, G., J. Immunol. 108:161, 1972;Taylor, R.B. and Wortis, H.H., Nature 220:927, 1968). T cells can also influence the subclass of IgG secreted by B cells (Slack, J. et al., J. Exp. Med. 151:853, 1980; Mongini, P.K.A. et al., J. Exp. Med. 153:1, 1981). In low density cell cultures in the presence of lipopolysaccharide (LPS), IgG secretion by murine B cells may not require T cells (Andersson, J. et al., J. Exp. Med. 147:1744, 1978; Andersson, J. et al., Eur. J. Immunol. 8:336, 1978; Kearney, J.F. et al., J. Immunol.

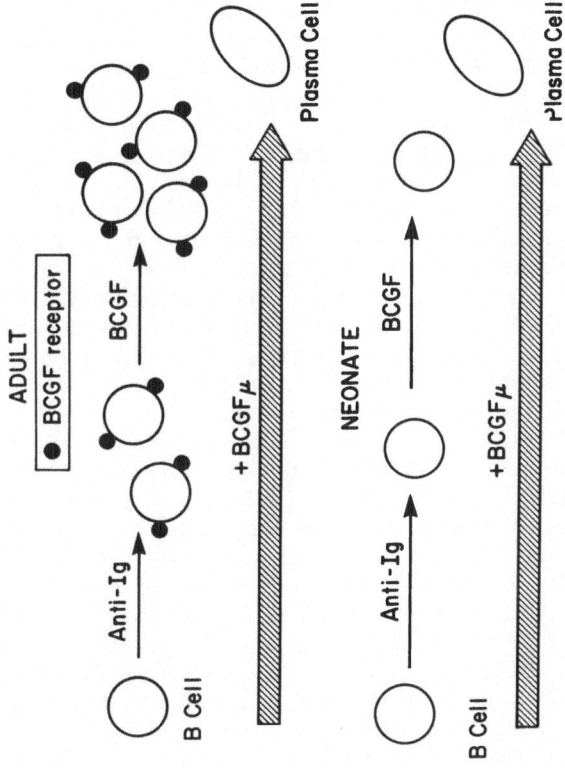

Figure 3. Model for the growth and differentiation of immature and mature B cells.

We have used B cells stimulated by LPS to investigate the effect of several monoclonal T cell-derived supernatants on isotype switching in normal B cells. As shown in Table III, two potent sources of $BCDF_u$ are the EL-4 and 7.1 supernatants. Neither supernatant affects the amount of IgM secreted in response to LPS (data not shown), but both increase the amount of IgG secreted, particularly when added one day after the initiation of the LPS culture.

$BCDF_{gamma}$ induces IgG secretion in both adult and neonatal B cells (not shown). Thus, like $BCDF_u$, $BCDF_{gamma}$ can act on immature cells which do not have the capacity to respond to BCGF, but can switch from IgM to IgG secretion. It appears that $BCDF_{gamma}$ is distinct from IL-2, TRF, and IFN-gamma since the 7.1 supernatant lacks these lymphokines (Farrar, J. et al., J. Immunol. 125:2555, 1980). By molecular weight analysis, $BCDF_{gamma}$ also appears to be different from $BCDF_u$ since $BCDF_{gamma}$ has a molecular weight of 15,000-20,000 whereas $BCDF_u$ is larger (Pure, E., Isakson, P., Krammer, P.H. and Vitetta, E.S., 1982, Submitted for publication). An analysis of the subclasses of IgG secreted following the addition of BCDF to LPS-stimulated B cells indicates a striking increase in IgG_1 secretion with a concomitant decrease in IgG_2 (Isakson, P., Pure, E., Krammer, P.H. and Vitetta, E.S., 1982, Manuscript in preparation). These results suggest that the $BCDF_{gamma}$ in both 7.1 and EL.4 supernatants may be subclass specific. $BCDF_{gamma}$ cannot, however, be absorbed with IgG_1 coupled to Sepharose (Isakson, P., Pure, E., Krammer, P.H. and Vitetta, E.S., 1982, Manuscript in preparation).

$BCDF_{gamma}$ induces IgG secretion in both adult and neonatal B cells (not shown). Thus, like $BCDF_u$, $BCDF_{gamma}$ can act on immature cells which do not have the capacity to respond to BCGF, but can switch from IgM to IgG secretion. It appears that $BCDF_{gamma}$ is distinct from IL-2, TRF, and IFN-gamma since the 7.1 supernatant lacks these lymphokines (Farrar, J. et al., J. Immunol. 125:2555, 1980). By molecular weight analysis, $BCDF_{gamma}$ also appears to be different from $BCDF_u$ since $BCDF_{gamma}$ has a molecular weight of 15,000-20,000 whereas $BCDF_u$ is larger (Pure, E., Isakson, P., Krammer, P.H. and Vitetta, E.S., 1982, Submitted for publication). An analysis of the subclasses of IgG secreted following the addition of BCDF to LPS-stimulated B cells indicates a striking increase in IgG_1 secretion with a concomitant decrease in IgG_2 (Isakson, P., Pure, E., Krammer, P.H. and Vitetta, E.S., 1982, Manuscript in preparation). These results suggest that the $BCDF_{gamma}$ in both 7.1 and EL.4 supernatants may be subclass specific. $BCDF_{gamma}$ cannot, however, be absorbed with IgG_1 coupled to Sepharose (Isakson, P., Pure, E., Krammer, P.H. and Vitetta, E.S., 1982, Manuscript in preparation).

To study the phenotype of the B cell responding to $BCDF_{gamma}$, B cells were stained with an anti-gamma reagent and negatively

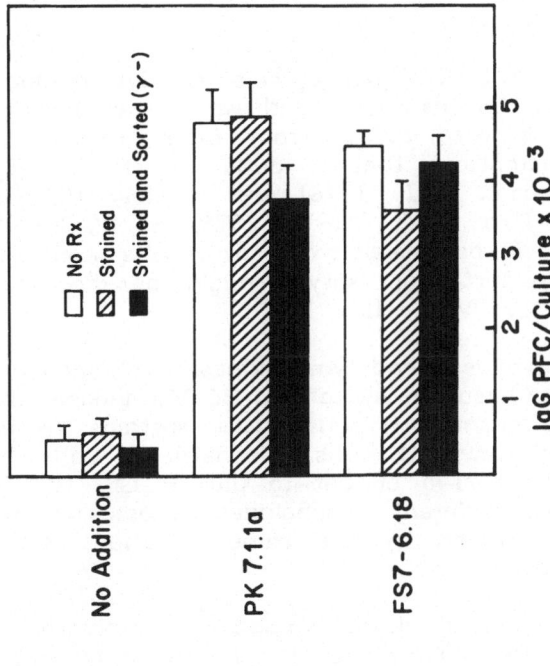

Figure 4. Induction of IgG secretion in sIgG⁻ cells cultured with T cell supernatants in the presence of LPS. B cells were stained with FITC-F(ab')$_2$ rabbit anti-IgG and positively stained cells were removed on the fluorescence activated cell sorter. Cells were cultured for 6 days at 2×10^5/ml with 20 ug LPS. IgG-secreting cells were enumerated by a PFC assay.

selected on the fluorescence activated cell sorter (Isakson, P.C. et al., J. Exp. Med. 155:734, 1982). The sIgG$^-$ cells were cultured in the presence of LPS and BCDF$_{gamma}$ (PK7.1.1a or FS7-6.18) and IgG secretion was assessed after 6 days. As seen in Fig. 4, the removal of sIgG$^+$ cells had no effect on the BCDF$_{gamma}$-induced IgG response, indicating that the precursors of the IgG-secreting cells lack sIgG at the initiation of the culture. Furthermore, an analysis of the precursor frequency of the BCDF$_{gamma}$-treated cells indicated that there was a significant increase in precursors secreting IgG$_1$ with little or no increase in their burst size (Isakson, P., Pure, E., Krammer, P.H. and Vitetta, E.S., 1982, Manuscript in preparation). These results support the notion that BCDF$_{gamma}$ induces a switch in isotype production by LPS-stimulated B cells. Whether or not these B cells are already committed to synthesize IgG, e.g. by appropriate rearrangement of DNA or by splicing of RNA is not known.

Our results suggest that BCDF$_{gamma}$ is a new lymphokine which differs from others thus far described and which can induce LPS-stimulated B cells to secrete IgG$_1$. From other reports in the literature, there are indications that T cells secrete BCDF$_{gamma}$ (Ishizaka, K., Adv. Immunol. 23:1, 1976) and possibly BCDF$_{gamma}$ (Elson, C.O. et al., J. Exp. Med. 14:632, 1979). If BCDFs for all classes and subclasses of Ig do indeed exist, or results would suggest that the switch to **any** particular isotype might be directed by a specific lymphokine secreted by T cells.

In summary, we have described lymphokines which induce B cell growth, differentiation, and isotype switching. BCDFs induce differentiation in both adult and neonatal B cells. BCGF sustains the anti-Ig-mediated proliferation of adult B cells. Neonatal B cells do not proliferate in response to anti-Ig or anti-Ig plus BCGF. BCDF$_u$ and BCDF$_{gamma}$ appear to be different lymphokines as assessed by their molecular weights. Furthermore, by the same criterion, BCGF and BCDF$_u$ appear to be different.

The mechanisms by which these lymphokines activate B cells remain to be determined. By analogy with T cell growth factors (Robb, R.J. et al., J. Exp. Med. 154:1455, 1981) and conventional hormones, it is likely that the lymphokines BCDF and BCGF act via specific receptors on the surface of either resting or activated B cells.

E. Möller: I fail to see that your tolerance induction scheme of exhaustive differentiation in immature cells would have an important biological significance, since the extremely high turn-over rate in the B cell system would very soon create new immunocompetent cells with probably very similar specificities.

Baltimore: You gain nothing from a process of neonatal tolerance because of new B-cell production in adults plus somatic mutation.

Coutinho: Let me just add two points from our experience with B cell-specific growth and maturation factors. First, neonatal B cells, in contrast to what was claimed here, respond to growth factors (BCGF) as well as adult B cells. They are certainly deficient, but rather in the ability to mature to high-rate secretion of Ig. A similar population of B cells appears to exist throughout life in the marrow. Secondly, I want to comment on the mutual interplay between growth and maturation factors. By using either selectively prepared conditioned media containing only one of those activities, or chemically separated fractions, it appears that the responses obtained from individual clones (proliferation versus maturation) depend upon the relative concentrations of each factor. Previous models based on a single factor (e.g. BRMF) do not account for this balance between growth and maturation in proliferating B cells.

Uhr: The results of Coutinho's absorption studies are provocative. To pursue them to a definitive conclusion, however, it would be important to use eventually a highly purified lymphokine rather than a supernatant containing a dozen different lymphokines many of unknown activity. Clearly, there must be receptors on at least one lymphocyte subset for the differentiation factors in question and the most likely subset(s) is a stimulated Lyb-5$^+$ one.

Coutinho: My main problem about maturation factors (BCMF) concerns their precise mechanism of action and of their recognition by target cells. I am thinking more precisely about the failure to absorb these factors on activated B cells (in contrast with BCGF (Leanderson et al., PNAS in press)) confirming the past experience on the failures to absorb TRF (also a maturation activity) with activated spleen cells. This situation is similar to that observed with CTL, which readily absorb T_kCGF but apparently fail to remove T_kCMI from conditioned media.

G. Möller: It is clear that different B cell populations exist characterized by different surface markers and activation properties. I have always thought about these subpopulations as being members of the same line. However, it is possible that B cells, as T cells, consist of parallell lines. Does Bill Paul have any evidence for or against one line versus parallell lines?

Paul: No definite evidence exists to distinguish the one or two lineage models. However, suggestive evidence is obtained from the study of nu/nu CBA/N mice. These animals have virtually no lymph node B cells and the relatively small number of splenic B cells they possess fail to mediate any detectable responses. They have very depressed serum Ig concentrations. This would suggest that the development of Lyb-5$^-$ B cells is dependent upon thymic influence. By contrast, "normal" nude mice (i.e. nu/nu CBA/Ca mice) express relatively normal B cell functions, including responses to type 2 antigens (i.e. responses of Lyb-5+ B cells). If the nu/nu defect precludes the development of functional Lyb-5- B cells but does not affect the development of functional Lyb-5+ B cells, it is very difficult to postulate that Lyb-5- B cells are the antecedents of Lyb-5+ B cells.

Benacerraf: Bill (Paul), can you comment on the properties of Ia.W39, a molecule expressed on B cells and macrophages and which function as a restrictive antigen presentation molecule.

Jones: I can answer to the question about the identity of Ia.W39. Brigitte Huber made antibodies in (CBA/N x B6)F_1 males (defective) against cells from B6 (normal) mice. This antibody reacts with I-A^b antigen indistinguishable by 2-D gels from normal I-A^b antigens, even though the producers of the antiserum has the **b** haplotype.

Benacerraf: This Ia.W39 does restrict immune response to certain antigens under Ia gene control as shown by Brigitte Huber. It is therefore a very important molecule, since it is very little different from I-A coded Ia molecules.

Ohno: Since the CBA/N mutation is X-linked, heterozygotes can be very informative. If a defect in a humoral factor, both B cells with a normal X and those with a mutant X should become Lyb-5+ in heterozygotes. If a defect resides within the cell, all Lyb-5+ cells in heterozygotes should be cells with a normal X. The introduction of X-linked markers such as PGK isozymes might be worthwhile.

Paul: Heterozygotes appear to be phenotypically normal. Joseph David and his colleagues have recently reported that in heterozygotes, those B cells which make responses of the IgG$_3$ type uniquely express the X chromosome of the normal parent, strongly implying that those with the X chromosome from the Xid parent are abnormal.

Uhr: Since we are placing considerable reliance on the CBA/N mouse as a useful model to help dissect out the normal B cell compartment, would you like to comment on the status of T cells in this strain?

Paul: In general, the T cells of Xid mice are normal with the exception that some "Th$_2$" cells, particularly those specific for the T-15 idiotype appear to be lacking. Bottomly and her colleagues have interpreted this as a secondary event flowing from the failure of Xid B cells to express T-15.

Svejgaard: 1. What are the differences between the immune deficiency in Xid mice and that in human with Brutton's agammaglobulinaemia?

2. Do Xid mice have abnormalities outside the immune system? If so, these abnormalities may point to a possible enzyme or other deficiency in these animals which might explain their immune deficiency.

Paul: The Xid defect in mice much more closely resembles the immunologic abnormalities of the Weiskott-Aldrich syndrome than of Bruton type agammaglobulinemia. This may be misleading, however, since when Xid is expressed together with other genes (i.e. nu/nu or an unidentified C3H gene) the phenotype changes quite dramatically.

Benacerraf: Bill (Paul), can you give us an idea which is the contribution of Lyb-5⁻ and Lyb-5⁺ to conventional immune response in adult animals, i.e. immune response to T dependent antigen and to T dependent antigens?

Paul: It is really quite difficult to provide an estimate of the fractional representation of Lyb-5⁺ and Lyb-5⁻ B cells in the in vivo antibody responses of **normal** mice to T-dependent antigens.

Uhr: The problem is the following: Polyclonal in vitro experiments indicate a major role for non specific T cell derived lymphokines. In contrast, in antigen induced cell cultures and in antigen induced adoptive transfer experiments, classical cognate recognition i.e. carrier specific, MHC restricted helper T cells appear to be crucial. In fact, at this point in time, we cannot state what the contributions of these 2 different pathways are to a physiological antibody response to a conventional thymic dependent antigen.

Cohn: What is type-2 thymus-independent antigens?

Paul: I do not believe that the differences between antigen classes are so difficult to account for and that the disjunction could not be made directly by B cells. In general, type-2 antigens are soluble polysaccharides which have large numbers of similar epitopes and which resist enzymatic degradation. Such molecules will, almost certainly, crosslink B cell membrane receptors quite differently than will conventional T-dependent antigens, which are easily degradable proteins expressing only 1, or only a few, copies of any given epitope. type-1 thymus-independent antigens appear to possess an innate activating signal, acting either directly on the B cell, or indirectly, but also allowing the B cell to appreciate the difference between epitopes on such carriers from those on either type 1 or TD carriers.

G. Möller: Is the Ig repertoir in Lyb-5⁺ and Lyb-5⁻ cells the same?

Paul: It is the same.

Cohn: According to the associative recognition model ("two signal" model) the first step in the induction of all antigen-sensitive cells (T or B) involves an interaction with a T-helper. This step is required in order to make the self/nonself discrimination and is mediated via a cell-cell interaction characterized by restrictive and associative recognition of antigen. Although the signalling mechanism is unknown, it must operate over synaptic distances and therefore cannot involve any of the known interleukins. The consequence of this interaction is an activated cell sensitive to interleukins which act in an intermediate distance range. The activated cell reacting with antigen and various interleukins now divides or differentiates to an end cell depending on the interleukins it encounters. The interleukins do not substitute for T_H-interactions with antigen-sensitive cells; they mediate division and differentiation in cells which have undergone and responded to the first and critical step of restrictive and associative recognition of antigen.

Coutinho: The model of B cell activation that you have presented can only apply if T-B cell interactions are not MHC restricted (antigen-dependent and direct induction of reactivity to helper factors produced upon T-macrophage interactions). Singer's experiments make in fact the claim that a subset of B cells can be induced in such an unrestricted way and you, therefore, limit your model to that subpopulation. There is a major problem, though, and this is the quantitative aspects of the argument. Thus, if about half of all B cells could be induced in this way (from the Lyb-5 phenotype and the direct cell cycle measurements you presented) Katz would have never discovered restriction of T-B cell interactions. If I am not mistaken both in those as in the more recent in vivo (J. Sprent) or in vitro (P. Marrack) experiments, the restriction is absolute. In other words, if that model applies, it concerns a very minor fraction of all cells.

Paul: I believe that data of Singer and his colleagues show clearly that Lyb-5$^-$ B cells are largely limited to "MHC-restricted" (cognate) T cell - B cell interactions. However, whether Lyb-5$^+$ B cells **cannot** display similar responses is not established, only that they are capable of "factor-mediated" interactions.

Sprent: I agree with Dr. Benacerraf that the secondary in vivo response to T-dependent antigens seems to involve mainly the Lyb-5$^-$ subset. In my hands the secondary response to sheep red cells in vivo is highly restricted at the level of T-B interaction, which implies that only the Lyb-5$^-$ cells and not the Lyb-5$^+$ cells are involved. Moreover, excellent responses are found with CBA/N B cells, i.e. cells which lack the Ly-b5$^+$ subset.

I have a question for Dr. Paul. Your finding that CBA/N nude mice have a few B cells in the spleen, but virtually none in the lymph node (LN) might imply that the production of LN-seeking (though not necessarily spleen-seeking) $Lyb-5^-$ cells is T-dependent. If so, in contrast to spleen cells, the proportion of $Lyb-5^-$ cells in the lymph nodes of non-Xid nude mice should be extremely low. Is this known?

Paul: We do not really know.

Uhr: It is important to emphasize to the non-B cell immunologists that there is a major gap in the available data concerning the function of the Ig receptors on B cells. The data we have discussed to date represents exclusively anti-Ig induced cross-linking of these receptors. We assume but no one has shown that polyvalent **antigen** can imitate anti-Ig. In other words, no one has demonstrated that in a population of $Lyb-5^+$ antigen-enriched cells, antigen can drive the cells to G_1 and together with BCGF and $BCDF_u$ induce Igh secretion. An additional reason for concern about this gap in the data is the stoichiometry of the anti-Ig effect. Although small amounts of anti-Ig are sufficient to make B cells enter G_1, very large amounts are needed to induce them to enter the S phase. The amounts needed in fact exceed those necessary for saturation of the B cell Ig receptors and this high level of anti-Ig must be present for a fairly long duration of time. This finding is not readily explainable and therefore adds impetus to the need to do experiments with specific antigen similar to the polyclonal experiments that we have discussed during this session.

I believe the major theme to emerge from this session is that B cells from normal lymphoid organs display marked heterogeneity apart from specificity to antigen. This heterogeneity is at the levels of antigen dependent and independent differentiation and results in the development of a large number of B cell subsets that have different requirements for activation, different surface phenotypes and different potential for secreting particular isotypes. We have not yet determined whether there is a single lineage during antigen-independent differentiation or whether there are branches. Because of this heterogeneity, we must use reductionist models using purified subsets and/or clones to determine the requirements for signalling these subsets and the relationship of one subset to another. Eventually, it will be necessary to determine how the whole system works in vivo.

Session VIII

B Cell Regulation I

Chairman: F. Melchers

THE DEGREE OF CLONAL ELIMINATION IN IMMUNOLOGICAL TOLERANCE AND REGULATION OF HEAVY CHAIN CLASS SWITCHES

Göran Möller, Susanne Bergstedt-Lindqvist, Carmen Fernandez and Eva Severinson

Department of Immunobiology
Karolinska Institute
Wallenberglaboratory
Lilla Frescati
104 05 Stockholm
Sweden

INTRODUCTION

Most concepts of the mechanism of lymphocyte activation and of tolerance induction are based on the interaction between antigen and the immunoglobulin (Ig) receptors. It is of importance, therefore, to study whether the entire clone is affected during the immune response or in tolerance induction, since the only common property of the clone is that all the cells have the same Ig receptor. It is already clear than an immune response does not involve all B cells in a clone. One example is given by Paul et al. in this symposium, when he shows that the Lyb-5 markers determine the ability to respond rather than the Ig receptors. However, it is less clear in tolerance induction and at least one theory of tolerance induction[1] actually predicts that tolerance results in clonal deletion and is the consequence of antigen interaction with the Ig receptors in the absence of a second signal.

In this paper we will analyze whether induction of tolerance leads to deletion of the entire B cell clone. We will also focuss attention on immunoglobulin heavy chain class switches and illustrate with some examples that the switch is probably regulated.

TOLERANCE

If it can be shown that a particular phenomenon of immunological unresponsiveness eliminates or irreversibly inhibits the entire B cell

233

clone it is highly probable that the mechanism of unresponsiveness is mediated by the Ig receptors. Contrariwise, if the entire clone is not eliminated, it is very likely that the mechanism does not directly involve the Ig receptors, but other receptors or properties of the B cells.

Methods to Study the Degree of Clonal Elimination

The most convenient way to establish whether a particular phenomenon of specific immunological unresponsiveness is due to clonal elimination or not is to use polyclonal B cell activators (PBA). These substances have the capacity to directly activate a large proportion of resting B cells to antibody synthesis without interacting with the Ig receptors[2]. Different PBAs act on different B cell subpopulations and the applications of several PBAs can therefore reveal the immuno-competence of most B cells belonging to a particular clone[3]. However, lipoplysaccharide (LPS) alone is usually sufficient, since this PBA can activate about 30% of the B cells. In certain cases it may be necessary to dissociate or remove the antigen from the Ig receptors before activating them with LPS, as will be described below. Thus, if a particular PBA can induce antibody synthesis against the relevant antigen, unresponsiveness cannot be due to a complete elimination of the clone.

A different approach utilizes thymus-independent and thymus-dependent forms of the same antigen. It is well known that these two types of antigens activate different B cell populations. If unrespon-siveness to a thymus-independent form of an antigen can be broken by thymus-dependent forms of the same antigen, unresponsiveness did not affect the entire clone of B cells.

Immunological Tolerance

Specific immunological tolerance can be induced by antigen doses that are considerably larger than those needed for an immune response. Tolerance to thymus-dependent antigens can affect helper T cells and B cells differently, whereas tolerance to most thymus-independent antigens does not involve T cells. Although several different mechanisms can lead to a state of specific unresponsiveness after antigen contact, we will limit our discussion to the classical tolerance phenomenon generally considered to represent a central defect of immunocompetence. We will define immunological tolerance to thymus-independent antigens as an inability of B cells to respond to the antigen because they have received an active signal leading to irreversible inactivation or elimination of the reactive B cells.

The Immune Response to Dextran

Native dextran B512 is a linear polymer of glucose in alpha 1-6 linkages. It is a thymus-independent antigen that gives rize to a mono- or pauciclonal immune response. The ability to respond is determined by one or several closely linked Igh-V gene(s) and mice that lack or do not express the gene cannot respond[3]. An important point in this connection is that non-responder mice cannot make use of other V genes to produce antibodies against the alpha 1-6 epitope, since non-responder mice remain unresponsive during their life time. In addition, young mice of high responder strains that possess the Igh-V gene do not express this gene or any other genes coding for antibodies against dextran for a long time period after birth[4]. Unresponsiveness in these two situations is not due to suppressor T cells or other suppressive cells or influences as shown by various types of mixing and transfer experiments described elsewhere[4].

Induction of Tolerance to Dextran

Immunogenicity of dextran B512 varies with the molecular weight[5]. Dextran preparations above 70.000 daltons are immunogenic and immunogenicity increases with the MW up to native dextran (MW $10 - 100 \times 10^6$). The ability of dextran to act as a polyclonal B cell activator also increases with molecular weight in parallel with immunogenicity[6].

Tolerance is regularly induced by injecting 5 - 10 mg/mouse of native dextran, e.g. 1000 times the optimal immunogenic dose and tolerance is complete and long lasting[7].

Tolerance is Caused by an Active Signal

We have shown before that tolerance is not induced immediately after injection of dextran into mice or after adding dextran to lymphocytes in vitro. More than 2 and less than 24 hours was required for tolerance induction[8]. In an attempt to study whether tolerance is caused by an active signal or passive events, such as blocking of immunoglobulin receptors, we compared tolerogenicity of native dextran with that of dextran MW 40.000, which is neither an immunogen nor a polyclonal B cell activator. Mice were given 10 mg native dextran or 100 - 150 mg of dextran 40.000 and thereafter both groups were immunized with an immunogenic dose of native dextran. There was no response to the alpha 1-6 epitope in any group. However, when the tolerized mice were given dextranase and thereafter immunized with native dextran, the animals given high doses of dextran MW 40.000 responded, indicating that they had not been tolerized, whereas those given 10 mg of native dextran, remained unresponsive even after dextranase treatment (Bergstedt-Lindqvist, Fernandez and Möller, unpublished data).

These findings indicate that non-immunogenic dextran preparations are non-tolerogenic[7], suggesting that tolerance requires a signal and cannot be explained by passive events such as immunoglobulin receptor blockade. However, if dextran was not removed by treating the animals with dextranase, the mice could not be immunized by native dextran, presumably because the immunoglobulin receptors on the specific B cells were blocked by the non-immunogenic dextran. Thus, the intact mice were phenotypically tolerant after treatment with high doses of dextran 40.000, although all their dextran-specific B cells remained in a resting state and could be activated by an immunogenic dextran preparation, provided their immunoglobulin receptors have been cleared from the dextran by treatment with dextranase.

Breaking of Tolerance to Dextran

It is well known that immunological tolerance to thymus-dependent antigens can be broken by the injection of cross-reactive antigens[9]. A common explanation for this phenomenon is that tolerance primarily affects T cells, but not B cells and therefore the cross-reactive antigen can interact with T cells directed against the new antigenic determinants[10]. Although this model is a sufficient explanation for breaking of tolerance to thymus-dependent antigens, it cannot be applied to thymus-independent antigens. Therefore, we studied whether tolerance to dextran could be broken by cross-reactive antigens.

Mice were tolerized with 10 mg of native dextran and at various times thereafter given dextranase. They were subsequently immunized, either with native dextran or with dextran conjugated to different protein antigens. The molecular weight of the dextran molecules conjugated to proteins varied from 7.000 (conjugated to the plant protein edestin) to 70.000 (conjugated to BSA, protein A, staphylococcus bacteria and others). It was shown that all the dextran-protein conjugates used were thymus-dependent.

It was consistently found that mice made tolerant to native dextran (and thereafter treated with dextranase) remained unresponsive when immunized with native dextran, but always gave an immune response to the thymus-dependent dextran-protein conjugates (Fig.1)[11]. This immune response was indistinguishable from that obtained with native dextran in non-tolerized mice. Since there appears to be only one or a few linked Igh-V gene(s) coding for antibodies to dextran and since other genes are not used (see above) it seems highly unlikely that the response to dextran-protein conjugates in tolerized mice could

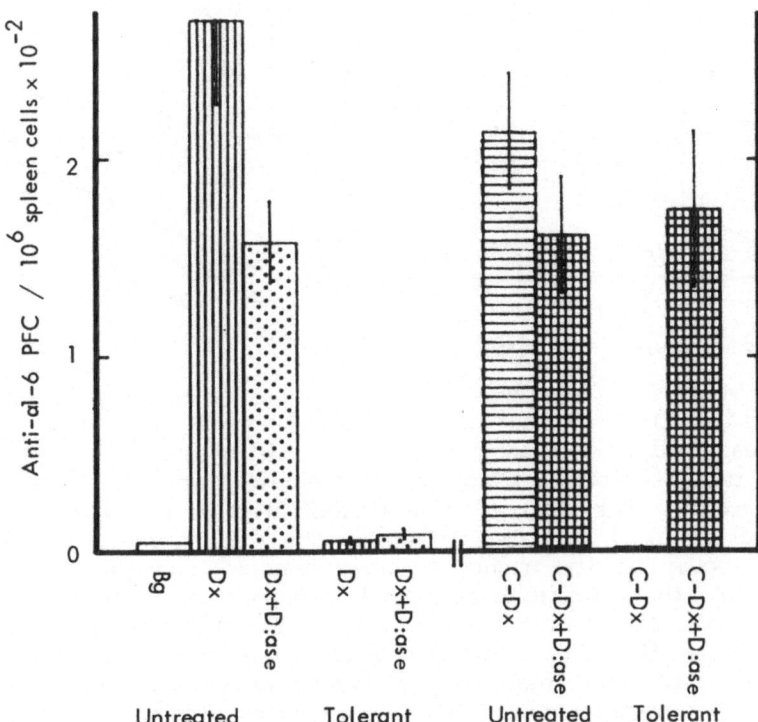

Fig 1. An immune response to the tolerogen can be obtained with dextran conjugates after dextranase treatment. C57BL mice were tolerized to native dextran by one injection of 10 mg. Five and 7 days later half of these mice as well as untreated controls were given injections of 20 units of dextranase. Three days later these mice and previously untreated controls were immunized with 2 ug native dextran or 0.2 ml of a 10% suspension of Cowan dextran. The direct PFC response was determined 5 days later. Three mice were used per group.

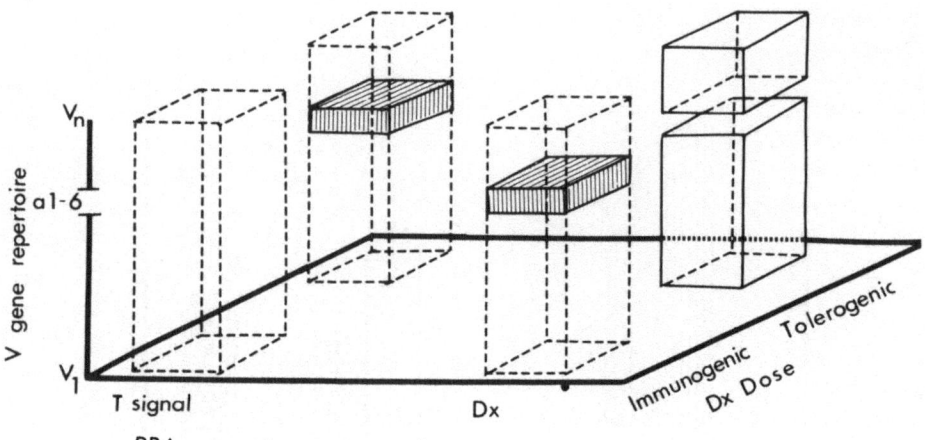

Fig. 2. Model for tolerance induction. The V-gene repertoire is indicated on the Y-axis, including the V gene for alpha 1-6 antibodies. Two B cell subpopulations are illustrated, one responding to thymus-dependent antigens (T signals) and the other to native dextran. The dextran dose is indicated in the Z-axis. The subpopulation of B cells responding to the PBA property of dextran is shown to the right. At immunogenic concentrations of dextran only the specific B cells in this subset are activated, the rest of the cells remain resting (broken lines), whereas at tolerogenic doses B cells with Ig receptors against alpha 1-6 are irreversibly tolerized (gap in the cube). However, immunogenic doses of thymus-dependent dextran conjugates are still competent to activate a specific alpha 1-6 immune response in the subpopulation responding to T signals (to the left). At immunogenic concentrations of dextran no cells in this subpopulation are activated.

be ascribed to antibodies of other affinities or specificities. It was actually shown that the anti-dextran antibodies possessed the same idiotype after immunization with BSA-dextran and dextran, respectively. The only tenable conclusion is that tolerance to a thymus-independent antigen did not affect all B cells with immunoglobulin receptors reactive with dextran. However, tolerance affected some B cells in this clone, since native dextran did not induce an immune response. It seems likely, therefore, that tolerance induction to native dextran affected the B cells that could be activated by native dextran given in immunogenic concentrations, but not the B cells that are activated by T cell help. Thus, tolerance only affects some of the B cells specific for the alpha 1-6 epitope of dextran, namely those having both activating and immunoglobulin receptors for dextran, whereas B cells with different activating receptors remain resting (Fig. 2). The latter B cells must be cleared from the dextran that have bound to their immunoglobulin receptors before they can be activated, as shown by the fact that no response occurred to thymus-dependent antigens if the tolerant mice had not been pretreated with dextranase, again indicating that blocking of immunoglobulin receptors can make the mice phenotypically unresponsive in spite of the fact that they possess immunocompetent B cells to the antigen.

We have also shown that lymphocytes from dextran tolerant mice can be activated into synthesis of antibodies against the tolerogen by polyclonal B cell activators such as LPS[12]. Again it was necessary to clear the cells from the tolerogen by giving dextranase or by adding them to serum-free cultures for 24 hours in vitro prior to contact with the polyclonal B cell activator.

REGULATION OF IMMUNOGLOBULIN CLASS SWITCHES

There are several findings that indicate that the immunoglobulin class switches do not occur randomly, but are regulated by as yet unknown mechanisms. We will describe some phenomena suggesting the existance of regulatory mechanisms.

The IgG Response to Dextran

Typical high responder strains to the alpha 1-6 epitope of dextran are CBA and C57BL. Both strains possess a V gene in the Igh locus coding for antibodies against dextran and both give a strong IgM response peaking at day 5 (Fig. 3). However, only C57BL mice give an IgG response[12]. It has never been possible to induce an IgG response in CBA mice using either thymus-dependent or thymus-independent dextran preparations, although both preparations give an IgG response in C57BL mice. The absence of an IgG response in CBA mice was not due to suppressor cells or other suppressive influences. CBA spleen cells transferred into irradiated C57BL mice still failed to make IgG anti-dextran antibodies, whereas C57BL cells similarly transferred into CBA mice gave IgG responses. It was also demonstrated that FITC-dextran induced an IgG anti-FITC response in both CBA and C57BL mice, indicating that dextran could serve as a carrier for the induction of IgG antibodies to conjugated epitopes.

Thus, it seems that CBA mice exhibit a determinant specific inability to make IgG antibodies to the alpha 1-6 epitope of dextran.

Different B Cell Activators Induce Different IgG Subclasses

Apart from apparent thymus-independent polyclonal B cell activation, it is possible to activate murine B cells polyclonally with thymus-dependent stimuli. Thus, T cells specific for determinants on B cells can act as polyclonal T helper cells for B cells in vitro[13,14]. Both thymus-independent and thymus-dependent stimulation will

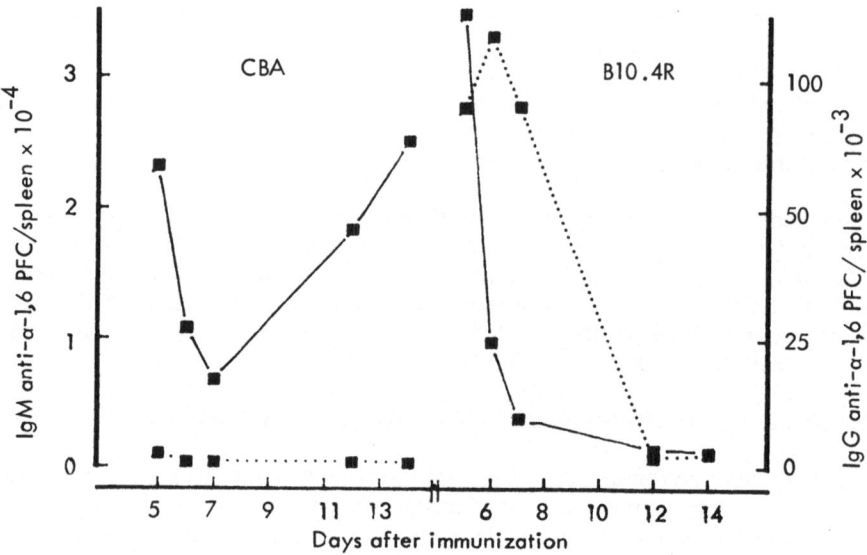

Fig. 3. Kinetics of the IgM (■———■) and IgG (■·······■) response against the alpha 1-6 epitope of native dextran B512 in CBA and B10.A(4R) mice. The IgG response represents the total number of PFC after addition of developing serum. The developing serum caused a 50-95% reduction of the number of IgM PFC.

activate B cells to proliferation, IgM secretion and switch to IgG secretion. There is, however, a difference in switch pattern between these two types of stimuli[13,15]. Thymus-independent stimuli, such as LPS, bacterial lipoprotein or LPS plus dextran sulphate activate B cells to switch to mainly IgG_{2b} and IgG_3[13,15-17]. On the other hand, thymus-dependent stimuli activate a switch to mainly IgG_1[13].

This seems to be a general phenomenon, since a similar switch pattern is observed after antigen stimulation[18,19]. Thus, IgG_3 is a thymus-independent IgG subclass, whereas IgG_1 is a thymus-dependent subclass.

We have recently described a factor which is similar to the B cell differentiation factor ($BCDF_{gamma}$) reported by Isaksson et al.[20,21]. We have used a T cell line developed by Coutinho, originating from the C3H/HeJ substrain, which was stimulated in vitro by irradiated C3H/Tif spleen cells. Supernatants from this line was collected one day after the addition of fresh medium plus stimulator cells. The supernatant was centrifuged twice and filtered to sterility and added to spleen cell cultures with or without LPS. In the absence of LPS, the supernatant had little effect on DNA synthesis or Ig secretion. When added together with LPS, the supernatant had no reproducible effect on cell proliferation or IgM secretion, but it enhanced IgG secretion. When the different subclasses of IgG was examined it was found that there was a selective enhancement of the IgG_1 secreting cells and that IgG_{2b} and IgG_3 responses were suppressed. We also found that the supernatant was most effective when added one day after onset of LPS activation and that the IgG_1 responses peaked on around day 6. At high concentration of the supernatant, the enhancement of the IgG response was approximately 100 fold, and the LPS induced IgG_{2b} and IgG_3 responses were reduced. We have preliminary evidence indicating that the activity can be partially absorbed on LPS blasts and Con A blasts, but less so on normal spleen cells. Furthermore, a T cell tumor (549) and a B cell tumor (BCL_1) could not absorb the activity.

Thus, there is evidence for the existance of a factor which regulates the switch to IgG_1. This factor could either in itself direct B cells to switch to IgG_1 or it could select cells that have already switch to membrane expression of IgG_1 to secrete this isotype.

However, it remains to be established whether the factor acts directly on B cells or on another cell type.

SUMMARY

The question whether the entire B cell clone is affected after immunization or induction of tolerance is of theoretical importance for the understanding of the mechanism of B cell triggering. It is now well established that immunization only affects a subpopulation of the antigen specific B cells, leaving others in a resting state.
In a system, where the immune response is controlled by an Igh-V linked gene, we have shown that tolerance also only affects a proportion of B cells. The implications of these findings for contemporary concepts of B cell activation is discussed,

Finally, it is shown by several examples that the switch from IgM to other IgG isotypes is carefully regulated and that different activating signals appear to determine/select the isotype to be expressed.

REFERENCES.

1. Bretscher, P.A. and Cohn, M. Science 169:1042, 1970.

2. Andersson, J., Sjöberg, O. and Möller, G. Transpl. Rev. 11:31, 1972.

3. Fernandez, C., Lieberman, R and Möller, G. Scand. J. Immunol. 10:77, 1979

4.   Fernandez, C. and Möller, G. J. Exp. Med. 147:645, 1978.

5.   Howard, J.G., Vicari, G. and Courtenay, B.M. Immunol. 29:585, 1975

6.   Howard, J.G., Vicari, G. and Courtenay, B.M. Immunol. 14:253, 1975

7.   Fernandez, C. and Möller, G. Scand. J. Immunol. 7:137, 1978.

8.   Weigle, W.O. J. Exp. Med. 116:913, 1962.

9.   Weigle, W.O., Chiller, J.M. and Habicht, G.S. Transpl. Rev. 8:3, 1972.

10.   Möller, G. and Fernandez, C . Scand. J. Immunol. 8:29, 1978.

11.   Fernandez, C. and Möller, G. J. Exp. Med. 146:308, 1977.

12.   Fernandez, C. and Möller, G. Scand. J. Immunol. 11:53, 1980.

13.   Martinez, A., Coutinho, A. and Augustin A.A. Eur. J. Immunol. 10:698, 1980

14.   Augustin, A.A. and Coutinho, A. J. Exp. Med. 151:587, 1980.

15.   Kearny, J.F. In "Developments in Immunology." Eds. M. Cooper, I. Sher and E.S. Vitetta. Elsevier-North Holland Inc. Amsterdam, p. 77, 1979.

16   Severinson-Gronowicz, E., Doss, C., Assisi, F., Vitetta, E.S., Coffman, R.L. and Strober, S. J. Immunol. 123:2049, 1979.

17   Bergstedt-Lindqvist, S., Fernandez, C. and Severinson, E. Scand. J. Immunol. 15:439, 1982.

18.   Rosenberg, Y.J. and Chiller, J.M. J. Exp. Med. 150:517, 1979.

19.   Perlmutter, R.M., Hansburg, D., Brites, D.E., Nicolotti, R.A. and Davie, J.M. J. Immunol. 121:566, 1978.

20   Isakson, P.C., Puré, E., Vitetta, E.S. and Krammer, P.H. J. Exp. Med. 155:734, 1982.

21   Bergstedt-Lindqvist, S. and Severinson, E. Submitted for publication 1982.

DISCUSSION

Jones: When you immunize with thymus-dependent dextran-protein conjugates after dextranase treatment, is the response of the usual idiotype?

G. Möller: Yes.

Cohn: Have you tried to see whether the tolerogenic and immunogenic form of the dextran compete to prevent the breaking of unresponsiveness?

G. Möller: No.

Paul: Can residual dextranase in the tolerant animal treated with dextranase degrade dextran and prevent a response to high molecular weight dextran?

G. Möller: No, that possibility has been tested and ruled out.

Coutinho: This is a proposal that has been championed by Max Cooper, namely that isotype switch is an inherent step in B cell differentiation which is, therefore, stimulation-independent and results in precommitment of individual B cells as to the isotype they can produce when stimulated. My question is: can we exclude such models if it is shown beyond doubt that the same clone of B cells, arising from an immunocompetent precursor, produces more than one non-IgM isotype?

G. Möller: We know that isotype switch is not stimulation independent, but that does not exclude precommitment. Nor do I think thats successive switches disprove precommitment.

Uhr: I think it is not possible from Göran Möller's data to distinguish whether the 2 subclasses of IgG are expressed by the same cell (i.e. that a switch was induced) or whether you have amplified a subset. It would be worthwhile, therefore, to use the cell sorter to purify the subset with the particular subclass of IgG on its surface and determine whether under your particular culture conditions, the additional subclass appears.

Coutinho: I want to make four points concerning isotype switch. These are conclusions from a large number of experiments performed by L. Forni at the Basel Institute for Immunology and collaborative efforts with R. Benner, C. Martinez and M. Björklund in my laboratory.

1. By studying over one thousand LPS-reactive B cell clones for all secreted isotypes, we can conclude that single B lymphocytes are not precommitted to the expression of a given non-IgM isotype, but rather that single clones of unprimed cells produce multiple isotypes. From this analysis, and making the assumption that only forward switches occur, we can derive the exact probability of switches for each isotype in single clones, under these conditions of stimulation and as to the secreted isotypes.

2. By studying single cells in double immunofluorescence detecting two isotypes, we can conclude that isotype switches are not single events in the B cell biography. Undoubtedly, a sizeable fraction of all cells produce more than one IgG isotype, indicating therefore gamma to gamma switches. In contrast, practically all cells expressing IgE or IgA also bear IgM, indicating direct M to E or M to A switches. These observations are in agreement with the S-region homologies described by Dr. Honjo. Interestingly, in case of double IgG isotype expression, one membrane associated and the other cytoplasmic, the secreted isotype is encoded 3' to that expressed as membrane.

3. The controls of membrane isotype expression are distinct from those for secreted isotypes. As an example, LPS stimulation which results in very limited production of IgG_1 plasma cells and IgG_1 secretion results in a large number of IgG_1 bearing, non-secretory blast cells, which constitute the predominant non-IgM isotype among membrane forms in these cultures. The intriguing observation in this respect is that the signals inducing terminal maturation is activated B cells and high-rate secretion of Ig appear to be isotype-specific. Thus, LPS is incompetent in inducing IgG_1 secretion but very efficient in activating both IgG_3 and IgG_{2b} secretion, while T helper cells are extremely inefficient in inducing IgG_3 secretion from IgG_3 positive blasts and are the stimulus of choice to activate high-rate secretion in IgG_1-bearing blasts.

4. Commitment of Ig isotypes is not the result of random "recombination and deletion" accompanying DNA replication and mitosis. Antigen-specific B cell clones followed for 9 consecutive weekly transfers in Göran Möller's original system, until clonal dominance was observed do not show an accumulation of produced isotypes towards the most 3' numbers in the C-gene cluster. Rather, the produced isotypes are fixed throughout the life of the clone, as long as the same conditions of stimulation are kept. A change in such conditions, however, as it can easily be done in vitro alters the typical thymus-independent to a thymus-dependent pattern, for example, demonstrating that isotype commitment is directly regulated by the quality of the stimuli driving clonal expansion and/or maturation..

All our data concern secreted isotypes. It is obvious, therefore, that our calculations on switch probabilities also apply to secreted isotypes only, and under the assumption that we detect all switches. It could well be for example that all clones undergo stepwise switches through all four gammas but we see then "jumping" one simply because they do not secrete that particular one. Immunofluorescence, on the other hand, also has limitations because of the narrow window in time, dependent upon half-life of message or protein, in which we can "freeze" single cells.

G. Möller: I have previously suggested that the observations that different antigens and polyclonal B cell activators give rize to different Ig subclasses could be explained by a non-antigen driven differentiation process resulting in parallel expression of certain activation receptors and specific switch enzymes. Now you say that your findings disprove this possibility. Can you elaborate on that?

Coutinho: If a single immunocompetent B cell gives rize to a clone which produce for example all four IgG subclasses, I conclude that the clonal precursor was not committed to the production of a single isotype or the chemistry of a defined unique switch event. These experiments, therefore, exclude in my opinion all precommitment hypotheses.

Milstein: Could you please define more precisely what do you understand are the differences between maturation and differentiation.

Coutinho: From the times in Basel with Jan Andersson and Fritz Melchers we need to distinguish differentiation - a process involving turning-on of gene(s) and expression of new product(s), from maturation - a process involving increased rates of synthesis of a product (such as Ig) which was already expressed before induction. In this sense, induction of high-rate Ig synthesis and secretion is not differentiation, as the resting B cell already expresses those genes.

E. Möller: I think what Cesar Milstein means is that these events imply clonal expansion and thus differentiation. Coutinho would claim that since these cells are still responsive to LPS as an activation signal they still belong to the same "maturation stage".

Severinson: I have two points to make with regard to Dr. Coutinho's comment. First, we have to define what we mean with a switch. Assuming that Dr. Honjo's hypothesis is correct, the switch would occur in two steps. The first step would be at the level of RNA and the second at the DNA level. If this was so, the IgG surface positive cells which Dr. Forni observe in LPS cultures, would have undergone the first but not the second event. The latter event could be directed by T cells. In any event, I think it remains to be proven whether LPS or T cells direct the switch in B cells in these in vitro systems. The second point regards the limiting dilution experiments and the idea of a continuous class or subclass switch. These experiments only say that one B cell can switch to different isotypes. However, there is as yet no evidence that the lineage of one cell can switch more than once.

Coutinho: I do not think, in fact, that helper factors - such as those "inducing" IgG_1 are "switch factors". These are simply maturation factors which induce high-rate secretion in cells that had previously switched - in the absence of the factors - to membrane expression of IgG_1. I also agree that this view depends on a definition of switch. I we adopt the frame of Honjo's model, one can say of course that such maturation factors directly induce DNA switch recombination (from cells producing membrane IgG_1 by differential splicing of long transcripts to cells transcribing at high rate a rearranged IgG_1 gene). From the point of view of cellular immunology however, such cells have already switched and, what is important, these factors fail to induce IgG_1 in any other cells. We have sorted membrane-positive IgG_1 cells in LPS cultures and added maturation ("switch") factor to both the depleted and enriched fractions: while, in less than 24 h, the majority of membrane-positive cells start secreting IgG_1 upon factor-dependent induction, no IgG_1 is recoverend from the depleted cell populations, demonstrating that such factors do not, in fact, induce a switch to the repression of IgG_1 in cells which did not produce it already.

G. Möller: I think we should limit the discussion to Ig secreting cells and not deal with Ig classes on membrane immunoglobulin. As mentioned by Honjo, it is likely that expression of membrane Ig occurs before DNA rearrangement, whereas Ig secretion occurs only after DNA rearrangement.

Wabl: I think we have formally proven that the heavy chain class switch can occur in a pure B cell line, that is before light chain is expressed, and before even the light chain locus has been rearranged. Thus, the switch can happen independently from antigen. However, I do not see any contradiction to the possibility that the switch can happen after antigen exposure.

Benacerraf: Are the switch events that occur, randomly in time and also randomly as to class? That is not directed e.g. on external stimulus. Does anyone have any data on this point?

Cohn: There are two models of class switch:
1) The switch is random
2) The switch is directed

In both cases the signal to switch from IgM to Ig other comes from the effective level of help to the given antigen.

If any relationship exists between the antigen contacted and the class of the response then the first model requires an isotype recognition mechanism while the second model requires a hormone inducing mechanism. The real problem is at the level of these required mechanisms.

Under the first model the cell switches randomly from IgM to anyone of the other classes and the isotype recognition mechanism (e.g. T cells specific for isotype, trapping device specific for isotype in tissues which permits homing, etc.) favours induction of a given class. Different antigens are distinguished by the isotype specific T cells they induce (not at all obvious how) or by where they lodge (not much of a categorization).

Given the problems of postulates relating a given antigen to a given isotype whether we consider models I or II, I wonder how general is the assumption that antigens do indeed induce specific Ig classes after the switch? To what extent can one classify the world of antigens into the Ig classes they preferentially induce?

Sachs: Dr. Baltimore, have you ever observed a reverse switch in your cell lines?

Baltimore: No, but we have not had the opportunity to select for them.

Leder: Is it clear that there have been no rearrangements in the DNA between u and IgG_{2b}?

Honjo: It is important to carry surface Ig as a marker of selection. There may be production of secreted Ig as well. The relative abundance of the surface- and membrane-forms may vary.

Wabl: One possibility for antigen preference for a certain class might be the preferential assembly of light chain to a certain heavy chain class. We have generated cells from the pre B cell line 18-81 which produce u, IgG_{2b}, and kappa synchronously, the kappa chain associated with IgG_{2b}, but not with u chain.

Smith: One could explain the IgG subclass expression by a certain B-cell that expresses every receptor for putative subclass-specific B cell differentiation factor (BCDF) by a selective secretion (by T cells) of a higher concentration of a subclass-specific factor. This, therefore, could explain a carrier-specific expression of one isotype.

Paul: I think it is possible to suggest that the apparent linkage between immunoglobulin class and the expression of antibodies of a given specificity may be the indirect consequence of the likelyhood that both may be preferentially expressed by a given B cell subset. For example, anti-carbohydrate antibodies are preferentially produced by Lyb-5+ B cells and such cells, under normal induction, particularly by type 2 antigens, are very likely to switch to IgG3 production. Thus, anti-carbohydrate responses would preferentially be of the IgG3 type, although there might be no **direct** link between the two. A complete explanation of this requires a reason for the likelyhood that anti-carbohydrate responses are preferentially made by Lyb-B5+ B cells. As a first approximation, this would be explained by the fact that carbohydrate epitopes are normally expressed on type 2 antigens, which can only activate Lyb-5+ B cells. In addition, environmental immunization could skew the expressed repertoire of Lyb-5+ and Lyb-5-B cells and, since only the Lyb-5+ B cells would respond to environmental polysaccharides, this would serve to increase the frequency of anti-carbohydrate precursors in Lyb-5+ B cells relative to that in Ly-b5- B cells.

Coutinho: The study of isotype commitment by means of polyclonal stimulation - either thymus-independent or with specific helper cells - offers the advantages of avoiding selection for combining site specificites and V-region-specific regulatory mechanisms, while providing systems where close to 100% of all reactive cells are stimulated and show the same selective patterns of isotype expression observed in specific antibody responses. Furthermore, as Davie's experiments have shown, the pattern of isotypes observed in specific responses is determined by functional properties of the "carriers" which are best studied at the polyclonal level.

Uhr: I question whether there is really no correlation between the surface isotype on a B memory cell and the isotype which that cell will produce after terminal differentiation. There is considerable experimental evidence that there is such a correlation and the concept makes biological sense.

Milstein: Is class switch or class expression carrier dependent? Paul and Coutinho think it may well be. If so, the class should be the same for all haptens on the same carrier. Is this so?

G. Möller: There are two types of what appear to be regulated switches. One is carrier dependent as examplified by polysaccharides inducing IgG3 and T help giving IgG1. These types of switches occur both in specific and polyclonal responses in vivo and in vitro.

The other type is determinant specific and the response to the alpha 1-6 epitope of dextran is (the only?) one example. In this case CBA mice do not switch, whereas C57BL switch to IgG. CBA do not give an IgG response to dextran whether the antigen is given in a TI or TD form, e.g. the response is carrier-independent. However, CBA mice give an IgG response to the FITC epitope conjugated to dextran. Thus, it appears that CBA mice specifically fail to switch to an IgG response against the alpha 1-6 epitope of dextran.

Honjo: If a V_H sequence selects a particular C_H sequence to terminate transcription it seems difficult to explain why all the B cell express the u chain at the beginning.

Baltimore: It would have to be that virgin cells can only make u and then a signal leads to a pre-determined switch.

Hood: There is one example where class switching is programmed and not random. The X sequence that always associates with the non expressed 5' region in IgA producing cells is such an example. Every IgA producer requires the X sequence be switched to the nonproductive chromosome.

Sachs: There are examples in several idiotype systems, including the NP system studied by Rajewski and collegues and our own anti-H-$2K^k$ system for induction of the same V_H gene expression by immunization of an animal with either antigen or anti-idiotype. Evidence that the same V gene is used is based not only on idiotype expression but also on analysis of heavy chain amino terminal sequences and iso-electric focussing data. In our case the heavy chain class induced is often different by the two different immunizations (i.e. IgG_2 following antigen, IgG_1 following anti-idiotype)

Melchers: I think the discussion has centerered around the following points and problems:

When a B cell switches the class of Igh chain that it expresses, two molecular mechanisms can be envisaged:

a) A B cell may transcribe the wole region of chromosome 12 (in the mouse) containing rearranged V_H, D_H, J_H segments and all exons and introns down to the domains for the alpha-chain in one large RNA molecule. RNA processing and splicing first ensures that mRNA molecules for membrane-bound and for secreted u heavy chains are made. Whatever induces the switch induces a change in the processing and splicing of this primary transcript RNA into mRNA molecules coding for other classes of Igh chains. This mode of class switching may occur in resting, antigen-sensitive B cells before stimulation, and in activated B blasts soon thereafter.

b). Switch recombination, which probably occurs by unequal crossing-over of sister chromatids, deletes a segment of the expressed chromosome 12 which carries information for all C_H domains expressed before the switching event and upstreams (5') gene which it expresses after switching. The suggestion is that this mode of class switching occurs more in Ig-secreting plasma cell.

Essentially nothing is known of the possible differences in conformations of DNA-, of chromosome- and of RNA structure, as well as of the enzymes and intracellular factors that regulate these molecular modes of H-chain switching. At present that makes it impossible for us to judge whether qualitatively different signals can really be recieved in one and the same B cell.

T-dependent stimulation via helper T cells, and T-independent stimulation via mitogens results in qualitatively different H-chain switches in B cells. Here, polyclonally distributed receptors for antigen-unspecific, H-2 unrestricted B cell replication and maturation factors are the best candidates for signal reception. Antigen-specific stimulation of the switching to a preferred class of H-chains, however, indicates that the specificity of Ig as the antigen-recognizing part of the B cell receptor may also influence H-chain class switching. The crucial issue remains whether the induction of such preferred H-chain class switching events is an instructive or selective process. I consider it to be instructive, if the different stimuli act on one and the same B cell. It is selective if these stimuli find, for reasons of inherent B cell differentiation of the system or of B cell memory of past experience, different B cell subsets as their targets.

Much is still to be learned of the behaviour of single, stimulated, replicating B cell clones. There is good evidence that after T-dependent more than after T-independent stimulation, IgM-positive resting B cell clones switch to the expression of other Igh chain classes in high frequencies. We know that this switch can occur after one, two or after 10 divisions, after which almost all B cell clones have ceased to replicate. Could all clones eventually switch to other Ig classes, if we only could clonally expand them long enough? The switch appears to be the individual event of one B cell in the clone, fixed in its descendents thereafter, rather than "the big bang" for every cell in the clone. A B cell which once switched may switch again. Is, threrefore, the final result of all switching the production and secretion of the last Igh class, i.e. of alpha chain? Or can even that be switched out to yield a plasma cell which has lost all Igh chain genes by deletion and, therefore, produces no more Igh chains?. The observed preference in the switching to a given heavy chain class other than alpha seems to argue against that. And finally, can switching occur without cell division, as the action of B cell matura-tion factors on resting B cells inducing IgM, but also IgG and IgA secretion seems to indicate?

What gives a B cell the signal to switch?. The major condidates are 1) Helper T cells and their specific cell-cell interaction molecules, such as the Ia specific ones and 2) Factors produced in the interaction of antigen, macrophages and helper T cells which replicate and mature B cells. It appears that different factors induce the maturation to the secretion of different classes of Ig. The heterogeneity of factors predicts a heterogeneteity of receptors for them.

I would conclude from the discussion that we can expect in the foreseeable future to understand the molecular mechanisms of class switching. We have, however, not even seen the tip of the iceberg that constitutes the cellular and physiological conditions of the immune system in which class switching occur and which control them.

Session IX

B Cell Regulation II

Chairman: M. Cohn

FACTORS DETERMINING VIRGIN AND POSTANTIGENIC REPERTOIRES

OF B CELL POPULATION AND ITS SUBSETS

Olli Mäkelä, H.O. Sarvas and I.J.T. Seppälä

Department of Bacteriology and Immunology
University of Helsinki
Haartmaninkatu 3, 00290 Helsinki 29

The repertoire of specifities (different Ig F_V pieces) that a population of B lymphocytes can produce is large but its size depends on what meaning is given to the word. Two meanings are important for this discussion (Table 1). One (the virgin repertoire) is the collection of F_V pieces in antigen-free individuals. The other repertoire includes all F_V structures that individuals of a certain genotype (say the BALB/c mouse) can produce when immunized with all possible antigens (the potential postantigenic repertoire). When it is discussed whether known mechanisms of diversity-generation are sufficient to explain the observed variability this potential postantigenic repertoire is often in the minds of the discussers.

Table 1.   B cell repertoires

1.   Virgin repertoire. All different F_V pieces
       in antigen-free animals of a certain genotype.
       (Either one individual or the whole strain.)

2.   Potential postantigenic repertoire. All
       different F_V pieces that animals of a strain
       collectively can produce when immunized with
       all possible antigens.

The virgin repertoire has been pruned from a larger repertoire by the self tolerization process, and an argument can be raised that rather than being virgin it is raped. The problem is that the truly virgin pretolerization repertoire cannot be studied. The

posttolerization repertoire can be studied e.g. by mitogenic stimulation, and therefore it makes sense to accept it as "virgin".

The main difference between the virgin and the postantigenic
repertoires is that the latter probably includes plenty of postantigenic somatic mutants but the former includes few. The important
finding of Gearhart et al.[1] that mutants are very common in IgG
antibodies but rare in IgM antibodies has given new credibility to
the early studies suggesting that postantigenic mutations are fairly
common in B cell clones[2].

The word potential is used because full repertoires hardly
exist in any single individual. This is certainly true of the postantigenic repertoire; no animal can be immunized by all possible
antigens. It may also be true of the virgin repertoire especially
in small animals.

There are six known factors that contribute to the generation
of the B cell repertoire (Table 2). The seventh factor has been
postulated, namely D-D joining[3]

Table 2.   Generation of the B cell repertoire

1. - Multiplicity of germ line loci for one V_L, J_L,
       V_H, D_H or J_H.

2. - Allelic differences can up to double the
       variability but not within an inbred strain

3. - Free combination of a V_L and a J_L to form
       an exon for the variable polypeptide of the
       I_g L chain. A corresponding combinatorial
       factor in the generation of VDJ_H.

4. - Minor inaccuracy in the site of the VJ_L
       joining (and probably in the joinings
       generating the VDJ_H)

5. - H-L combinatorial pairing

6. - Somatic mutations

The number of F_V-structures that the mechanisms of Table 2
are able to produce can be estimated only roughly. If we assume
that there are 200 V_L-gene segments, 100 V_H segments, 20 D segments,
and 4 J gene segments for both chains[4] the germ-line can generate
the maximum of 8000 different $V_H DJ_H$ combinations. If we assume
that ten different mutants can be generated from each germ line

sequence the number of potential L-chain sequences is 8000 and that of H chain sequences 80 000. The potential number of different F_V structures would then be 640×10^6. This calculation does not include the contribution of factors 2 and 4 of Table 2.

The B cell repertoire must cover all potentially pathogenic microbes and variants that the microbes routinely develop to avoid antibodies. One of two strategies could have been adopted to meet these requirements. One is conservative. The germ-line repertoire and its somatic mutants cover the structures that today's microbes either carry or can easily develop by mutation. Such a repertoire would have to evolve continuously since microbes evolve continuously. The other possible strategy is the strategy of saturation: The repertoire is so huge that all structures conceivably generated by any future microbes are already covered. The main advantage of the conservative strategy would be economy, and the main advantage of the saturating strategy would be safety. It is impossible to tell which strategy prevails, even an intermidiary strategy is possible. Animals can produce antibodies to almost any synthetic compounds, and this may suggest that the saturation strategy has been adopted by Nature.

Simple rules may dictate the generation of the B cell repertoire as suggested in Table 3. It can be built up from random combinations of the five subunits V_L, J_L, V_H, D and J_H and their somatic mutants. The only other factors may be the elimination of cells that are specific for self structures, and stimulation by antigens, often modified by T_H cells or T_S cells.

Are we permitted to entertain this minimun hypothesis or is there strong evidence that prove it inadequate? The objection, that these mechanisms cannot possibly generate a large enough repertoire does not look compelling in view of the arguments discussed above.

There is specific evidence suggesting that the recruitement of different V-gene segments does not happen at random but is "programmed". B-cells of newborn mice cannot produce antibodies to phosphocholine[5] or α-1-6-dextran[6] while they can produce antibodies to DNP or FITC[5,6]. Newborn mice should have the genes for the production of at least anti-phosphocholine (PC) since the product

Table 3. Minimum hypothesis about virgin B cell repertoires

- Virgin repertoires are determined by the six elements of Table 2 in a lottery-like manner. The only other factor is self-tolerization.

  Objection: V genes are recruited according to a programme.

of a germ-line kappa chain gene and germ-line H chain gene can
make up an adequate anti-PC antibody[1].

It may still be possible to postulate that newborn mice do
not have an inherent shortage of B cells specific for PC or α-1-6-
dextran. Their failure to repond could be due to a combination
of two things: the low number of Lyb-5 positive B cells in newborn
mice[7] and the uniformly low affinity of IgM antibodies to the PC
hapten. The six IgM anti-PC hybridoma proteins studied had affinities varying from 0.34 to 5.7 million l/M although the spleen cell
donor had been immunized for 1-2 months[1,8]. The affinities are low
compared with affinities of three IgM hybridomas studied by Péterfy
et al. (unpublished). They were 0.15, 27 and 115 million l/M. The
spleen cell donors had been immunized only 14 days before the sacri-
fice, thus there was little time for selection of high-affinity
clones.

Let us make still two assumptions, one (ad hoc) that the
Lyb-5 positive B cells are more easily triggerable than Lyb-5
negative B cells and the other (reasonable) that low-affinity
antigen-binding causes a less efficient triggering than high-
affinity binding. Then it is possible that Lyb-5 negative B cells
cannot be triggered by the low-affinity binding that is inherent to
anti-PC antibodies, at least not in the absence of T cell help.
This triggering can happen with the low-affinity binding in the
Lyb-5 positive subset. The corresponding explanation could be
valid for the anti-1-6-dextran response although antibody affinities
are unknown. A problem remains, however, since LPS activation did
not induce the production of anti-α-1-6 dextran antibodies by newborn cells[6]. This finding appears to prove that programming is
involved or that distant V-gene segments are recruited later than
proximal ones as Möller et al. suggested[6]

Biased repertoires in different subsets of B cells?

There are antigens (e.g. phosphocholine, PC, and α-1-6 dextran)
to which newborn mice and CBA/N mice of any age respond very
weakly[9,10]. This has been taken to mean that the repertoire in the
subset(s) that these mice have (Lyb 5 negative B cells) is limited.
Another explanation has been discussed above, that the repertoire
is complete also in the Lyb 5-negative subset but these B cells are
not as easily triggered by antigens as the Lyb 5-positive B cells.
Since anti-PC antibodies (at least in virgin B cells) never have
high affinities, PC antigens can only trigger B cells in the Lyb 5+
subset, not in the Lyb 5-negative subset(s).

Another phenomenon potentially belongs to this discussion;
some antigens induce antibodies that belong predominantly to one
subclass of IgG, e.g. murine anti-polysaccharide antibodies tend to
be IgG3[11-13]. There are at least three possible explanations for

Table 4. Possible explanations why antibodies to
certain antigens exhibit an isotype preference
(murine anti-polysaccharide antibodies have a
preference for IgG3 etc.)

1. A priori repertoires are identical in IgG3 and IgG1
committeed subsets but an antigen triggers one or
the other <u>selectively</u>. Polysaccharides trigger IgG3
cells.

2. A certain antigen <u>induces</u> the switch to a certain
isotype (polysaccharides - IgG3).

3. A preference exists already in the virgin repertoire
(there is an excess of IgG3 in anti-polysaccharide
antibodies because B cell clones that bear a
rearranged VDJ gene specific for a carbohydrate tend
to switch to the gamma-3 C-gene)

subclass preferences (Table 4). One of them postulates that antigens select B cells from a pool of lymphocytes that are at least
partially committed to one isotype.

At least two mechanisms can be imagined that could lead to a
selective immunization of, say IgG1 or IgG3 B cells. According to
one an antigen (say a polysaccharide) has a tendency to home in a
certain part of the body and IgG3 B cells home in the same region.
Antibodies induced are then predominantly IgG3. Alternatively,
one can postulate that there are T helper cells that help IgG1 B
cells preferentially, and these T cells only recognize antigen B,
not A. Anti-B is then predominantly IgG1.

The second possibility is that antigens <u>induce</u> B cell clones
to switch to the production of non-IgM isotypes as suggested by
Hurwitz et al.[14] and Martinez-Aloso et al.[15]. To explain subclass-
preferences this induction would have to be selective. There is
evidence that T_H cell factors favour the production of IgG[15]
but whether this effect is inducive or selective is still unknown.

The third explanation denies any real role of the antigen in
the subclass preferences. It postulates that there is an excess of
IgG3 in anti-polysaccharide antibodies because B cell clones that
bear a rearranged VDJ gene specific for a carbohydrate tend to
switch to the gamma 3 C-gene. The third possibility would mean
that the subset of IgG3 B cells has a non-random fraction of the
total virgin repertoire.

The antigen-induction and the antigen-selection hypothesis
would predict that any subclass prediction that is associated with a

particular antigen is valid for all determinants of the antigen.
A likely candidate for the hypothetical factor that induces a switch
is a factor produced by a T cell that is activated by the same
antigen as the B cell. The B cell then is an efficient target for
the factor because it is brought close to the T cell by the antigen
bridge. B cells should then be switched regardless of the epitope
via which they are brought to the association. The same argument
is valid if the T cell effects are selective rather than inductive
or if the subclass-preferences are based on selective homing of
cells and antigens.

We have studied responses to protein and polysaccharide conjugates of haptens by separating isotypes with protein A columns[16].
Responses to the protein conjugates were strong (> 3.6 mg/ml,
Table 5) and more than 90% of anti-hapten antibodies and of anti-
protein antibodies were IgG1 (came off the protein A column at pH
5.5). Comparing the antibody concentrations and O.D. values we
came to the conclusion that more than 50 per cent of the protein
was specific antibody. We did not believe our sums, absorbed the
fraction with a NIP-sorbent and an irrelevant sorbent,and measured
optical densities after absorption. The results confirmed our
sums[17].

The responses to the polysaccharide conjugates were much
weaker than the responses to protein conjugates, only one per cent
measured by antibody concentrations. Still they were more than 3
times (anti-CHO) or more than 4 times (anti-hapten) higher than
the background titre[18].

Of anti-polysaccharide antibodies one half was IgM or IgA,
25% IgG3 and the remaining 25% was accounted for by the other subclasses of IgG. Anti-hapten antibodies that had been measured from
the same protein A fractions were 58% IgM 22% IgG1, and the remaining
18% was covered by IgG2 and IgG3. The isotype distribution of anti-
hapten antibodies was thus different from anti-hapten antibodies
induced by protein conjugates. The excess of IgG3 in antibodies
to polysaccharides has been earlier found by other investigators
but earlier reports about isotypes of anti-hapten antibodies induced
by polysaccharide conjugates were conflicting[11,13,19].

The simplest explanation for the very strong response to the
hapten-protein conjugate is an efficient T cell help. Milligram
concentrations of a specific antibody on day 14 cannot be achieved
without such help. We would like to explain also the extreme IgG1
predominance in the same way. T cell help would then either induce
switches preferentially to IgG1 or preferentially help the subset
of B cells that express IgG1. Consistent with this is that T cell
depletion causes a greater concentration drop of IgG1 than of other
subclasses of IgG (discussed in ref. 17), and nonspecifically administered T cell help induces more IgG1 reverse plaques than reverse

Table 5.   Isotype distribution of anti-hapten and
            anti-carrier antibodies in sera of mice
            that had been immunized 14-15 days previcously
            with a hapten coupled to a protein or to
            a polysaccharide. The bottom part of the table
            is modified from reference 18. Serum pools
            (1.5 ml) were introduced into a protein A
            column (4.5 ml) and protein was eluted by
            decreasing the pH stepwise[17]. The antibodies
            in the passed fraction (pH 8.0) are called
            IgM + IgA, those in pH 5.5 fraction IgG1, in
            pH 5.0 fraction IgG2a, in pH 4.5 fraction
            IgG3 and pH 3.5 fraction IgG2b. Further
            justification for these names is in ref. 18.
            The Farr assay was used for anti-polysaccharide
            antibodies, and one ml of anti-ficoll sera bound
            16-38 μg of the antigen. Anti-pneumococcal
            CHO-type 14 (S14) sera had an ABC of 1400-
            5800 μg/ml of serum. A solid phase radio-
            immunoassay was used for the other antibodies,
            and the concentrations of anti-NIP antibodies
            varied from 16 to 40 μg/ml in antisera to
            NIP-polysaccharide conjugates. It was 3600
            μg/ml in the anti-NIP-CGG serum. We did not
            have a useful standard for anti-CGG or anti-
            TNP antibodies.

Antigen	NIP-CGG		NIP-ficoll, TNP-ficoll or NIP-S14	
Antibody, day 14	α-CGG	α-NIP	α-CHO	α-hapten
No of pools separated	1	1	5	6
Proportion on (%) of antibody activity in each fraction				
IgM + IgA	2.5	1.1	45	58
IgG1	96	93	13	22
IgG2a	0.65	3.2	10	6.0
IgG3	0.04	0.4	25	5.6
IgG2b	0.4	0.4	5.6	6.5

plaques of IgG2 or IgG3 subclasses[15]. If the T cell effect is
selective we only have to postulate that T cell factors induce IgG1
B cells to a vigorous multiplication and Ig-production. If the
T cells induce switches to IgG, we must postulate an additional

proliferative effect to explain the high antibody concentration. Both alternatives predict the observed IgG1 predominance in anti-hapten and anti-carrier antibodies.

The isotype distribution of anti-hapten antibodies induced by hapten-polysaccharide conjugates roughly corresponds to the synthetic rates of different isotypes, and does not require a special explanation. It becomes interesting when it is compared with the isotype distribution of anti-polysaccharide antibodies. It namely excludes simple explanations for the anti-polysaccharide antibodies ("polysaccharides home to the parts of the body where IgG3 cells reside" or "there is a T helper cell that helps IgG3 B-cells preferentially, and these T cells recognize polysaccharides preferentially"). These explanations would have predicted that anti-hapten antibodies induced by polysaccharide conjugates are predominantly IgG3 which was not the case.

We seem to be left with an explanation 3 of Table 4, which postulates a biased virgin repertoire in the subset that produces IgG3. This explanation has a problem, however, it would mean that the mechanism which switches a clone from μ-production to $\gamma 3$ production recognizes not only the μ and $\gamma 3$ switch sequences but also the V gene that is kilobases up the stream. It is difficult to see how this is possible, and therefore we would like to consider a fourth explanation. It has much in common with the explanation that we offered for the unresponsiveness of CBA/N mice or newborn mice of any strain to phosphocholine or 1-6-dextran: We postulated that only Lyb 5-positive cells are triggered by these antigens because the interaction of the antigen and the receptor antibody has a low affinity.

There is (weak) evidence that antibodies to carbohydrates also have low affinities[20-22]. Again only Lyb-5-positive cells may be triggered. Since IgG3 is predominantly produced by IgG3 B cells[23] any antigen that induces only Lyb-5-positive cells is likely to induce IgG3 antibodies preferentially.

CBA/N mice have defective responses not only to polysaccharides but also to haptens coupled to polysaccharides[19]. This looks like an evidence against our hypothesis since anti-hapten antibodies (IgG) were mainly IgG1. The weight of this objection is reduced by the finding of Press[24] that CBA/N mice have a general immuno-deficiency. As a further test of our hypothesis wer are carefully comparing anti-NIP and anti-ficoll responses of CBA/N mice to NIP-Ficoll. The prediction is that anti-NIP responses are less defective than anti-ficoll responses although both are defective.

In summary we propose that there is no compelling evidence against the hypothesis of Table 3; even if it is extended to say that all subsets of B cells have random samples of the total repertoire.

REFERENCES

1. P. J. Gearhart, N. D. Johnson, R. Douglas, and L. Hood, IgG
    antibodies to phosphorylcholine exhibit more diversity than
    their IgM counterparts, Nature, 291:29 (1981).
2. A. J. Cunningham, Evolution in microcosm: the rapid somatic
    diversification of lymphocytes, in: "Symposia on Quantitative
    Biology," Cold Spring Harbor Laboratory, New York (1977).
3. Y. Kurosawa and S. Tonegawa, Organization, structure, and
    assembly of immunoglobulin heavy chain diversity DNA segments,
    J. Exp. Med., 155:201 (1982).
4. P. J. Gearhart, Generation of immunoglobulin variable gene
    diversity, Immunology Today, 3:107 (1982).
5. N. H. Sigal, P. J. Gearhart, J. L. Press, and N. R. Klinman,
    Late acquisition of a germ line antibody specificity, Nature,
    259:51 (1976).
6. C. Fernandez and G. Möller, Immunological unresponsiveness to
    native dextran B512 in young animals of dextran high
    responder strains is due to lack of Ig receptor expression.
    Evidence for a nonrandom expression of V-genes, J. Exp. Med.,
    147:645 (1978).
7. A. Ahmed, I. Scher, S. O. Sharrow, A. H. Smith, W. E. Paul,
    D. H. Sachs, and K. W. Sell, B-lymphocyte heterogeneity:
    development and characterization of an alloantiserum which
    distinguishes B-lymphocyte differentiation alloantigens,
    J. Exp. Med., 145:101 (1977).
8. In: "Idiotypes - Antigens on the Inside" page 18, I. Westen-
    Schnurr, ed., F. Hoffmann-La Roche & Co, Basle (1982).
9. J. J. Mond, R. Lieverman, J. K. Inman, D. E. Mosier, and
    W. E. Paul, Inability of mice with a defect in B-lymphocyte
    maturation to respond to phosphorylcholine on immunogenic
    carriers, J. Exp. Med., 146:1138 (1977).
10. C. Fernandez and G. Möller, Immunological unresponsiveness to
    thymus-independent antigens: two fundamentally different
    genetic mechanisms of B-cell unresponsiveness to dextran,
    J. Exp. Med., 146:1663 (1977).
11. R. M. Perlmutter, D. Hansburg, E. Briles, R.A. Nicolotti, and
    J. M. Davie, Subclass restriction of murine anticarbohydrate
    antibodies. J. Immunol.,121:566 (1978).
12. G. P. D. Der-Balian, J. Slack, B. L. Clevinger, H. Bazin, and
    J. M. Davie, Subclass restriction of murine antibodies. III.
    Antigens that stimulate IgG3 in mice stimulate IgG2c in rats,
    J. Exp. Med., 152:209 (1980).
13. P. K. A. Mongini, K. E. Stein, and W. E. Paul, T cell regulation
    of IgG subclass antibody production in response to T-inde-
    pendent antigens, J. Exp. Med. 153:1 (1981).
14. J. L. Hurwitz, V. B. Tagart, P. A. Schweitzer, and J. J. Cebra,
    Patterns of isotype expression by B cell clones responding
    to thymus-dependent and thymus-independent antigens in vitro,
    Eur. J. Immunol., 12:342 (1982).

15. C. Martinez-Alonso, A. Coutinho, and A. A. Augustin, Immuno-
    globulin C-gene expression. I. The commitment to IgG sub-
    class of secretory cells is determined by the quality of
    the nonspecific stimuli, Eur. J. Immunol., 10:698 (1980).
16. I. Seppälä, H. Sarvas, F. Péterfy, and O. Mäkelä, The four
    subclasses of IgG can be isolated from mouse serum by using
    protein A-Sepharose, Scand. J. Immunol. 14:335 (1981).
17. H. O. Sarvas, I. J. T. Seppälä, T. Tähtinen, F. Péterfy, and
    O. Mäkelä, Mouse IgG antibodies have subclass associated
    affinity differences, Submitted to Molecular Immunology.
18. H. Sarvas, L. Aaltonen, F. Péterfy, and O. Mäkelä, IgG sub-
    class distributions in anti-hapten and anti-polysaccharide
    antibodies induced by haptenated polysaccharides, Submitted
    to J. Immunol.
19. J. Slack, G. P. Der-Balian, M. Nahm, and J. M. Davie, Sub-
    class restriction of murine antibodies. II. The IgG plaque-
    forming cell response to thymus-independent type 1 and type
    2 antigens in normal mice and mice expressing an X-linked
    immunodeficiency, J. Exp. Med., 151:853 (1980).
20. W. Schalch, J. K. Wright, L. S. Rodkey, and D. G. Braun,
    Distinct functions of monoclonal IgG antibody depend on
    antigen-site specificities, J. Exp. Med., 149:923 (1979).
21. W. Schalch, J. K. Wright, L. S. Rodkey, and D. G. Braun,
    Clonal dominance of low-affinity antibodies in rabbit hyper-
    immune anti-streptococcal group A-variant polysaccharide
    antisera, Eur. J. Immunol., 9:145 (1979).
22. S. T. Shulman and E. M. Ayoub, Qualitative and quantitative
    aspects of the human antibody response to streptococcal group
    A carbohydrate, J. Clin. Invest., 54:990 (1974).
23. R. M. Perlmutter, M. Nahm, K. E. Stein, J. Slack, I. Zitron,
    W.E. Paul, and J. M. Davie, Immunoglobulin subclass-specific
    immunodeficiency in mice with an X-linked B-lymphocyte defect,
    J. Exp. Med., 149:993 (1970).
24. J. L. Press, The CBA/N defect defines two classes of T cell-
    dependent antigens, J. Immunol., 126:1234 (1981).

DISCUSSION

G. Möller: I have three comments to make:

1. There is now much evidence against the existence of self tolerance at the B cell level. It was first demonstrated that polyclonal B cell activators could induce self reacting B cells to the synthesis of autoantibodies (Primi et al., Cell. Immunol. 32:252, 1977) a finding later substantiated in several different systems.

2. The role of somatic mutation in B cells may not be very great in some cases. This is illustrated by the response against the alpha 1-6 epitope of dextran. Non-responder strains lacking the V_H gene for antibodies against dextran remain unresponsive for their life time, suggesting that other V genes could not mutate to give rize to antibodies against dextran. In this system various suppressive influences were excluded.

3. To your suggestions why young mice to not respond to PC and the alpha 1-6 epitope of dextran, I only want to add the experimental finding that polyclonal activation of B cells by LPS, known to induce 30% of the B cells, failed to reveal any antibodies against alpha 1-6, although all other specificities tested were detected. Therefore, your suggestion concerning differential activation of Lyb-5$^+$ versus Lyb-5$^-$ cells appears less likely.

Mäkelä: I happen to believe that there is at least a degree of self-tolerization affecting the B cell repertoire, but this is not an essential part of the minimum hypothesis. The hypothesis is made still simpler if the virgin B cell repertoire is not affected by the self-tolerization.

Coutinho: I would like to make two comments which are both related to the "completeness" of antibody repertoires, a point of major importance, in my understanding at least. They argue against G. Möller's interpretation that there are "non-responder" mice to dextran which, therefore, do not carry V-genes that can make up a combining site fitting that molecule. I would submit that any mouse can make antibody molecules to fit any "antigen" with more or less precision. This is, after all, the basis for the selective theories of antibody formation and the result of degeneracy in antibody-antigen reactions. Even in the classical examples, such as the alpha-1,3 dextran, the "low responders" do make reasonable amounts of antibodies. And even if a given test would not reveal antibody activity, I would still say that the mouse is making specific antibodies with an affinity below the threshold of detection in the test employed. In other words, there are no "blanks" in the antibody repertoires.

Moreover, such a completeness appears to be redundant, that is, each mouse is complete several times and has always at its disposal multiple ways of generating combining sites for the same molecules. H. Köhler and J. Kearney have just shown, for example, that mice immunized with a thymus-dependent form of dextran alpha-1,3 utilize clonal precursors carrying kappa light chains and negative for the very dominant J558 idiotype. In essence, I cannot agree with the idea that there are "non-responders" at the level of antibody repertoires.

Sachs: Do you get heteroclitic antibodies with thymus-dependent and independent antigens.

Mäkelä: Yes, NP-ficoll induces heterolytic anti-NP antibodies.

Cohn: Given our present knowledge of how the Igl- and Igh-loci are expressed, I doubt that the findings of Klinman and Möller on the late appearance of germline encoded activities reflects an ordered expression of V-genes. Similar findings were reported by Silverstein some years ago and at the time I interpreted them as due to tolerance. If the library of self components changes as the animal undergoes ontogeny then the order found in the expression of germline V-genes might not be due to an inherent ontogenetic program for their expression but to the elimination by tolerance of B cells expressing certain of these genes.

In rare cases the response to a given determinant might occur late because it takes many steps of mutation and selection to recognize it. However, in the case of anti-PC or anti-alpha(1,6)Dex the recognition is germline encoded. In both cases, the determinants are self-components, PC being present on lecithin which is a major component of cell membranes and alpha(1,6)glucose is a linkage found in glycogen. The adult is not tolerant to these self-components because they are cryptic and never encounter the immune system. PC is on the inside of the membrane and glycogen is an intracellular metabolite. However, this might not be true during ontogeny and the immune system born tolerant to them, might lose tolerance when the tolerogen disappears or becomes cryptic as the animal matures. Whether or not this explanation is correct in detail for these two determinants, the principle is surely involved.

Mäkelä: The results of Silverstein can be explained in several ways, and one of these is that the response to "strong" antigens emerges early but the response to "weak" antigens emerges late. "Strong" can mean a high number of different antigenic determinants and "weak" a low number. For this reason I consider the late emergence of anti-PC and anti-1-6 dextran responses more relevant for this discussion than the results of Silverstein.

Doherty: The problem in interpreting the old experiments with sheep red cells is, that at the stage that the early responses are seen the lymphoid tissue contains very few cells. The apparent hierarchy of response might thus as readily reflect differences in processing, or handling, of diverse antigen, rather than graded emergence of a predetermined repertoire.

G. Möller: The old findings on different expressions of antibodies in ontogeny by Silverstein were based on injection of different antigens into fetal lambs. This method could not distinguish between T and B cell maturation (which were not known at that time) and differences in assay systems. Now we can use various polyclonal B cell activators for the direct activation of B cells. This approach has shown that most antibodies are expressed within a week after birth in the mouse, but there are notable exceptions, such as T15 and the alpha 1-6 epitope of dextran.

One possibility of explaining the differential timing of expression of various V_H genes is that the position of the genes somehow determines its expression. It seems that the T15 and alphaT-6 gene are rather close to each other and both these genes appear late in ontogeny. Maybe the translocations necessary for gene expression is to some extent controlled by the gene localizations.

Cohn: I have proposed that the immunoglobulin loci are selected upon during germline evolution for specificities of survival value at birth. Some of these are known: anti-alpha(1,3)Dex; anti-alpha(1,6)Dex; anti-phosphorylcholine; anti-myxovirus (influenza); anti-galactan; anti-levan, etc. This selection maintains the germline V_L- and V_H-genes optimally functional. V-genes which are not sufficiently selected upon because there are too many copies become pseudogenes. About 30-40% of the V-gene pool is functionless as would be predicted. As an aside there is no hint that the germline is selected upon for its anti-idiotypic specificity as often proposed and in fact it makes no biological sense that it should be thus selected.

This raises the question then of the precise role of combinational joining and chain (LH) complementation in contributing to the repertoire. Clearly, as an extreme, if this source of amino acid diversity contributed the major part of the repertoire there could be no evolutionary selection possible for diversification by somatic mutation on the one hand or maintaining given germline encoded specificities on the other. The usual discussions of diversity which begin by casually multiplying combinatorially are sentimental attempts to reinvent the germline model and run into the same arguments that made it untenable in the first place. Without the temper of appropriate fudge factors, the calculations involving multiplication of nV_H x mD_H x qJ_H x pV_L, etc. do not provide meaningful numbers in discussing functional repertoire size.

What role does this source of amino acid diversity play? We need precise answers. One role of combinatorial joining and complementation would be to increase the dispersion in the initial B cell pool from which somatic mutants are derived such that one step already gives a significant repertoire. In other words, this source of diversity is only a variation on a germline theme. This suggestion would permit a maintenance of the germline by selection for specificity on the one hand and an optimization of the germline for somatic diversification on the other.

Hood: You can select on only one of the many possible combinations for the V_L and V_H's in combinatorial joining. This way you could place selective pressures on each V and still generate the vast repertoire of combinatorial joining.

G. Möller: Do you want to comment on Dresser's finding that about 50% of the B cell repertoir was directed against the Fc part of immunoglobulins and the findings by Lunningham and Cox that around 50% was directed against autologous bromelein treated red cells.

Cohn: A large proportion of B cells are in the activated or B^*-state normally in an animal. The activation is due in large measure to induction by effete self components as red cells and immunoglobulin. This may well represent a normal pathway for ridding this material and for this reason I avoid the word "autoimmune". This antibody response in the mouse is revealed by interactions with bromelein-treated red cells (not normal cells) and Fc or protease clipped Ig (not normal Ig). It is quite possible that the same antibody specificities are involved in both these activities.

The anti-bromelein mouse RBC, crossreacts with sheep RBC and accounts for the high reactivity to SRBC in so-called primary responses. This same antibody seems also to react with isologous and heterologous Fc accounting for high reactivity to xenogeneic Ig. In fact, the polyclonal activation by LPS affecting about 30% of B cells must involve this population since interaction with antigen (Signal (1)) is required for LPS induction (Signal (2)) of B cells to PFC.

Paul: What is your exact meaning of B^* cells?

Cohn: The importance of the existence of activated T^* and B^* cells in the unmanipulated cell populations is often unappreciated. These are the cells which have undergone a T^H-interaction **in vivo** and as a consequence are responsive by proliferation and differentiation to interleukins and antigen. As I pointed out earlier, most of these activated B^* cells are specific for effete self components as red cells and immunoglobulin; others are in the process of induction by foreign antigens. On an average, this later is the non-majority population.

In the **absence** of T helpers, the B^*-population in spleen would show two properties:
1) it would proliferate and differentiate when given appropriate interleukins and antigen. The PFC response of splenic B cells to Con A or cell line supernatants plus sheep RBC is one example. Another example is the bystander response to horse RBC when an ongoing response to sheep RBC generates interleukins.
2) it would give a "polyclonal" PFC response to Type 1 substances like LPS (Signal (2) substitutes) because of the cryptic presence of antigen and LPS generated interleukins.

This opens two comments:
1) The many studies showing that restrictive and associatie recognition of antigen by T^H and B is **not** required (Step 1) are incorrectly analyzing the B^*- not the B-state.

2) The known interleukins are **not** the Signal (2) transmitters. They do **not** substitute for T^H-cells in the associative and restrictive interaction with antigen-sensitive T or B cells. Interleukins only act on the activated antigen-sensitive cells (T^* and B^*) which have undergone the first step of .induction by interaction with T^H. If the T^H-interactions function via a synapse, then this transmitter has yet to be identified.

The physiological requirement for this is obvious. The T^H-interaction is what makes the self-nonself discrimination and regulates the class of the response. The antigen-sensitive cell anti-nonself is now activated and divides. Since T^H is an end cell and acts monogamously, the immune response would be unable to increase exponentially if the requirement for a cell-cell interaction were not now substituted for by a hormone (interleukin) which acts at "intermediate" range and permits free division and differentiation.

However, it is still important that the production of this hormone (interleukin) be strictly under the control of the state of responsiveness of the immune system, i.e. be autogenously regulated. Its production must be turned on and off by the presence or absence of the invading antigen and the T^H-cell recognizing it. If the interleukins were expressed like insulin or ACTH, i.e. under the outside control of an endocrine organ, then any leakiness in the first step requiring a T^H-interaction that resulted in the activation of a single anti-self cell would be lethal.

Wabl: I would like to propose a model for allelic and isotype exclusion. As C. Milstein presented yesterday and was also concluded by G. Köhler, heavy chain in absence of light chain seems to be toxic for the cell. The problem then arises, how pure-B cells survive. We have found a protein which binds to heavy chain in the absence of light chain. We postulate that this protein prevents the toxicity of the heavy chain. If heavy chain is toxic to the cell, and for that reason there is a protein to neutralize its toxicity, why do the cells then blast with heavy chain, and not with light chain? I suggest that there is a connection to allelic exclusion: I postulate that the maximum amount of binding protein that a cell can make is sufficient to neutralize one heavy chain but not two heavy chains. For many people it seems difficult to accept that the amount of binding protein is well controlled to not reach low equivalents of heavy chains. Results of G. Köhler concerning hybridomas of $H_1 H_2 L_1 L_2$ and $H_1 H_2 H_3 L_1 L_2 K_3$ type show that only when there are three light chains present, loss of one light chain prior to heavy chain is allowed. Therefore L chain synthesis is equivalent to 1,5 heavy chains, but not 2 heavy chains. I am proposing the same type of control for the binding protein. Thus, cells which rearrange both H chain loci to yield normal H chains will die because there is not enough binding protein. When there is one, and only one H chain made, rearrangement at the L chain locus will take place. When an L chain is made which can displace the binding protein on the heavy chain, thus forming a complete Ig molecule, the rearrangement process stops. By this mechanism allelic and isotype exclusion for the L chain loci is accomplished.

Session X

Immune Networks

Chairman: D. Sachs

IS THE NETWORK THEORY TAUTOLOGIC?

A. Coutinho, L. Forni, D. Holmberg and F. Ivars

Department of Immunology
University of Umeå, Sweden
Basel Institute for Immunology, Switzerland

INTRODUCTION

Amongst many divergencies, there is at least one point in which Wittgenstein and Popper not only agree but use the same rhetoric example. When explaining tautologies, Wittgenstein writes "For example, I know nothing about the weather when I know that it is either raining or not raining"[1]. Popper, elaborating on falsifiability, rather than verifiability, as a criterion of demarcation for admitting a system as empirical or scientific writes: "Thus, the statement "It will rain or not rain here tomorrow" will not be regarded as empirical, simply because it cannot be refuted; whereas the statement "It will rain here tomorrow" will be regarded as empirical"[2]. Those who know well all the writings of Niels K. Jerne, cannot avoid to recall the last sentence in the Introduction to the 1977 Annual Report from the Basel Institute for Immunology: "... immunology may turn out to be like meterology: we know all the basic elements, but we cannot foretell the weather tomorrow in Basel"[3].

Experiments and interpretations of the idiotypic "network" have in fact turned out like this: any given manipulation may sometimes suppress and others induce, what is true with a monoclonal antibody may well be false with the next, it will rain or not rain, and every result is apparently accommodated by the postulates of the network theory. As Lindenmann once pointed out, immunologists in the post-network era are like trapeze flyers of fancy circuses who always work over a net: they can produce nearly any experimental result

273

and the net(work) is always there to protect them in case of miscalculation.

It may be argued, of course, that the essential characteristics of the immune system embodied by a network of idiotype-paratope interactions which are degenerate and largely generated by random somatic variation would impose precisely those meteorologic conditions. Yet, we believe that much of the research effort produced ever since the presentation of the theory has aimed at forcing open doors, as it has attempted to verify idiotype-anti-idiotype reactions rather than to falsify the basic postulates of the theory. The result is manifested by the present crisis in this area, when the existence of an idiotypic network is still a matter of belief and where most experiments though complicated, beatiful and of very skilful performance tell us little or nothing on the basic rules of the immune system. Historically, we are in the rococo period of this research, and as for the architectural counterpart, this is a dead-end in development. All what these experiments show is that vertebrates produce antibodies against any molecular pattern whatsoever if conveniently immunized. This, we know since Landsteiner.

Again, the experimentalists may argue that the theory itself is already baroque and contains the germ for the fatal rococo development. In its original form, they may say, the network theory is not falsifiable: in an enormously high degree of complexity, it leaves open all possibilities. If this were true, the network theory is a tautology and it cannot be accepted as a scientific exercise.

THE ATTRACTION OF NETWORK PERSPECTIVES AND THE PROBLEMS THEY POSE

The milestones of modern immunology were shaped by Jerne with increasing complexity: from the degeneracy in antigen-antibody reactions and the natural selection in antibody responses[4] to the somatic origin of diversity and the significance of MHC polymorphisms[5], the immunological theory reaches unprecedented levels of elegance and completeness with the idiotypic network ideas[6] [7]. It is now possible to consider immune systems, rather than unorganized collections with various sizes of independent clones of immunocompetent cells. Natural antibody production and the whole inner life of the system, its dynamic properties and stability, are now understandable, and it is even acceptable to consider them quite independent of environmental pressures both ontogenically and phylogenetically. In other words, even the Prometheic paradox in the evolution of immune diversity and recognition[8] can find its logical

explanation in the completeness of the idiotypic repertoire, that
disposes of the rather unappropriate requirements for incomplete
collections of antigens on common pathogens to drive the evolution
of antibody completeness.

Furthermore, internal recognition allows for the selection of
available antibody repertoires to take place (as it must) before
exposure to antigens. Such selection is strictly necessary because,
at any point in their lifetime, individuals can never express more
than 0.1-1 % of the potential antibody repertoire, guaranteed by the
multiplicity of germ line sequences encoding V-regions and the
somatic processes necessary for, or accompanying their expression.
Without selection, the generation of available repertoires would be
entirely based upon the probabilities of physico-chemical DNA
recombination (and mutation) events, which are necessarily ordered
along a hierarchy, determined by primary sequences and/or relative
positions in the chromosome. It would follow that some antibody
clones would be produced very frequently while most of the others
would never "make it " to the 1 % possible in the available
repertorie. This, in turn, would condemn the corresponding genes to
nonsense drift and the germ line repertoires to marked unstability,
for which there is no evidence so far. The requirement for selection
is further reinforced by the enormous turn-over in the B lymphocyte
compartment throughout life (5-10 % a day). While teleologically
justifiable by the size limitations in the available repertoire,
this continuous renewal does not allow for solutions based on the
mere persistance of rare clones. As argued elsewhere[9], an idiotypic
network containing self-reactive antibodies to cellular structures
which control growth of B lymphocytes, and to V-region markers of
antibody clones provides the tools that continuously select for
diversity, as well as the internal stimulation necessary to the
expansion and turnover in the B lymphocyte compartment.

To many immunologists, the attraction in network concepts has
been the possibility of explaining old phenomenology, such as
"clonal dominance", and various other aspects of regulation. While
accepting that idiotype-directed mechanisms provide the only way to
understand immune regulation based on properties other than affinity
to the ligands used as antigens, as well as the intricacies of
paratope-idiotype relationships in populations of antibody
molecules, we do not consider these as fundamental aspects of the
theory. Most often, however, this type of experiments are used as
the major support for network perspectives in quite superficial
analyses of phenomenology, dissociated from the ultimate
significance of the findings.

To us, the essential contribution of the network theory is the possibility of "connecting" B and T cell repertoires, both in the individual immune systems and in the evolution of germ line polymorphisms in the species. Considering that qualitatively different evolutionary requirements have imposed distinct repertoires of antibodies and T cell receptors, as we do, an idiotypic network may provide the unique solution to a unifying perspective of the immune system.

For classical immunological thinking, however, the network ideas have probably posed more problems than those they solved. First of all, by making idiotypic repertoires "complete" (from the point of view of antibody combining sites) the theory abolishes the distinction between self and nonself antigens, unifying both sets in the same universe of molecular patterns, recognizable with greater or lesser precision, by a complete combining site repertoire. This, of course, makes "clonal abortion" an unacceptable cataclism, and revives old fears of "horror autotoxicus".

For simple minds, network ideas may actually transmit the basic repulsion that pre-hellenic labyrinths raised in the barbarian invaders. In fact, immune responses lose the linear simplicity of rabbits producing the "right" high affinity antibodies because a given bacteria was injected: the anti-polysaccharide antibody may well be specific also for the variable regions of an antibody against alloantigens, or even "look like" bovine serum albumin. Even the corner stone of modern immunology can be thought to be threatened: the basic rule of one antigen - a few specific clones is no longer valid, because any perturbation of the immune steady state is expected to have consequences to the whole system, involving many clones which display no specificity to the inducing ligand.

Finally, the idiotypic network was presented as a necessary consequence of immune diversity, almost as a curse let upon the system by its own requirements for universal recognition. It is just there, and there were no suggestions as to where it had come from (specificity of germ-line antibody genes and its evolution from primitive, small immune systems).

All together, the network theory does not make predictions that can be tested by the experimentalist who, in addition, feels it as an impossible task to describe all the unique interactions amongst many millions of different antibody molecules or lymphocytes that all can, in one way or another, influence any other.

ANALYSIS OF THE FALSIFIABILITY OF THE NETWORK THEORY

The reading of the two papers in which the network theory was presented and developed reveals a picture quite different from that currently taken as correct. The reasons for this are many. The theory became rapidly fashionable , not always taken with the necessary rigor and precision. To start with, its name was popular before its content, and a variety of "networks" immediately flourished, made up of all sorts of cell types and "factors" supposed to suppress, amplify or stimulate some other ones, and demonstrating all thinkable "patterns of restriction". Jerne's theory has of course nothing to do with all this, as it applies to interactions between variable regions regardless of the functional properties of the molecules or cells carrying them. For example, the network theory is properly applicable to isolated B lymphocyte or antibody collections. Unavoidably, therefore, hundreds of contributions were, and will continue to be added to the initial formulation, in particular by those wanting to use "network(s)" to explain their findings. As a result, the "network theory" has spread unformed, to become the tautology we described above.

Very clearly, however, Jerne's theory contains only a single, fully falsifiable postulate, namely, the existance of an idiotypic network: the large diversity of antibody variable regions must result in internal recognition, and the degeneracy of antibody recognition must establish a multiplicity of interactions involving each individual molecule, resulting in the composition of a formal idiotypic network with unknown levels of "connectance". The stability of such network can perhaps be taken as the other proposition in the theory, but neither the completeness of the idiotypic repertoire nor the functionality or relevance of the network were ever postulated by Jerne. In 1976, he was still asking whether or not "... every antibody is an anti-idiotypic antibody", questioning therefore that completeness. And "Even granted that the immune system is a network, does that have important functional consequences or does it just happen to be a network?". Even more explicit: "Is the network of idiotypes and anti-idiotypes the essential feature of the immune system, or is this an illusion?"[10] And in 1981, "Does the set (of V-genes) have no logic at all except that it should maximize antibody diversity?"[11]

It is surprising, therefore, that after 8 years not one experimentalist has decided to directly test the validity of that single postulate, and not one experiment has aimed at investigating

the very existence of a formal idiotypic network. We have instead
spent our time describing the phenomenology of idiotypic
manipulations, not even attempting to study and describe the
properties of the putative network.

     Much was left to be developed from the original propositions
of Jerne. Soon afterwards, Adam and Weiler[12] added another step
towards a complete formulation of the theory, by introducing a new
postulate which makes clear predictions about germ-line repertoires.
Adam and Weiler proposed that antibody clones expressed in early
ontogeny immediately engage in idiotype-paratope interactions,
making it very likely that an idiotypic network is germ-line encoded
and that the determinants driving the evolution of germ-line
sequences are the idiotypic profiles of the other members in the
set. They further postulate the functional relevance of such
interactions which result in expansion of the B cell compartment and
in the generation of antibody diversity, by the selection of
variants into the available repertoires. Here again, the
propositions appear within the reach of experimentation, in
particular the existence of a formal network in early ontogeny, and
the functional properties of "early" antibodies in the development
of B cell clones. Adam and Weiler's postulates complete Jerne's
propositions by defining one characteristic of the germ-line
repertoire, namely, its internal complementarity: the basic
specificity of germ-line antibodies is not the set of MHC antigens
of the species (as previously proposed by Jerne), but rather the set
of idiotypic determinants in the same collection of antibodies.
Furthermore, they underline the necessity of providing an internal
driving force for the expansion and turn-over in the B lymphocyte
compartment, and propose the general principles controlling the
selection of available repertoires.

     In our opinion, these are the postulates thus far available
on the network theory. As already pointed out, they are clear and
testable, and carry the enormous attraction of all potentialities
they suggest. On the other hand, they propose no solution to a
number of fundamental questions and do not consider that, whatever
functional consequences we can expect from these V-region
interactions, they depend on the performance of lymphocytes and,
consequently, the theory must necessarily consider (and it does not
so far) the physiology of lymphocytes. In its present form, the
network theory applies to molecules only, and exclusively to one
single set of molecules. It appears to us that the next step
forwards must bring in the cells which perform and ensure the
putative functionality, much in the same way as the "clonal
selection theory" represented the next step to the "natural

selection theory" of antibody formation.

WHERE THE NETWORK THEORY IS INCOMPLETE

We shall analyse now the problems left unsolved by the original propositions of the theory. As already pointed out, the network theory does not consider the question of self-nonself discrimination. The theory proposes that self and nonself antigens are equally well represented in the immune system itself by the diversity of idiotypes, but it includes no solution to the functional discrimination determining health and disease. Further analysis of this point clarifies the nature of the problem. By postulating internal recognition of self determinants (which may vary in serum concentrations by orders of magnitude), the original propositions are formally incompatible with deletion of self-recognizing antibodies and, therefore, imply that such fundamental discrimination cannot be based on the range of antibody specificities present in the available repertoire. It follows that, if antibody recognition does not provide the means to discriminate (determine whether or not auto-antibodies are produced and self-reactive B cells activated), antibody receptor recognition cannot be discriminatory in the functional process of B cell activation (paralysis versus induction). As previously pointed out[9], it is precisely this functional aspect of the theory which is the least developed, but its postulates are sufficiently clear to be mutually exclusive with all hypotheses on B cell activation which ascribe discriminatory properties to immunoglobulin receptors (e.g.,the "two signal hypothesis"[13]). In contrast, the original network postulates not only are compatible with alternative perspectives on the mechanisms of B lymphocyte activation ("one signal hypothesis"[14]), but they merge with, and raise to higher levels the implications derived from these models[9 15].

Another consequence of the lack of cell-biological perspectives, both in the original network postulates and in current interpretations of the theory, is manifested by our present ignorance on the basic rules controlling selection of available repertoires and the functionality of idiotypic interactions. In turn, the final consequences of any V-region-directed manipulation of the system is, currently, quite unpredictable. The selection of available repertoires is, perhaps, the central question in immunology, related as it is to self-nonself discrimination and to the protective role of the immune system. It is not sufficient, however, to postulate continuous selection for diversity and completeness, as antibody collections have the property of being complete in thousand and one different ways[16][17]. Here again, the present difficulties arise from the lack of clear postulates on the physiology of lymphocyte precursors and immunocompetent cells, on the receptors they use to be turned on or off, and on the set of mechanisms controlling the growth and terminal maturation to high-rate antibody secretion. If one anti-idiotype stimulates and the next suppresses, if one idiotype requires complementary helper cells for "dominance" while others do not, this cannot be all left as indications that the "network functions", and it must be due to the fact that the specificities and interactions we are analysing (between antibody molecules) are not the basis for their functional properties. In fact, from the dozens of genes encoding the functions and receptors which make a B lymphocyte different from a neuron or a liver cell, we only know of one type, and this, perhaps, makes us forget that combining sites and idiotypes on antibody molecules may well interact with many cellular structures other than antibody receptors. Obviously, the solution of immunology requires the basic knowledge on those non-immunoglobulin genes and of their products'physiology in the cells using them, and this will take time. It is our conviction, however, that the present crisis in the idiotypic research is largely due to the exclusion from the "network" of everything else but antibodies and T cell receptors. Astonishingly so, because it is the essence of the theory that idiotypes may "look like" anything else and that specificities must be available in the combining site repertoire against functionally relevant receptors of lymphocytes, whatever these might be.

The third and perhaps more important limitation in the original network postulates is central to the essential aims of the theory itself: a unifying perspective of the immune system. We referred above to this question as the "connection" between B and T cell repertoires which, thus far, are thought to communicate as mature sets, but are left quite isolated (independent) evolutionarily and ontogenically. Having proposed the anti-MHC specificity of germ-line antibody genes a few years earlier, Jerne did not address this question in the frame of the network theory. Meanwhile, lymphocytes were divided in T and B cells and the rightness of the 1971 hypothesis in what respects T cell repertoires could only be compared to the increasing conviction that B lymphocytes and antibodies did not appear particularly preoccupied with MHC. In parallel, Adam and Weiler explicited that an idiotypic network in the mature immune system must start from a "germ-line network" (implying anti-idiotypic specificity of germ-line genes), and the prevalent belief that B and T cells shared V-region genes slowly faded away. We are then left with two quite independent immune

systems and no unifying concept. Perhaps more aware than anybody
else, Jerne has pointed out the problem and actually suggested a
solution. In the same Introduction to the 1977 Annual Report, he
writes "Do idiotypes relate to MHC? An answer to these questions is
needed for developing a unified theory of immunology".

A FEW MORE POSTULATES PORSUING NETWORK PERSPECTIVES

It is not our ability or intention to delineate that unified
theory of immunology. We will simply add to the basic postulates a
few propositions derived from our perpectives directly bred on
studies of lymphocyte physiology. We will elaborate on the three
basic points in which the network theory is not explicit, letting it
clear that our current experiments aim, primarily, at testing the
existence of an idiotypic network altogether.

We will consider three sets of receptor molecules and
respective gene families, displaying, perhaps, different degrees of
diversity in vertebrate immune systemns, but all three fundamental
to the specificity and function of lymphocytes: (a) antibodies; (b)
T cell receptors (for simplicity, and because the basic rules are
common, only one class of T cells is considered, although cytotoxic
and helper lymphocytes should be distinguished in any detailed
analysis); (c) receptors controlling activation from the resting
state in mature B lymphocytes, and their growth and differentiation
as precursors (this set is also likely to include different families
of receptors in precursors and immunocompetent cells; they are here
included in one category only, because of their unique functional
properties). It should not pass unnoticed that we do not postulate
an equivalent set of activation receptors for T lymphocytes. As
analysed below, this is because induction of T cells must take place
via clonally distributed receptors for reasons of self-nonself
discrimination and, consequently, set (b) ensures simultaneously
immunological specificity and functional reactivity.   Recent
experiments do support this identity[18].   Precisely the opposite
aplies to B lymphocytes, carrying a complete recognition repertoire
as antibody receptors. The detailed argumentation of these
postulates has been previously presented[9 15 17]. Finally, we will
not consider in this analysis the cell type-specific polyclonally
active growth or maturation factors and respective receptors,
necessary for expansion of induced lymphocytes. As Jerne says:
"...for grass to grow, many conditions must be fulfilled, though
they do not determine what kind of grass".

We postulate that all three gene families have evolved from

primitive systems in intimate connection with, and submitted to the evolution of the gene complex ensuring individuality in species which reproduce sexually, within which self must be learned ontogenically. The central gene family in the evolution of immune systems is, therefore, the most ancient and perhaps the most polymorphic: the major histocompatibility complex.

We next postulate that, evolutionarily, sets (b) and (c) branched very early, while antibodies, the (a) set, are of much later acquisition. (We will not engage in alternative considerations of convergent evolution of these gene families if independent origins are postulated, even though we recognize the validity of this exercise.) The original set of genes controlling reactivity to nonself was thus duplicated and specialized in: set (b), recognizing similar-to-self structures, namely, MHC antigens of the species; and set (c), recognizing very-different-from-self structures, e.g. bacterial products. Both sets of receptors are fully competent in functional discrimination, that is, they regulate induction of cells from the resting state. Set (b) is complete (recognizes all MHC allotypes in the species) but, as previously argued[9], such completeness is only apparent and inbuilt in the type of driving forces provided by self-complementarity which ensure the ontogenic development of immune systems. Set (b) and MHC genes have, therefore, evolved in interdependence as mirror images, provided with some of the properties of immune recognition - crossreactivity and lack of precision. This apparent evolutionary "completeness" of the germ-line set (b) ensures the internal driving forces for ontogenic expansion and, consequently, the possibilities for somatic selection of available repertoires and for inactivation of self-reactive cells. Once again, this is only possible because receptors of set (b) are discriminatory. The result is the partial, incomplete repertoire displayed by the immunocompetent T cell compartment and its self MHC-dependence, recognizing and reacting with a range of variations from self markers but ignoring, for example, bacterial lipopolysaccharides.

The germ-line set (c), on the other hand, can be let to evolve exclusively on the basis of environmental pressures which can never be "confused" with self (e.g., endotoxin, rather than the antigenic determinants of variant polysaccharides). This set, therefore, need not show extensive polymorphism across species, in contrast with set (b) which must follow whatever MHC consequences of speciation events. Because of their functional ability as receptors and the corresponding danger of auto-aggression, set(c) genes must evolve for precision rather than for degeneracy of recognition. Most importantly, the cellular expression of these genes (surely anti-nonself) requires no ontogenic modification or "learning", and this results in another fundamental property of set (c) genes, namely, their polyclonal expression. In contrast, there is an obvious advantage in the clonal expression of set (b) genes. The selection and maintenance of set (c) genes appears quite straightforward, except on one point, namely, their dependence upon environmental nonself for ontogenic cellular expansion and turnover.

We then postulate the evolutionary advantage of internal recognition: any product of set (c) which will happen to "look like" an MHC product will be selected for, as it will be maintained by complementary set (b) specificities, even in the absence of "symbiosis" with external pathogens. The selection of idiotypic profiles of set (c) products, and therefore, of this germ-line collection of genes is then an indirect consequence of the primordial selection for MHC-set (b) complementarities.

The appearance of effector molecules such as antibodies brings in fine tuning, new types of complementarities and the final degree of complexity. Because their production can only be initiated by discriminatory steps in which they do not participate, antibody repertoires can evolve for universality of recognition and degeneracy without endangering self-nonself discrimination. Individuals may then contain a complete recognition set of combining sites (produce antibodies against any molecular pattern), but neither complete functional ability (e.g., high and low responders) nor B cell reactivity to all substances (e.g., thymus-dependent and -independent antigens; haptens and immunogens). This dicotomy between antibody recognition and B cell activation also imposes the strict necessity of ensuring clonality in the expression of antibodies. It is perhaps not very profitable to consider from which set, (b) or (c), or none of these, did set (a) evolve, because the final result is completeness. It may be necessary, however, to explicit the postulates that guarantee the functional conditions for these evolutionary requirements. Thus, three orders of internal complementarities are now possible in the system: between sets (b) and (c) as before, but also between sets (b) and (a), and (a) and (c) as well. Combining sites of set (c) are not involved in any internal recognition, because of their evolutionary selection for nonself. Their "idiotypic" profile, however, can be recognized by set (b) as before, but also by set (a) and the same postulate can be made again, for the advantage of retaining anti-set (c) antibody specificities. Such combining sites are ultimately crossreactive with MHC, in view of the evolution of set (c) idiotypes. In parallel, the interactions between sets (b) and (a), bring us to a complementary solution. Thus, set (b) will select for complementary members in the (a) set, in other words, for idiotypic profiles "resembling" MHC products. It follows that set (a) is the result of two simultaneous but independent selective pressures: positive selection for a set of "anti-MHC" (anti-set (c)) combining sites and positive selection for a set of idiotypes reproducing MHC from the "point of view" of set (b). These two subsets are complementary within set (a) itself, resulting in an idiotype-paratope network in the collection of germ-line antibodies.

An equivalent process can certainly be postulated to occur in ontogeny. These properties of antibody repertoires also result in the important (?) advantage of making the B lymphocyte system (carrying both sets (a) and (c)) independent of the presence of set (b), also from the functional and developmental points of view.

In summary, our propositions are as follows, when applied to the mammalian immune system:

1. Set (b) (T cell receptors) is predominantly anti-MHC, while set (c) (polyclonal B cell receptors for induction) is predominantly similar to MHC in its idiotypic profile. Set (a) is a network, developed around fundamental specificities which are complementary MHC-like-anti-MHC specificities.

2. Paratopically, set (a) is complete, on the basis of degenerate recognition. Somatic diversification and continuous selection for variants results in the generation of larger repertoires with much greater precision of recognition for any particular pattern randomly selected. B lymphocytes expressing antibody receptors with specificities for nonself and self determinants (except those recognized by members of set (b)) are generated and decay at similar rates. Self-nonself discrimination is ensured by the specificity of: I) polyclonally expressed receptors of set (c) which are germ-line encoded, recognize very-different-from-self molecules, and do not vary somatically; II) receptors of set (b), which are ontogenically selected against anti-self specificities.

3. Internal driving forces provided either by (a) anti-(c), by (b) anti-(c), or both types of complementarities lead to expansion of B cell precursors and ensure B cell turnovers. The unequal distribution of (c) receptors in B cell populations and their precursors, together with the clonality of (a) molecules ensure

selection for variants of (a) as a continuous somatic process. Two sites and mechanisms of somatic selection are postulated. One, basically T cell-independent and mediated by antibodies, which operates at the level of precursor cell expansion and bone marrow output of competent B lymphocytes. It provides the eigen-behaviour of the immune network, as the available collection of circulating antibodies selects for a given available repertoire of immunocompetent cells. Another, basically T cell-dependent, which operates in the periphery and selects, from the available pool of specificities carried by short-lived immunocompetent B cells, those which will persist and terminally differentiate to "natural" antibody production.

4. The only functionally relevant interactions in the idiotypic network are those involving these three sets of germ-line encoded specificities. The majority of the idiotype-paratope interactions, therefore, are of no particular systemic significance and result from the portion of randomness in the process of somatic generation of higher diversity (any collection of 10^6 different proteins will necessarily show a given degree of "connectance").

REFERENCES

1. L. Wittgenstein, "Tractatus Logico-Philosophicus", Rontledge and Kegan Paul, London (1961).
2. K. R. Popper, "The logic of Scientific Discovery", Hutchinson, London (1959).
3. N. K. Jerne, Introduction, in "Basel Institute for Immunology, Annual Report 1977", Basel Institute for Immunology, Basel (1978).
4. N. K. Jerne, The natural selection theory of antibody formation, Proc. Natl. Acad. Sci. USA, 41:849 (1955).
5. N. K. Jerne, The somatic generation of immune recognition. Eur. J. Immunol., 1:1 (1971).
6. N. K. Jerne, Towards a network theory of the immune system. Ann Immunol. (Inst. Pasteur), 125C:373 (1974).
7. N.K. Jerne, The immune system: a web of V-domains, Harvey Lectures, Series 70, Academic Press, New York (1976).
8. S. Ohno, The significance of gene duplication in immunoglobulin evolution (Epimethean natural selection and Promethean evolution), in "Immunoglobulins", G. W. Litman and R. A. Good, eds., Plenum Medical Book Company, New York (1978)
9. A. Coutinho, The self-nonself discrimination and the nature and acquisition of the antibody repertoire. Ann. Immunol. (Inst. Pateur), 131D:235 (1980).

10. N. K. Jerne, in "Idiotypes: What they said at the time", Basel
    Institute for Immunology, Basel (1980).
11. N. K. Jerne, in "Idiotypes: Antigens on the inside", Editiones
    "Roche", Basel (1982).
12. G. Adam, and Weiler, E., Lymphocyte population dynamics during
    ontogenetic generation of diversity, in "The generation
    of antibody diversity", A. J. Cunningham, ed., Academic
    Press, London (1976).
13. P. Bretscher and Cohn, M., A theory of self-nonself
    discrimination. Science, 169:1042 (1970).
14. A. Coutinho and Möller, G., Immune activation of B cells:
    evidence for "one nonspecific triggering signal" not
    delivered by the Ig receptors. Scand. J. Immunol. 3:133
    (1974).
15. A. Coutinho, The theory of the "The nonspecific signal" model
    for B cell activation. Transpl. Rev., 23:49 (1975).
16. L. Forni, and Coutinho, A., Individuality of immune systems:
    the thousand ways and one way of being complete, in "The
    Immune System", C.S. Steinberg and I. Lefkovitz, eds.,
    vol. 1, Karger, Basel (1981).
17. A. Coutinho, Forni, L., and Bernabe, R.R., The polyclonal
    expression of Immunoglobulin variable region determinants
    on the membrane of B cells and their precursors. Springer
    Sem. Immunopathol., 3:171 (1980).
18. E.-L. Larsson, Gullberg, M., Beretta,.A., and Coutinho, A.,
    Requirement for the involvement of clonally distributed
    receptors in the activation of cytotoxic T lymphocytes.
    Immunol. Rev., 68:in press (1982).

DISCUSSION

Sachs: The present session has been titled "Immune Networks" by the organizers, and how controversial this title may be depends rather heavily on its definition. In the broadest sence "immune network" would include all of the cellular and humoral interactions by which immune reactivity is controlled. From this view point we must all agree that immune networks exist, since it is an empirical fact that all immune sequences are subject to regulation and control. In addition it is clear from genetic studies in murine models that multiple genetic loci are involved in this control. Thus, even in response under demonstrable H-2 linked to Ir gene control, over-all levels of antibody produced are regulated precisely by background (non-H-2) genes. There would obviously be room for many types of inductive and suppressive immune interactions in such a definition of "network".

However, the more common interpretation of "immune network" at present is restricted to the net of idiotype-anti-idiotype interactions proposed by Jerne and others to form the basis of immune regulation. While the existence of such interactions has now been demonstrated in numerous systems, it remains controversial whether or not they play a physiological role in regulation of immune responses. In addition, even among those who support the concept of idiotype network regulation there is debate as to whether networks exist prior to perturbation by antigen or are only set in motion as regulatory elements following antigen exposure.

In this session we have already heard from Dr. Antonio Coutinho, who discussed the concept of the idiotype network.

I believe Dr. Mel Cohn has a few comments to clarify his own views on this question. I shall then show a few examples from work in my own laboratory indicating that refardless of whether or not idiotype network interactions are of physiological significance they can be used experimentally to manipulate the immune response following exogenous administration of anti-idiotype. Drs. Möller and Coutinho then also have some brief results bearing on the idiotype network to present within the discussion which will hopefully follow these presentations.

Cohn: There is in my mind a difference between a postulate (or a guess) and a theory. Most so-called theories in immunology are guesses at various levels of generality. Whether they are right or wrong is not in question. What is in question is whether they are reasoned from a set of **a priori** principles, whether they can be tied into the bracketing levels of organization and whether they can select for analysis the fundamental properties of the system and then deal with them.

Classic postulates (or guesses) are the so-called "instructionist" theory, "self-marker" theory, "altered-self" theory, "germline" theory and "network" theory. Each is a statement about immune behaviour without a reasoned reductionist tie to other levels of organization. These postulates or (guesses) can be compared to an "astrological" theory of the immune system, i.e. the position of the planets determines responsiveness in the immune system. Given possible effects on circadian rhythms, etc. it is as informative, defensible and disprovable as the above guesses. I am surprised that it is not more popular.

If, as Coutinho argues, the **only** point that Jerne has made concerning network interactions via the idiotype is that they are inevitable or **a priori** necessary or a logical necessity, we would have little to discuss since that assertion is easily falsified. However, even if it were true, this postulate alone provides no theory of immune regulation since it cannot deal with any aspect of immune behaviour, e.g. the self-nonself discrimination or regulation of class of the response, without many additional assumptions. Clearly, postulates must be added concerning the configuration and functional consequence of each type of network interaction.

In fact, however, in the Jerne 1974 paper you are referring to, the unstated additional assumptions were used to account for a series of observatios, e.g. low zone tolerance, 7S-inhibition, antigenic competition, the Oudin-Cazenave enigma, unspecific response, etc.

Did the network postulate permit Jerne to select, pose and deal with fundamental questions? Let us compare it to associative recognition theory.

In 1967, the associative recognition theory permitted us to face the self-nonself discrimination (essentially still ignored by network theory) and select out of a morass of data three phenomena.

1. The Landsteiner phenomenon or the hapten-carrier relationship. A non-immunogenic substance must be coupled to an immunogenic one to induce antibody to it.

2. The Mitchison phenomenon.
The establishing of tolerance (negative unresponsiveness) is antigen-dose dependent whereas the maintaining of tolerance is antigen-dose independent.

3. The Weigle phenomenon.
The breaking of tolerance by cross-reacting immunogens is prevented by the presence of the tolerogen i.e. there is competition between

tolerance and induction at the level of the antigen-sensitive cell.

These are the cornerstones of cellular immunology showing that, in order to induce, two determinants linked on an antigen must be recognized associatively, one by the antigen-sensitive cell and the other by a T-helper. Recognition of one determinant by an antigen-sensitive cell must lead to tolerance by inactivation.

The associative recognition theory was then extended by Bretscher and by myself to include the problem of the regulation of class and the phenomenon of suppression was placed in that context. Further, as Langman and I showed, restrictive recognition could be easily understood as the mechanism of associative recognition.

What has network theory added?

It cannot deal with the self-nonself discrimination until a **reasoned** postulate is added as to how the immune system distinguishes self-idiotopes from all other self-epitopes. It cannot deal with the regulation of Ig class because all Ig classes have the same idiotopes and suppression which is required (but never analyzed) by network theory for the self-nonself discrimination cannot be used for regulation of class.

The assumption that suppression determines tolerance only puts the problem of the self-nonself discrimination at the level of induction and tolerance in the suppressor population. Who has dared to tackle that problem? In addition, some statements about which class of immune response is suppressed (and by "whom") is required. I have pointed out why suppression (positive unresponsiveness) cannot be the mechanism of the self-nonself discrimination. If unresponsiveness to self components on the surface of antigen-sensitive cells were maintained by suppression, they would be unresponsive to all antigens. If suppression maintained tolerance, in order for antigen-sensitive cells to respond to foreign antigens, tolerance would have to be broken to self antigens. The network provides no role for restrictive recognition of antigen because the cell-cell interactions are disassociative ("abnormal") via the idiotype not the antigen.

Further, the above three phenomena selected by associative recognition theory would have been ignored by network theory. In fact, they form an embarrassment for network theory as Jerne's 1974 paper shows. Consider, for example, how the hapten-carrier relationship would be explained! Or ask yourself if 7S-inhibition, antigenic competition, unspecific response, etc. are primary or secondary phenomena compared to the Landsteiner, Mitchison or Weigle phenomena. And in any case, are they adequately explained?

The best test of a guess vs. a theory is that a guess does not tell you which experimental observations to be suspicious of. For example, the Oudin-Cazenave observation if it were general could not be understood under associative recognition theory. I am referring to the generalization that, if two unrelated determinants, H_1 and H_2, are linked together on one molecule of a given carrier (C) (H_1-C-H_2) then the antibodies induced to them, anti-H_1 and anti-H_2, will express crossreactive idiotypes. However, if they are on separate given carrier molecules (H_1-C+H_2-C) then the antibodies induced to them, anti-H_1 and anti-H_2, will not express crossreactive idiotypes. Observed once, I would define it as a fortuity; observed more than once, associative recognition theory would require the explanation that it is an artefact. Under network theory there are no grounds for suspicion and the heroic explanation proposed by Jerne (using many additional guesses) illustrates my point although by calling it an "enigma" he shows that his instincts are good.

This leads to my last point. Most investigators will soon start taking a middle road by arguing that both associative and network recognition are important. Here you are absolutely correct. Associative recognition of antigen trivializes (makes second order) any possible contribution of network recognition as a useful regulatory mechanism. Given that "associative recognition" and "network" theory are incompatible, the choice between the two must be made by experiment and reason and not by arguing that "since Jerne has always been right" (?), the possibility that his network "postulate is wrong is **a priori** disregarded".

If the network postulates turns out to be wrong (or even second order for immune regulation), in what context would we analyze all of the data interpreted under the umbrella of "suppressor" and "helper" circuits **obligatorily** operating via recognition of the self-idiotype? Should't we be preparing for that?

Coutinho: Mel (Cohn), whatever considerations we may draw over it, it remains for me as the most important point that the network theory (which I consider a theory and not wishful thinking, as you do) is formally incompatible with all hypotheses ascribing a discriminatory role to antibody recognition in self-nonself discrimination. We both agree that the network theory did not solve self-nonself, but also that network and two-signal hypotheses are incompatible and at least one must be wrong.

Cohn: All theories of immune regulation must account for autoimmunity. The existence of autoimmunity does not, however, permit the argument that any given class of antigen-sensitive cell, e.g. B, is not tolerizable. And, above all, it does not permit, without a blush, two conclusions:

1. "Two signal" postulates are now untenable, for they would

impose the elimination of the complete repertoire of antibodies".

2. "Since the same Ig can be both an idiotype (recognizing antigen X) and an anti-idiotype, the "Two signal" theory would lead to an empty immune system completely paralyzed by natural tolerance".

It is a source of wonder to me how man can use his common sense to invent such uncommon nonsense.

First, even if you reject the associative recognition model (two-signal) hypothesis at the level of the B cell, you will be forced to reinvent it at the level of the regulatory T cell. Think it through!

Second, the direct evidence today (Glasebrook for LPS (1982); Julius for anti-Ig (1982)) that B cells receive signals via their Ig receptors is too strong to be ignored above all in the absence of a **conceptual** argument as to why not!

Third, the animal lives in a sea of immunogens which crossreact with self-tolerogens. Yet, normally it only responds to the unshared determinants (X_F), i.e. the Weigle phenomenon of competition between tolerogen and immunogen at the level of the antigen-sensitive B and T cell. How do you account for that?

Fourth, tolerance can be broken when the competition favours induction, e.g. in the absence of the tolerogen or in the presence of sufficiently high effective levels of help. This is the origin of autoimmunity.

Where do the T and B cells anti-self come from?

The T and B cells anti-self and anti-nonself are generated continously throughout life. This is an inevitable consequence of the generation of diversity. The anti-self cells because of an insufficiency of T^H anti-self are eliminated by tolerance (negative unresponsiveness). The antigen-sensitive cells anti-nonself accumulate and turnover in a steady state, antigen-independent, until they encounter the selective pressure of an immunogenic stimulus. It is possible to divert an anti-self cell from a tolerogenic to an inductive pathway (the Weigle phenomenon). The fact that this is possible does not tell us the B cells are not tolerizable. It only tells us that at no stage are they tolerizable only. The same must be and is true for the T cell.

Doherty: Antonio Coutinho raises the question as to whether a new formulation of network theory is needed. Cohn points out that, to include T cell specificity and MHC restriction, we would end up with a global theory which would, in fact, encompass all of immunology. Thus, though one does not doubt the usefulness of experiments concerned with idiotype-anti-idiotype interaction, can one really argue that this is telling us about the nature of a network.

Sachs: I would like now to show some recent work by Drs. Bluestone and coworkers in my laboratory indicting that in vivo administration of anti-idiotype to mice can have a profound effect on the repertoire of antibodies produced in response to subsequent antigen exposure.

Our system involves the anti-H-2K^k response, and we have used several monoclonal antibodies directed against H-2K^k as a source of anti-K^k receptors for production of anti-idiotypic reagents. The purified hybridoma antibodies were prepared by sequential immuno-absorptions of the xenogeneic antisera. In each case studied, the anti-idiotype produced recognized a relatively "private" idiotype, i.e. an idiotype detectable only rarely and at very low levels, in the normal response of mice to the H-2K^k alloantigen on a skin graft on lymphoid cells. This, by the way, is in contrast to the idiotype of one of our anti-Ia monoclonals, 14-4-4, studied by Dr. Epstein in my laboratory, which we have recently reported to constitute a common or "public" idiotype, detectable in anti-I-Ek sera of all mice with appropriate H-2 and allotype (J. Exp. Med. 1981).

When purified anti-idiotypic antibodies to one of the anti-H-2K^k monoclonals, 11-4.1, were injected into BALB/c mice (H-2^d), about 20% of the animals began to make detectable anti-K^k antibodies bearing 11-4.1 idiotypic determinants as detected by specific binding inhibition. This phenomenon was seen regularly following adminstration of 50 ug of anti-Id in saline i.p. on days 0 + 3.

Animals treated in this way were then given C3H (H-2^k) skin grafts. As mentioned above, the 11-4.1 idiotype is seen only very rarely and at low levels following skin grafts to untreated animals. However, in animals pretreated with anti-Id, 30-80% of the anti-K^k antibodies produced following skin grafts bore 11-4.1 idiotypic determinants as detected by binding inhibition. This induction of 11-4.1-like anti-K^k antibodies was seen in 50-80% of treated animals, rather than only in the 20% which were already making anti-K^k antibodies prior to skin grafting. Thus, it would appear that treatment with xenogenic anti-idiotypic antibodies is capable of converting a private idiotype to a public one in the response to H-2K^k. This is likely, therefore, to represent exogenous manipulation of V_H gene repertoire expression by the use of anti-id antibodies.

In very recent experiments we have also been able to transfer this change of repertoire expression by adoptive transfer of T cells from anti-Id treated mice to lightly irradiated untreated host. The adoptive hosts, like anti-Id treated animals, produced the 11-4.1 idiotype as a major component of their humoral response to H-2K^k

skin grafts. These results suggest that the mechanism by which exogenous anti-Id influences V_H repertoire expression may involve a network of immune interactions including both T cells and B cells and both idiotypic and anti-idiotypic receptors.

E. Möller: Is there any effect by pretreatment with the anti-idiotypic antibody on the actual skin graft survival time?

Sachs: To date we have not observed any effect of anti-idiotype treatment on skin graft survival. It should be noted, however, that each anti-K^k monoclonal antibody would react with only one epitope of the K antigen. In the case of the 11-4.1 antibody, the skin grafts from C3H differed from BALB/c at I and D regions as well as at non-H-2 loci and at other epitopes of K^k. It is therefore probably not surprising that manipulation of the response to the 11-4.1 determinants did not affect the overall response. Even in the case of our 36-7-5 antibody (A.TL anti-A.AL) in which the skin grafts differed only at H-2K, only the response to one K^k epitope would have been altered. We are now attempting studies in a system involving the H-2K^b mutants (28-13-3 reacts with C57BL/6 but not with the bM10 mutant) in which we hope that with a single epitope difference we may stand a greater chance of detecting an effect. Of course, it would have been nice if modification of the response to one epitope had produced an effect on the skin graft survival times, and I am sure that had that happened we could have found equally cognant arguments to explain the results!

Svejgaard: Would a subsequent skin graft (after the animal has developed anti-idiotype antibodies) have prolonged survival?

Sachs: The anti-K^k antibodies produced following anti-Id treatment were predominantly of the IgG_1, while anti-K^k antibodies following conventional immunizations are generally presominantly IgG_2. In vitro these IgG_1 antibodies do indeed block cytotoxicity presumably since they bind but do not fix complement. They are thus "blocking antibodies". However, in vivo, as mentioned earlier, we have not yet observed any effects on skin grafts.

Cohn: I will make two points:
First an (AB to A) chimera will reject B skin. The reason is that the B skin expresses a polymorphic differentiation antigen, Sk^b, which induces an immune response in the chimera. I would imagine that the rejection is due to humoral antibody, anti-Sk^b, because the chimera restricted to A could not eliminate the B skin by a T cell (T anti-A anti-Sk^b) restricted in its effector function. It is argued by some that B skingrafts break tolerance to B in the chimera and the **in vivo** rejection is by an allo-T anti-B respone. I rather doubt that this occurs as the animal survives the rejection of the graft, although I am aware of the studies that allo-T anti-B can be induced **in vitro** in the primed spleen from an animal rejecting a skin graft.

Second, the mechanism by which xenogeneic anti-Id induces a humoral response Id^+ anti-X is straight forward under an associative recognition model. The complex formed in the animal couples an immunogenic foreign carrier (xeno anti-Id) to a nonimmunogenic self-component (self-Id). This does two things. It lowers the concentration of self-Id (tolerogen/non-immunogenic) to a point where it cannot compete in the breaking of tolerance by the immunogenic complex (the Weigle phenomenon). Since anti-self cells (T and B) are generated continuously, the immunogenic complex diverts the anti-self Id cells from a tolerogenic to an inductive pathway. We should remember that the T^H anti-xeno Ig could be quite high in animals due to an ongoing response ridding effete Ig and RBC. In any case, the carrier xeno anti-Id is quite immunogenic.

The outcome is induction of RII restricted T^H anti-Id. When antigen X is now presented to the animal, this disassociative source of help, anti-Id, plus the associative source of help, anti-X, favours the induction of B cells which are Id^+ anti-X.

This need not be the only outcome of the administration of anti-Id. If the carrrier anti-Id is administered under conditions where the effective level of help to it is low, then T^S anti-Id could be induced and in that case the induction of Id^+B cells anti-X would be disfavoured.

The principles in breaking tolerance to the self-Id are the same whether, as an outcome, as suppressive or inductive mode dominates. In addition, they are the same whether a self-idiotope or any other self-epitope is involved. In this regard, there is nothing special about self-idiotopes.

I have found no phenomenon discussed in the framework of an idiotype network that cannot be more precisely and meaningfully analyzed in the framework of associative recognition.

Sprent: The paradox that anti-idiotypic antibodies primes both C.B20 and BALB/c T cells, whereas only BALB/c B cells produce the idiotype (ID), is only a paradox if the T cells are indeed Id^+. Why not invoke antigenic mimicry and argue that a portion of the anti-Id antibody "resembles" antigen (K^k)? One could argue that the (Id) T cells recognize this antigen (anti-Id) after typical processing by macrophages and presentation in association with self Ia. These T cells then collaborate with B cells to produce anti-K^k antibody. In this case of BALB/c B cells these T cells would be expected to preferentially stimulate Id^+ B cells, i.e. B cells with the closest specificity for the antigen used to prime the T cells, i.e. anti-Id. The key question obviously is whether anti-Id plus C' would kill both C.B20 and BALB/c specific T cells.

Sachs: CB-20 animals make very low levels of 11-4.1 Id in response to anti-Id treatment. However, this Id appears to be entirely of the Id' variety - i.e. it bears idiotopes but does not have anti-K^k binding activity. Presumably, the CB-20 does not make antibodies containing sufficient 11-4.1 idiotopes to also bind antigen. The idiotopes it does produce, however, could be sufficient to induce anti-Id T cells and this may be why they also worked in the adoptive transfer system.

Forman: Your data supports the idea of a feedback loop rather than a network. How can we use your data to go further and support a network theory?

Paul: I would like to point out that the simple existence of B cells and/or antibodies capable of mutual reactivity does not establish that they are actually in contact with one another. Their concentrations may be so low that the chance they may form complexes would be correspondingly low. This would be akin to a spider web containing nodes without threads joining these nodes.

G. Möller: Carmen Fernandez and I have tried to investigate the role of autoanti-idiotypic antibodies in the regulation of an immune response. We found that autoanti-idiotypic antibodies appear spontanously in the course of an immune response to the alpha 1-6 epitope of dextran (Proc. Nat. Acad. Sci. 76:5944, 1979). The immune response to dextran is characterized by a very rapid increase of IgM antibodies that peak on day 5 and of IgG antibodies (in certain strains) that peak on day 6. Thereafter, there is a marked decrease of the response and no plaque forming cells can be detected at days 10-12 (Fig.3 in my presentation in Session VIII).

Another characteristic of the immune response to dextran is that it is not possible to induce a secondary response to the antigen (Scand. J. Immunol. 11:53, 1980). Actually, there is no response at all after the primary, even if the mice are treated with dextranase and the interval between the first and second antigen injection is more than 20 weeks. This suppression is determinant specific and does not affect another epitopes conjugated to dextran.

Suppression was found to be mediated by autoanti-idiotypic antibodies and could be passively transferred to untreated recipients. Furthermore, it was found that the appearance of these autoanti-idiotypic antibodies was thymus dependent. Thus, nude mice do not develop autoanti-idiotypic antibodies and nude mice give a response to a second injection with dextran, which is similar to the primary response.

The important question is whether the rapid decline of the

plaque-forming cells that occurs in the primary response was due to endogenous regulation by autoanti-idiotypic anibodies. This can be studied by comparing the response in normal and nude mice or T cell depleted animals. We found that there was no difference between these mice, indicating that autoanti-idiotypic antibodies do not normally regulate the primary immune response.

Mäkelä: What turns off the response in the nude mice?

G. Möller: There are many regulatory mechanisms that could operate. Antibody feed-back suppression would be the most likely candidate.

Coutinho: I want to report on experiments carried out by Dan Holmberg and Fredrik Ivars in our laboratory, which aim at testing the existance of a formal idiotypic network in the pool of "natural antibodies". We think this is the only postulate in the network theory and it is fully testable. We attempted to study this point in immune systems which are as little as possible influenced by environmental priming, and therefore, closest germline. We are preparing collections of hybridomas from normal newborn mice and screening such antibodies for mutual interactions. This work is still in progress but I could perhaps discuss a few results obtained in the original screening from primary cultures. I must underline that all these have yet to be confirmed by isolation of the hybridoma Igs.

We have also tested a simple hypothesis on the basis of the selection determining the choice of "background", natural plasma cells: if alloreactive helper cells are available in the internal environment, it is reasonable to suppose that they will engage in productive inter-actions with normal B lymphocytes expressing Igs displaying an idiotypic profile which mimics also MHC antigens. It could be expected, therefore, that natural antibodies contain a set of idiotypes that can be recognized by anti-MHC antibodies. We have, therefore, screened one such collection, obtained in Balb/c mice, for reactivity with a set of 7 monoclonal anti-MHC IgG_{2a} antibodies. The first surprise was that more than half of these natural, newborn antibodies reacted with at least one of the test antibodies. Preliminary analysis, however, has shown that the majority of the reactions involve the C-regions of IgG_1 and as many as 15% of all hybridomas display rheumatoid factor specificity. The significance of this is far from clear. On the other hand, we have also identified specific reactions which are certainly due to variable region interactions at a frequency which is fully compatible with the above hypothesis. In particular, we have isolated a natural IgM antibody that appears to be an "internal image" of Ia7. This line of experimentation therefore not only reveals a wealth of interactions in the developing immune system, but it might also bring the clues to the functional relationships between the two major sets of "diverse" elements in immune systems: MHC antigens and Ig idiotypes, closing in the same network T and B cell repertoires.

Melchers: In a collaborative effort with Walter Gerhard from the Wistar Institute in Philadelphia, we have made approximately 600 cloned hybridomas of X63AG8 myeloma cells with polyclonally activated fetal liver cells (cultured and activated with LPS as described by Melchers, F., Eur. J. Immunol). The hybridoma proteins, about 95% of IgM class, were tested for binding with a range of bacterial and viral antigens as well as the common haptens, such as NP, DNP, TNP, PC and such. Binding was found to be highly cross-reactive for many related antigens, with no exquisite specificity for only one or a given set characteristic of specific hybridomas, indicating that the random fetal liver repertoir does not contain highly specific antibodies for the antigens tested. A strange reaction of one given hybridoma with others and with many myeloma proteins was observed, indicating some kind of "network-like" stickiness of IgM's to each other. For some of these crossreactions these sticky binding reactions have now been confined to the V_H portion of these IgM's, by preparing V_H from these IgM's,

PARTICIPANTS

David Baltimore | Center for Cancer Research, Massachusetts Institute of Technology, 77 Massachusetts Avenue, Cambridge, Mass. 02139, USA

Baruj Benacerraf | Department of Pathology, Harvard Medical School, 25 Shattuck Street, Boston, Mass. 02116, USA

Melvin Cohn | The Salk Institute, Post Office Box 85800, San Diego, Calif. 92138, USA

Antonio Coutinho | Avdelningen för Immunologi, Umeå Universitet, 901 87 Umeå, Sweden

Peter Doherty | The Wistar Institute, Thirty-sixth Street at Spruce, Philadelphia, Pa 19104, USA

James Forman | Department of Microbiology, Southwestern Medical School, University of Texas, Harry Hines Blvd., Dallas, Texas 75235, USA

Göran Holm | Department of Clinical Immunology, Huddinge Hospital, 141 86 Huddinge, Sweden

Tasuku Honjo | Department of Genetics, Osaka University, Medical School, 3-57 Nakanoshima, -Chome Kita-ku, Osaka 530, Japan

Leroy Hood | Division of Biology, California Institute of Technology, Pasadena, Calif. 91125, USA

Patricia P. Jones | Department of Biological Sciences, Stanford University, Stanford, Calif. 94305, USA

Jan Klein   Abteilung Immungenetik, Max Planck
                                   Institute, Correnstrasse 42, D-7400
                                   Tübingen 1, West Germany

Philip Leder   Department of Health and Human Services,
                                   Public Health Service, NIH, Bethesda, Md.
                                   20205, USA

Frank Lilly   Department of Genetics, Albert Einstein
                                   College of Medicine of Yeshiva Uni-
                                   versity, 1300 Morris Park Avenue, Bronx,
                                   N.Y. 10461, USA

Fritz Melchers   Basel Institute for Immunology, Gren-
                                   zacherstrasse 487, 40 58 Basel, Switzerland

Jacques Miller   Walter and Eliza Hall Institute for Medical
                                   Research, Royal Melbourne Hospital,
                                   Melbourne, Victoria 3050, Australia

Cesar Milstein   MRC Laboratory of Molecular Biology,
                                   University Postgraduate Medical School,
                                   Hills Road, Cambridge, CB2 2QH, England

Olli Mäkelä   Department of Serology and Bacteriology,
                                   University of Helsinki, Haartmaninkatu 3,
                                   Helsinki 29, Finland

Erna Möller   Department of Immunobiology, Wallenberg-
                                   laboratory, Karolinska · Institute, 104 05
                                   Stockholm, Sweden

Göran Möller   Department of Immunobiology, Wallenberg-
                                   laboratory, Karolinska Institute, 104 05
                                   Stockholm, Sweden

Marcus Nabholz   Swiss Institute for Experimental Cancer
                                   Research, CH-1066 Epalinges S, Lausanne,
                                   CH. des Boveresses, Switzerland

Susumu Ohno   Division of Biology, City of Hope Research
                                   Institute, 1450 East Duarte Road, Duarte,
                                   Calif. 91010, USA

William E. Paul   Laboratory of Immunology, National
                                   Institute of Allergy and Infectious
                                   Diseases, NIH, Bethesda, Md. 20205, USA

Per A. Peterson   Department of Cell Research, Wallenberg-
                                   laboratory, 751 22 Uppsala, Sweden

David H. Sachs

Transplantation Biology Section, Immunology Branch, National Cancer Institute, NIH, Bethesda, Md. 20205, USA

Elizabeth Simpson

Transplantation Biology Section, Clinical Research Centre, Walford Road, Harrow, Middlesex HA1 3UJ, England

Kendall A. Smith

Hematology Research, Dartmouth Medical School, Hanover, New Hampshire 03755, USA

Jonathan Sprent

Department of Pathology, School of Medicine, University of Pennsylvania, Philadelphia, 19104, USA

Jack L. Strominger

Biology Laboratories, Harvard University, 16 Divinity Avenue, Cambridge, Mass. 02138, USA

Arne Svejgaard

Vaevstypelaboratoriet, Rigshospitalet, Blegdamsvej 9, 2100 Köpenhamn Ö, Denmark

Jonathan W. Uhr

Department of Microbiology, Southwestern Medical School, University of Texas, 5323 Harry Hines Blvd., Dallas, Texas 75235, USA

Ellen Vitetta

Department of Microbiology, Southwestern Medical School, University of Texas, 5323 Harry Hines Blvd., Dallas, Texas 75235, USA

Matthias Wabl

Friedrich-Miescher-Laboratorium der Max-Planck Gesellschaft, P.O. Box 2109, Tübingen 1, West Germany

Martin Weigert

The Institute for Cancer Research, 7701 Burholme Avenue, Philadelphia, Pa 19111, USA

Hans Wigzell

Department of Immunology, Box 582, 751 23 Uppsala, Sweden

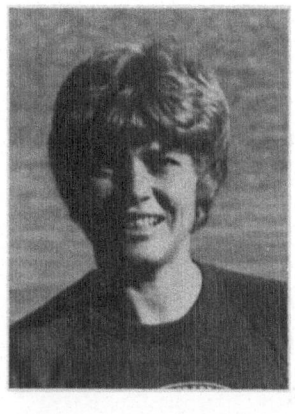
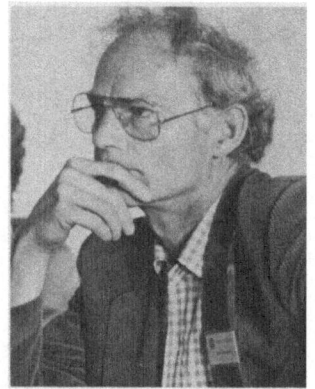
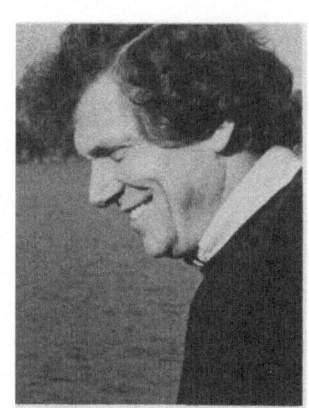

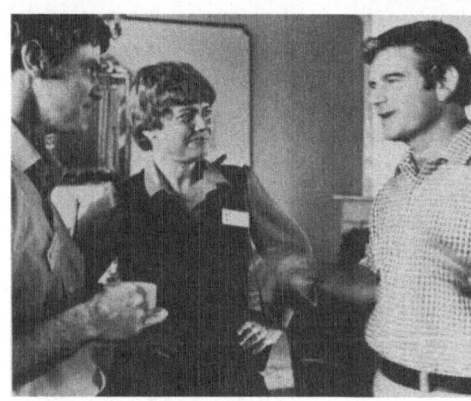
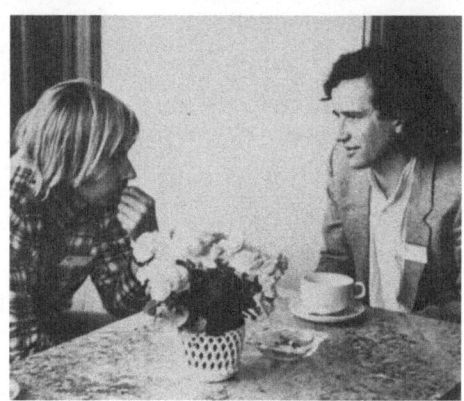

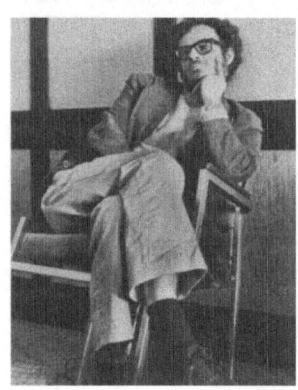
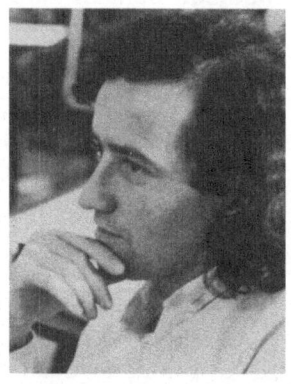
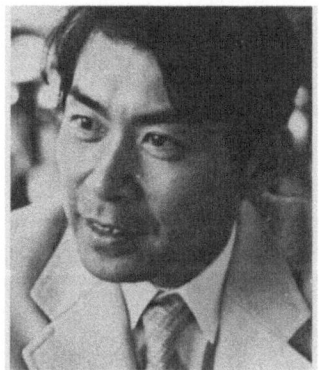

First row: E. Möller; A. Svejgaard; F. Melchers.
Second row: L. Hood, E. Möller and D. Sachs; H. Wigzell and M. Wabl.
Third row: J. Sprent; M. Wabl; T. Honjo.

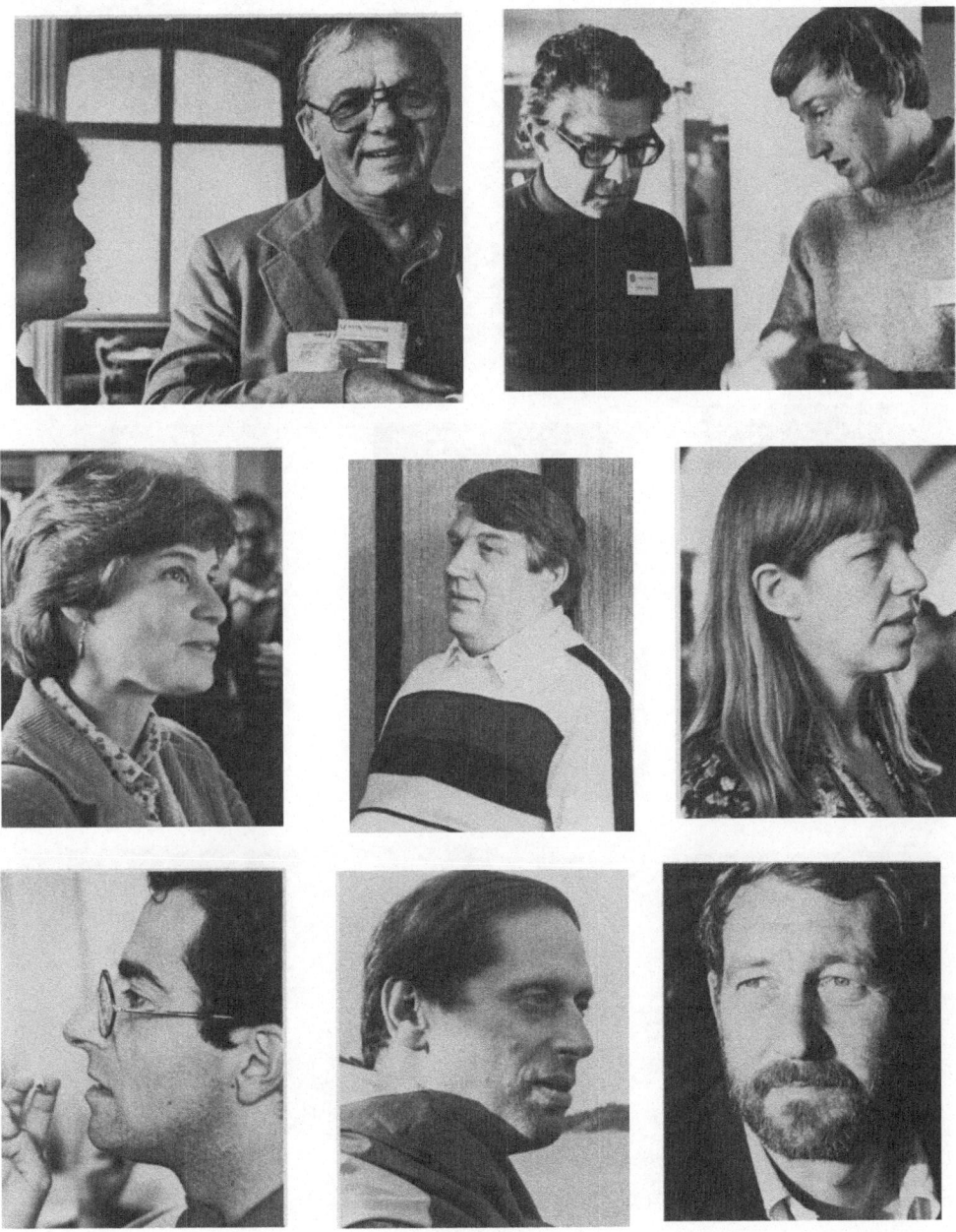

First row: P. Jones and J. Strominger; J. Miller and P. Doherty.
Second row: P. Jones; J. Klein; E. Simpson.
Third row: A. Coutinho; W. Paul; M. Weigert.

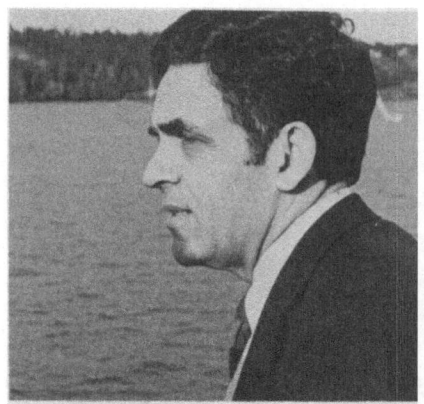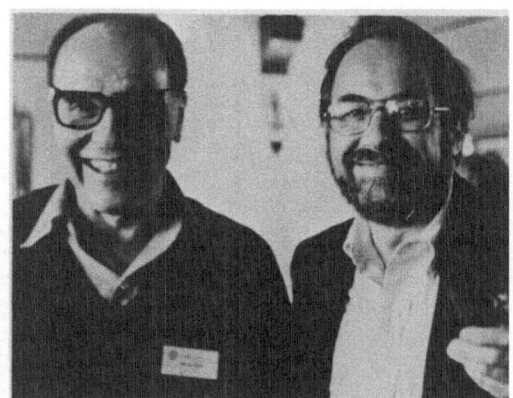

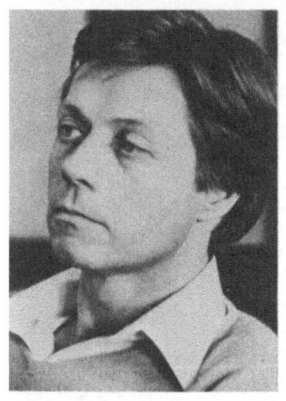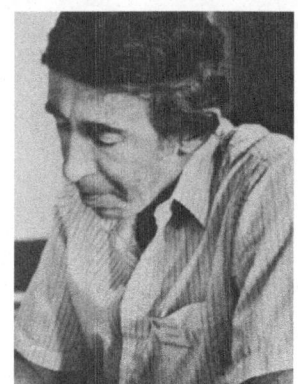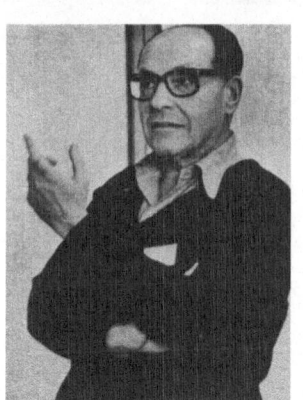

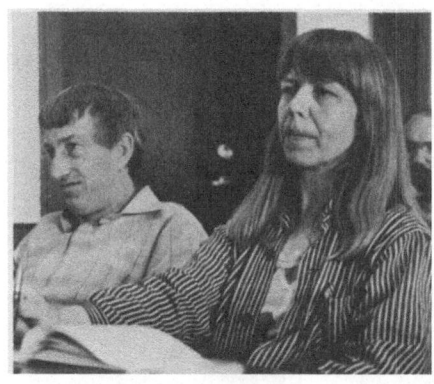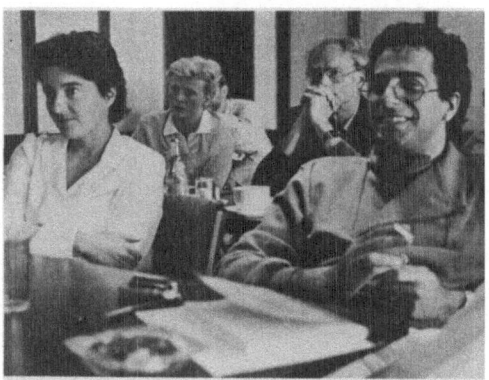

First row: P. Leder; M. Cohn and D. Baltimore.
Second row: K. Smith; J. Uhr; M. Cohn.
Third row: P. Doherty and E. Simpson; T. Ramos, E.-L. Larsson, A.
          Svejgaard and A. Coutinho.

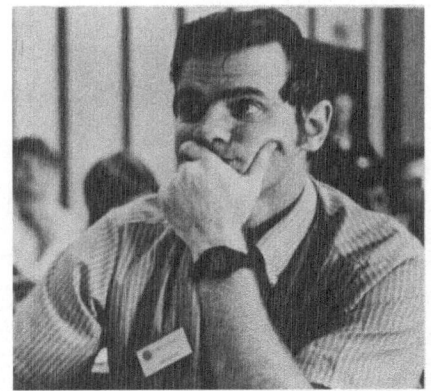
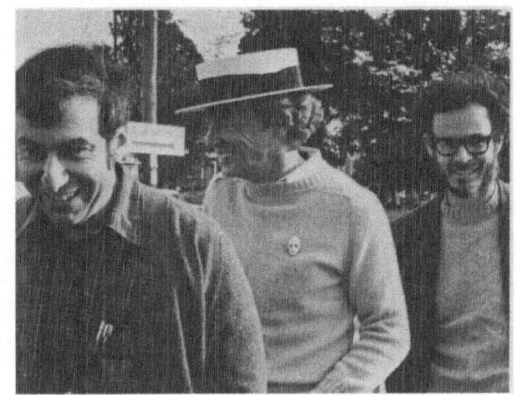

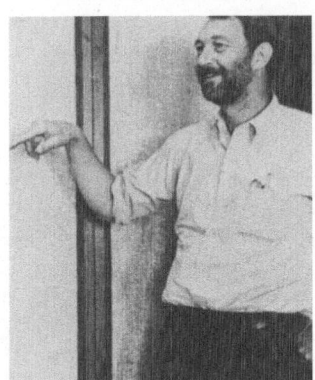
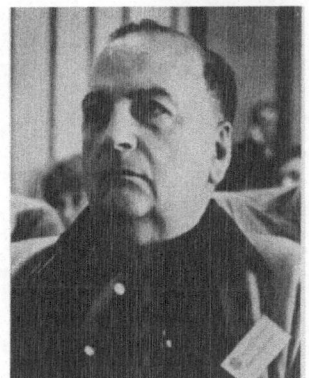
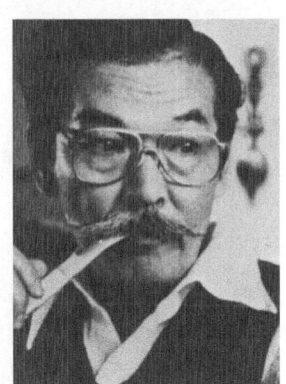

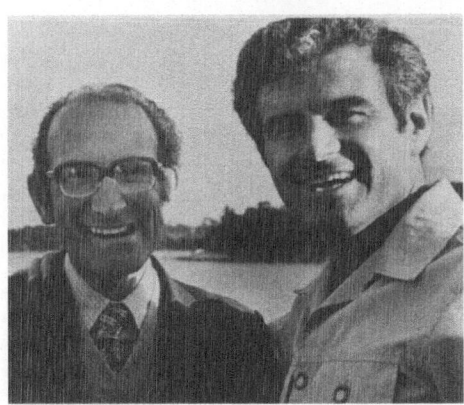
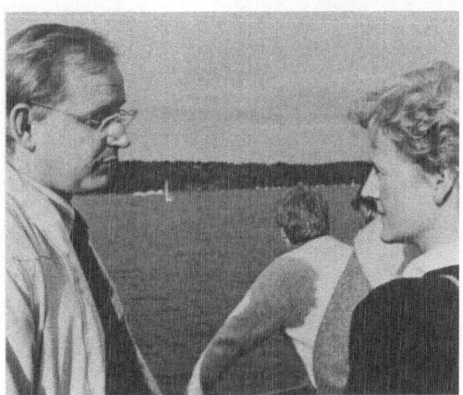

First row: L. Hood; J. Forman, F. Lilly and J. Sprent.
Second row: M. Weigert; B. Benacerraf; S. Ohno.
Third row: C. Milstein and D. Sachs; P. Peterson and E.-L. Larsson.

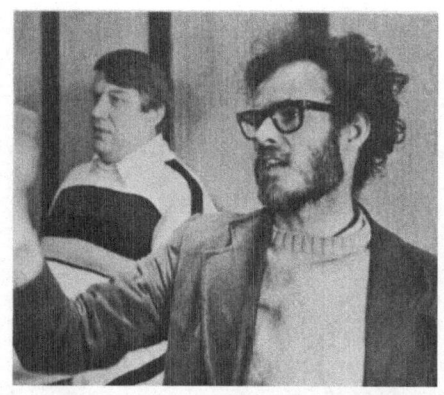 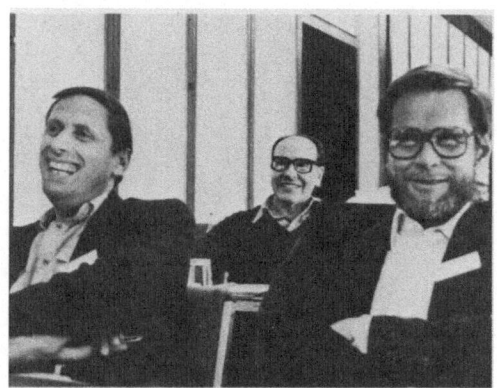

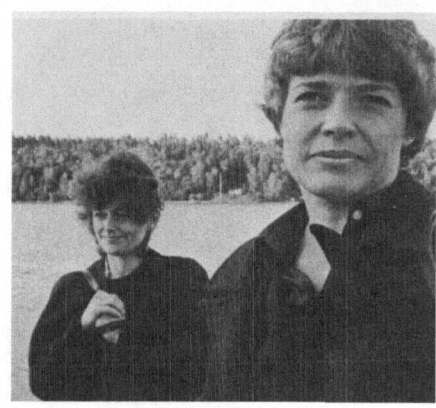 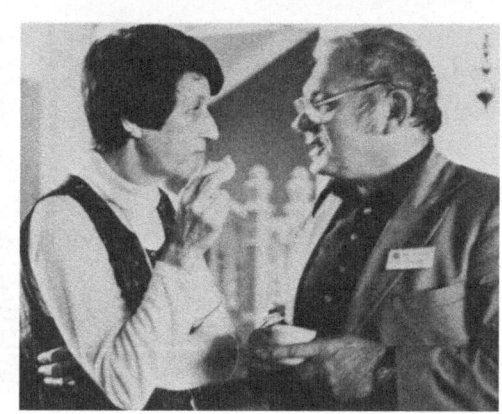

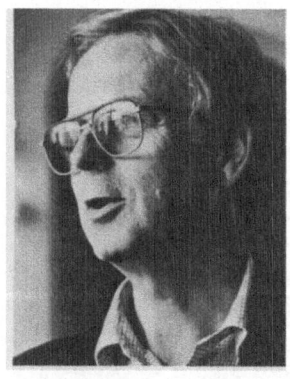 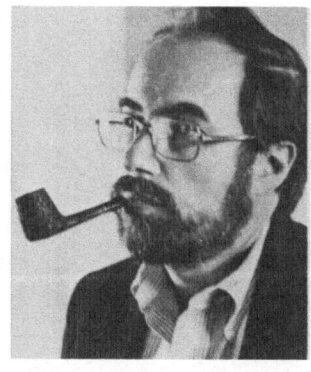 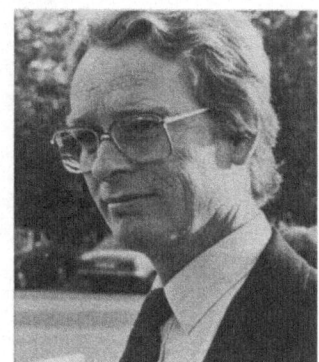

First row: J. Klein and J. Sprent; W. Paul, M. Cohn and O. Mäkelä.
Second row: E. Severinson and E. Möller; A. Benacerraf and J. Stro-
    minger.
Third row: G. Holm; D. Baltimore; G. Möller.